A Text Book Of

PHARMACEUTICAL ENGINEERING

As Per PCI Regulations

SECOND YEAR B. PHARM.
Semester III

Dr. Ashok A. Hajare
M. Pharm. Ph.D.
Professor and Head,
Department of Pharmaceutical Technology,
Bharati Vidyapeeth College of Pharmacy,
Kolhapur, Maharashtra, India

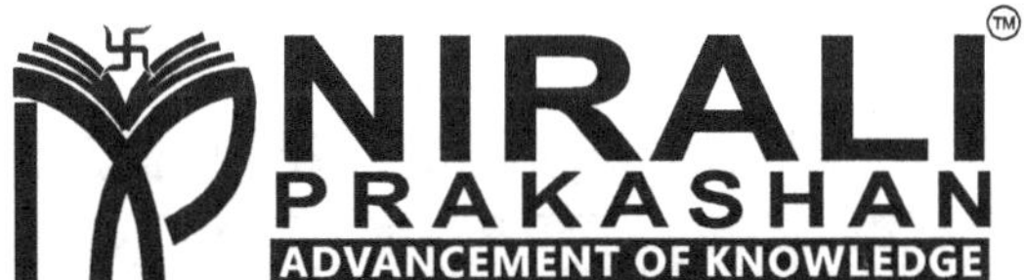

N3956

Pharmaceutical Engineering   **ISBN 978-93-89533-53-8**

Second Edition : February 2020

©   : **Author**

Published By :
NIRALI PRAKASHAN
Abhyudaya Pragati, 1312, Shivaji Nagar,
Off J.M. Road, PUNE – 411005
Tel - (020) 25512336/37/39, Fax - (020) 25511379
Email : niralipune@pragationline.com

➢ ## DISTRIBUTION CENTRES

PUNE

Nirali Prakashan : 119, Budhwar Peth, Jogeshwari Mandir Lane, Pune 411002, Maharashtra
(For orders within Pune) Tel : (020) 2445 2044, Fax : (020) 2445 1538; Mobile : 9657703145
Email : niralilocal@pragationline.com

Nirali Prakashan : S. No. 28/27, Dhayari, Near Asian College Pune 411041
(For orders outside Pune) Tel : (020) 24690204 Fax : (020) 24690316; Mobile : 9657703143
Email : bookorder@pragationline.com

MUMBAI

Nirali Prakashan : 385, S.V.P. Road, Rasdhara Co-op. Hsg. Society Ltd.,
Girgaum, Mumbai 400004, Maharashtra; Mobile : 9320129587
Tel : (022) 2385 6339 / 2386 9976, Fax : (022) 2386 9976
Email : niralimumbai@pragationline.com

➢ ## DISTRIBUTION BRANCHES

JALGAON

Nirali Prakashan : 34, V. V. Golani Market, Navi Peth, Jalgaon 425001, Maharashtra,
Tel : (0257) 222 0395, Mob : 94234 91860; Email : niralijalgaon@pragationline.com

KOLHAPUR

Nirali Prakashan : New Mahadvar Road, Kedar Plaza, 1st Floor Opp. IDBI Bank, Kolhapur 416 012
Maharashtra. Mob : 9850046155; Email : niralikolhapur@pragationline.com

NAGPUR

Pratibha Book Distributors : Above Maratha Mandir, Shop No. 3, First Floor,
Rani Jhanshi Square, Sitabuldi, Nagpur 440012, Maharashtra
Tel : (0712) 254 7129; Email : pratibhabookdistributors@gmail.com

DELHI

Nirali Prakashan : 4593/15, Basement, Agarwal Lane, Ansari Road, Daryaganj
Near Times of India Building, New Delhi 110002 Mob : 08505972553
Email : niralidelhi@pragationline.com

BENGALURU

Nirali Prakashan : Maitri Ground Floor, Jaya Apartments, No. 99, 6th Cross, 6th Main,
Malleswaram, Bengaluru 560003, Karnataka; Mob : 9449043034
Email: niralibangalore@pragationline.com

Other Branches : Hyderabad, Chennai

niralipune@pragationline.com | www.pragationline.com

Also find us on 🅕 www.facebook.com/niralibooks

Preface

Pharmaceutical industry is mainly divided into manufacturing of bulk drug and intermediates and finished pharmaceutical formulations. In both these areas in pharmaceutical industries various unit operations are involved to perform various day to day activities. Personnel dealing with these activities need to have thorough knowledge of unit operations to perform their duties in most appropriate manner.

The current curriculum implemented by Pharmacy Council of India New Delhi as Regulation 2014 has Pharmaceutical Engineering subject at Semester III of second year of the B. Pharm. course. There are few books available for this subject in the pharmacy educational sector in India that fulfill and cover all the contents prescribed in the syllabus for the subject. Taking this as an opportunity author has tried his level best to overcome the difficulties and limitations of the books already published and are available to the readers.

This book has in all FIVE Units with each unit has different number of chapters. Each chapter is covered in depth as per requirement taking into consideration the students knowhow at second year. Efforts have been taken to elaborate basic concepts of engineering issues of various equipments and techniques employed in most simple and lucid language. This is supported by giving flow diagrams, figures, equations and data tables. Unit operations are described by giving enough examples from industries to understand various unit operations described in syllabus. At the end of each chapter review questions are given that well help the readers to assess the knowledge gained after reading this book.

As an author I would like to acknowledge my sincere students, fellow teacher colleagues and my teachers who always remained a force for me in writing books.

I am indeed very grateful to my GURU Prof. Dr. Shivajirao Kadam, Pro-Chancellor, Bharati Vidyapeeth Deemed University, Pune for his consistent motivation and Dr. Vishwajit Kadam, Secretary Bharati Vidyapeeth, Pune for encouragement and cheerful support. I honestly extend our gratitude to Dr. H. N. More, Principal Bharati Vidyapeeth College of Pharmacy Kolhapur for giving me freedom to work. I am thankful to Mrs. Snehal Patil Librarian and Mr. P. D. Sawant for their co-operation during literature work. My special thanks to Mrs. Suvarna, Master Digvijay and my parents for sustained support, encouragement and for their forbearance.

I am thankful to Mr. Jignesh Furia, Ilyas Shaikh, Roshan Khan, Anjali Muley of Nirali Prakashan, Pune and Staff of Nirali Prakashan for bringing out nicely printed book.

Dr. A. A. Hajare

Syllabus

UNIT I   **(10 Hours)**

- **Flow of Fluids:** Types of manometers, Reynolds number and its significance, Bernoulli's theorem and its applications, Energy losses, Orifice meter, Venturimeter, Pitot tube and Rotometer.

- **Size Reduction:** Objectives, Mechanisms and Laws governing size reduction, factors affecting size reduction, principles, construction, working, uses, merits and demerits of hammer mill, ball mill, fluid energy mill, edge runner mill and end runner mill.

- **Size Separation:** Objectives, applications and mechanism of size separation, official standards of powders, sieves, size separation, principles, construction, working, uses, merits and demerits of sieve shaker, cyclone separator, air separator, bag filter and elutriation tank.

UNIT II   **(10 Hours)**

- **Heat Transfer:** Objectives, applications and Heat transfer mechanisms. Fourier's law, Heat transfer by conduction, convection and radiation. Heat interchangers and heat exchangers.

- **Evaporation:** Objectives, applications and factors influencing evaporation, differences between evaporation and other heat process. Principles, construction, working, uses, merits and demerits of Steam jacketed kettle, horizontal tube evaporator, climbing film evaporator, forced circulation evaporator, multiple effect evaporator and economy of multiple effect evaporator.

- **Distillation:** Basic Principles and methodology of simple distillation, flash distillation, fractional distillation, distillation under reduced pressure, steam distillation and molecular distillation

UNIT III   **(08 Hours)**

- **Drying:** Objectives, applications and mechanism of drying process, measurements and applications of Equilibrium Moisture content, rate of drying curve. principles, construction, working, uses, merits and demerits of Tray dryer, drum dryer spray dryer, fluidized bed dryer, vacuum dryer, freeze dryer.

- **Mixing:** Objectives, applications and factors affecting mixing, Difference between solid and liquid mixing, mechanism of solid mixing, liquids mixing and semisolids mixing. Principles, Construction, Working, uses, Merits and Demerits of Double cone blender, twin shell blender, ribbon blender, Sigma blade mixer, planetary mixers, Propellers, Turbines, Paddles & Silverson Emulsifier,

UNIT IV (08 Hours)

- **Filtration:** Objectives, applications, Theories and Factors influencing filtration, filter aids, filter medias. Principle, Construction, Working, Uses, Merits and demerits of plate & frame filter, filter leaf, rotary drum filter, Meta filter and Cartridge filter, membrane filters and Seidtz filter.

- **Centrifugation:** Objectives, principle and applications of Centrifugation, principles, construction, working, uses, merits and demerits of Perforated basket centrifuge, Non-perforated basket centrifuge, semi-continuous centrifuge and super centrifuge.

UNIT V (07 Hours)

- **Materials of pharmaceutical plant construction, Corrosion and its prevention:** Factors affecting during materials selected for Pharmaceutical plant construction, Theories of corrosion, types of corrosion and there prevention. Ferrous and non-ferrous metals, inorganic and organic non-metals, basic of material handling systems.

Contents

UNIT - II

4.   HEAT TRANSFER   **4.1 - 4.20**

UNIT - III

10. CENTRIFUGATION

UNIT - V

11. Materials of Pharmaceutical Plant construction, Corrosion and its Prevention

UNIT - I

Chapter ... **1**

FLOW OF FLUIDS

♦ **OBJECTIVES** ♦

This chapter contains some basics of fluid dynamics and is outlined to discuss and describe pressure measuring devices. More specifically, the difference between Newtonian and Non-Newtonian fluids as well as Reynolds Number to characterize the transition between laminar and turbulent flow in a fluid and Bernoulli's theorem to investigate the distribution of pressure in moving incompressible fluids. In addition, students will learn various factors responsible for energy losses during flow of fluid as well as devices used to measure flow rates of wide variety of fluids under different conditions and their applications in pharmaceutical filed. Thus the objectives are,

- To introduce fundamental aspects of fluid flow behaviour.
- To understand properties of fluid and its behaviour under internal and external flows.
- To develop energy balance equation for fluid flow systems and estimate pressure drop in fluid flow systems.
- To determine performance characteristics of fluid flow rate measurement devices.
- To develop and grasp the basic ideas of turbulence.
- To learn basic laws and equations used for analysis of static and dynamic fluids.
- To inculcate the importance of fluid flow measurement and its applications in pharmaceutical industries.
- To determine the losses in a flow system, flow through pipes, boundary layer flow and flow past immersed bodies.

1.0 INTRODUCTION

Fluid is a substance such as a gas or a liquid that has no fixed shape and flows easily upon application of external pressure. Flow is defined as the action of moving along in a steady, continuous stream. Thus, fluid flow is a part of fluid mechanics that deals with fluid dynamics and is a motion of gases and liquids. The motion of a fluid is due to unbalanced forces, and this motion continues as long as unbalanced forces are applied.

For example, if you are pouring a water from a beaker, the velocity of water is very high over the edge, moderately high approaching the edge, and very low at the bottom of the beaker. The unbalanced force is gravity, and the flow continues as long as water is available and the beaker is tilted.

Fluid flow has all kinds of aspects such as they can be steady or unsteady, compressible or incompressible, viscous or non-viscous, and rotational or irrotational. These characteristics reflect properties of the liquid itself, and others focus on how the fluid is moving. As mentioned earlier, fluid flow can be steady or unsteady and it depends on the fluid's velocity. In steady fluid flow, the velocity of the fluid is constant at any point where as in case of unsteady, the fluid's velocity can differ between any two points. Viscosity is a measure of the thickness of a fluid, and very gloppy fluids such as motor oil or shampoo are called viscous fluids.

The volume of fluid replaced in a given interval of time is called the fluid flow rate. It is expressed as

$$\text{Mass flow rate} \ = \ \rho AV \qquad\qquad\qquad \text{.... (1.1)}$$

Where, ρ = density, V = Velocity and A = area.

Thus, $\qquad\qquad\qquad$ Flow rate $\ = \$ Area $\times$ Velocity $\qquad\qquad\qquad$ .... (1.2)

Both gas and liquid flow can be measured in volumetric or mass flow rates, such as L/sec or kg/sec, respectively. Fluid flow measurements are related by the material's density. The density of a liquid is almost independent whereas for gases, the densities of which depend greatly upon pressure, temperature and to a lesser extent, composition. There are several types of flow meter that works, either by measuring the differential pressure within a constriction, or by measuring static and stagnation pressures to derive the dynamic pressure.

1.1 TYPES OF MANOMETERS

The term manometer is derived from the ancient Greek words 'manós', meaning thin or rare, and 'métron' meaning measure. A manometer works on the principle of hydrostatic equilibrium and is used for measuring the pressure (static pressure) exerted by a still liquid or gas. Hydrostatic equilibrium states that the pressure at any point in a fluid at rest is equal, and its value is just the weight of the overlying fluid. The manometer is the simplest instrument used for gauge pressure (low-range pressure) measurements by balancing the pressure against the weight of a column of liquid. The action of all manometers depends on the effect of pressure exerted by a fluid at a depth. Following are the advantages of manometeters:

(i)   Simple and time proven.

(ii) They have high accuracy and sensitivity.

(iii) Availability of a wide range of filling fluids of varying specific gravities.

(iv) It has reasonable cost.

(v)   There are suitable for low pressure and low differential pressure applications.

The different types of manometers are discussed below.

1.1.1 Simple U-tube Manometer

A manometer is a device to used measure pressures. A common simple manometer consists of a U shaped tube of glass filled with some liquid. In its simplest form, this type of manometer consists of an incompressible fluid like water or mercury. Typically it is mercury because of its high density.

Consider a U shaped tube whose both ends are open to the atmosphere is filled with a liquid. The points A and B, Fig. 1.1 (a), are at atmospheric pressure and at same vertical height. In another case, Fig. 1.1 (b), consider that the left arm of U-tube top end is closed and there is a sample of gas in the closed end of the tube. The right side of the tube remains open to the atmosphere. The point A, then, is at atmospheric pressure. The point C is at the pressure of the gas in the closed end of the tube. The point B has a pressure greater than atmospheric pressure due to the weight of the column of liquid of height h. The point C is at the same height as B, so it has the same pressure as point B. Thus, pressure at point C is equal to the pressure of the gas in the closed end of the tube. The pressure of the gas trapped in the closed end of the tube is greater than the atmospheric pressure by the amount of pressure exerted by the column of liquid of height h.

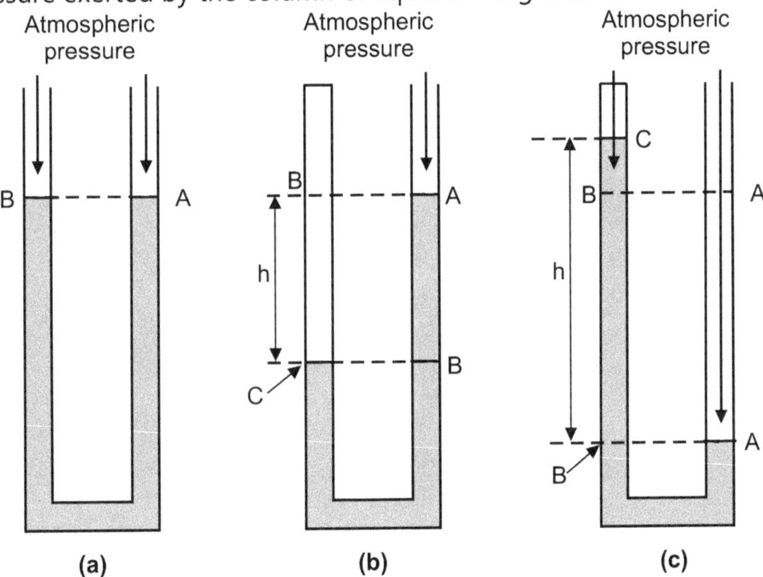

Fig. 1.1: Liquid and Gas at Atmospheric Pressure in U-tube Manometer

Another possible arrangement of the manometer where the top of the left side of the tube is closed and the closed end of the tube contains a sample of gas or it contains a vacuum, Fig. 1.1 (c). The point A is at atmospheric pressure. The point C is at some pressure if it contains gas in the closed end of the tube. Since the point B is at the same height as point A, it is at atmospheric pressure. But the pressure at point B is also the sum of the pressure at point C and the pressure exerted by the weight of the column of liquid of height h in the tube. Thus, it can be concluded that pressure at point C is less than atmospheric pressure by the amount of pressure exerted by the column of liquid of height h. If the closed end of the tube contains a vacuum, then the pressure at point C is zero, and atmospheric pressure is equal to the pressure exerted by the weight of the column of liquid of height h. The U-tube manometer is inexpensive and does not need calibration.

Pressure is defined as the force per area. The SI unit for pressure is the pascal, which is N/m^2. Another common unit for measuring atmospheric pressure is mm of mercury, whose value is usually about 760 mm. If the closed end of the tube, Fig. 1.1(c), contains a vacuum, the height h is about 760 mm. In many situations, measuring pressures in units of length of the liquid in the manometer is perfectly adequate.

The pressure measurement in manometer is calculated by considering a cylinder of liquid of height h and area A. The weight of the cylinder is its mass 'm' times the acceleration due to gravity 'g'. This is the force exerted by the cylinder of liquid on whatever is just below it. It is expressed as :

$$F = m g \qquad\qquad .... (1.3)$$

The pressure 'P' is this force divided by the area 'A' of the face of the cylinder and is expressed as :

$$P = \frac{F}{A} \qquad\qquad .... (1.4)$$

The mass of the cylinder is the density of the liquid 'ρ' times the volume 'V'.

$$m = \rho \times V \qquad\qquad .... (1.5)$$

The volume is the area 'A' of the face of the cylinder times its height 'h'.

$$V = A \times h \qquad\qquad .... (1.6)$$

So, the pressure P is: $\qquad\qquad P = \dfrac{F}{A}$

$$P = \frac{m \times g}{A}$$

Since, $m = \rho \times V$; $\qquad\qquad P = \dfrac{\rho \times V \times g}{A}$

$$P = \frac{\rho \times A \times h \times g}{A}$$

$$P = \rho \times h \times g \qquad\qquad ... (1.7)$$

1.1.2 Differential U-tube Manometer

A differential manometer is a device that measures the difference in pressure between two places. They can range from simple to complex digital equipment. Standard manometers are used to measure the pressure in a container by comparing it to normal atmospheric pressure. Differential manometers are also used to compare the pressure of two different containers. They are used to know which container has greater pressure and how large the difference between the two is.

The simplest differential manometer is a U-shaped tube with both ends at the same height. A liquid usually used is water or mercury and it rests at the bottom of the tube. If one end of the tube is in a place with higher air pressure, the pressure will push down the liquid on that side of the tube. By measuring the difference between the heights of liquid, it is possible to calculate the difference in pressure. To calculate the difference in pressure, difference in height is multiplied by the density of the gas and the acceleration due to gravity.

There are two types of differential manometer namely;

(i) U-tube differential manometer.

(ii) Inverted U-tube differential manometer.

There are two types of U-tube differential manometers.

(a) U-tube differential manometer at the same level.

(b) U-tube differential manometer at the different level.

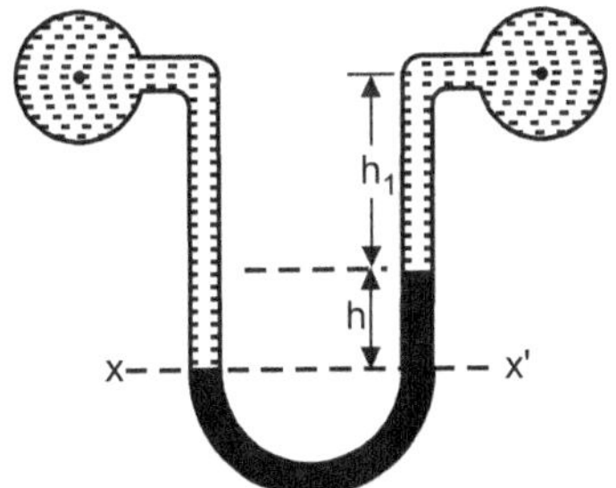

Fig. 1.2: U-Tube Differential Manometer at the Same Level

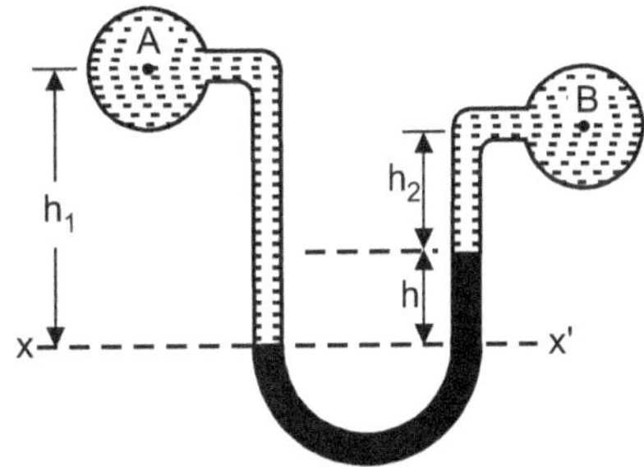

Fig. 1.3: U-Tube Differential Manometer at the Different Level

The first type of manometer has two pipes in parallel position, Figure 1.2. This type of manometer is used for measuring the fluid pressure difference between these two pipes arranged at same level. The second type of manometer, Fig. 1.3, is used where two pipes are at different place and are not in parallel condition. This type of manometers is used for measuring the fluid pressure between these two pipes arranged at different levels. Differential manometers have a wide range of uses in different disciplines. One example is that they can be used to measure the flow dynamics of a gas by comparing the pressure at different points in the pipe.

1.1.3 Inverted U-tube Manometer

The inverted U-tube differential manometer is reciprocal of U-tube differential manometer at the different level. This type of manometers is used to measure accuracy of small difference if pressure is increased. Inverted U-tube manometer, Fig. 1.4 is used for measuring pressure differences in liquids. The space above the liquid in the manometer is filled with air. In order to adjust the level of the liquid in the manometer a tap at the top is provided that admits or expels the air. The pressure at the same level in a continuous body of static fluid is equal.

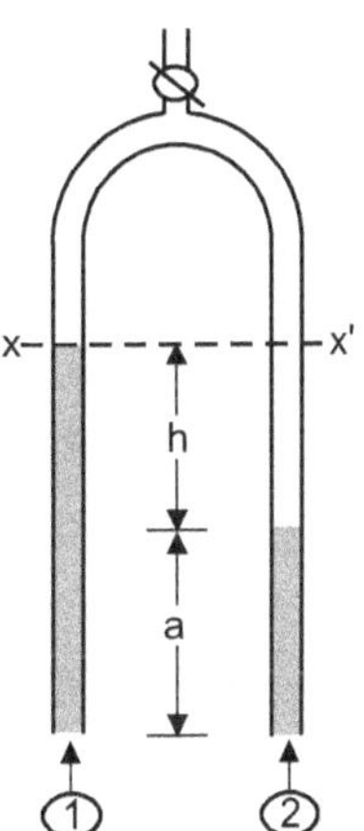

Fig. 1.4: Inverted U-tube Manometer

The pressure at the level XX' is equated as follows:

For the left arm of manometer:

$$P_x \;=\; P_1 - \rho\, g\,(h + a) \qquad\qquad \dots (1.8)$$

where, P_x is pressure in left arm at point X, P_1 is pressure in the left arm fluid, ρ is density of the air and g is gravitational force.

For the right arm of manometer:

$$P_x^{'} \;=\; P_2 - (\rho\, g\, a + \rho_m\, g\, h) \qquad\qquad \dots (1.9)$$

where, ρ_m is density of mercury.

$$\text{Since,} \qquad\qquad P_x \;=\; P_{x'} \qquad\qquad \dots (1.10)$$

$$P_1 - \rho\, g\,(h + a) \;=\; P_2 - (\rho\, g\, a + \rho_m\, g\, h)$$

$$P_1 - P_2 \;=\; (\rho - \rho_m)\, g\, h \qquad\qquad \dots (1.11)$$

If the manometric fluid is chosen in such a way that $\rho_m \ll \rho$ then,

$$P_1 - P_2 \;=\; \rho\, g\, h \qquad\qquad \dots (1.12)$$

For inverted U-tube manometer the manometric fluid is usually air.

1.1.4 Micro Manometer

A micromanometer is used for the accurate measurement of extremely small pressure differences. The micromanometer is another variation of liquid column manometers based on the principle of inclined tube manometer. The meniscus of the inclined tube is at a reference level as shown in the Fig. 1.5, viewing through a magnifier provided with cross hair line. This is done for the condition, $P_1 = P_2$. The adjustment is done by moving the well up and down a micrometer. For the condition when $P_1 \neq P_2$, the shift in the meniscus position is restored to zero by raising or lowering the well as before and the difference between these two readings gives the pressure difference in terms of height.

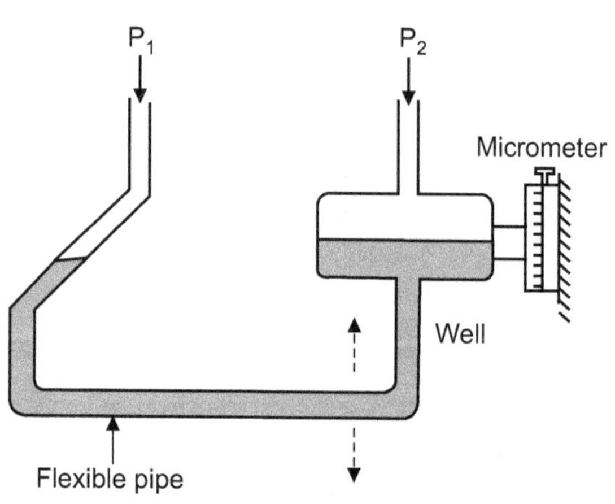

Fig. 1.5: Micromanometer

Micromanometer is a static fluid pressure difference measuring device. Its dynamics can rarely be ignored. Considering manometric fluid as a free body, the forces acting on it are

  (i) The weight distributed over the entire fluid.

  (ii) The drag force due to its motion and the corresponding tube wall shearing stress.

  (iii) The force due to differential pressure.

  (iv) Surface tension force at the two ends.

1.1.5 Inclined Manometer

For accurate measurement of small pressure differences by an ordinary U-tube manometer, it is essential that the ratio of density of mercury (ρ_m) to density of water (ρ_w) should be close to unity. This is not possible if the working fluid is a gas. A manometric liquid of density very close to that of the working liquid and giving at the same time a well defined meniscus at the interface is not always possible. For this purpose, an inclined tube manometer is used.

If the transparent tube of a manometer, instead of being vertical, is set at an angle 'θ' to the horizontal, Fig. 1.6, then a pressure difference corresponding to a vertical difference of levels 'x' gives a movement of the meniscus $s = \dfrac{x}{\sin\theta}$ along the slope. If 'θ' is small, a considerable magnification of the movement of the meniscus may be achieved. Angles less than 50° are not usually satisfactory, because it becomes difficult to determine the exact position of the meniscus. One arm of this manometer is usually made large in cross-section

than the other. When a pressure difference is applied across the manometer, the movement of the liquid surface in the wider arm is practically negligible compared to that occurring in the narrower arm. If the level of the surface in the wider arm is assumed constant, the displacement of the meniscus in the narrower limb needs only to be measured, and therefore only this arm is required to be transparent.

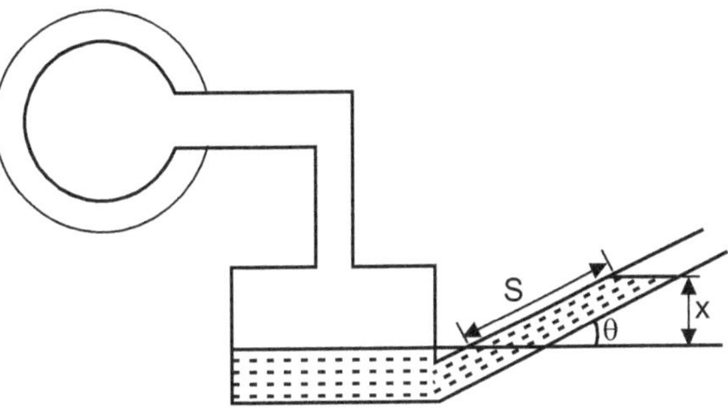

Fig. 1.6: Inclined Tube Manometer

1.2 REYNOLDS NUMBER AND ITS SIGNIFICANCE

The non-dimensional parameter called Reynolds number was discovered by an Irish engineer and physicist Osborne Reynolds in 1883. He identified the fundamental dimensionless parameter that characterizes the behaviour of flowing fluids known as Reynolds number. It was the ratio that shows the effect of viscosity in a given medium which governs the transition between laminar and turbulent flow. Before this invention it was believed that turbulent flow occurs in pipe of large cross-sectional dimensions and flows at high velocities, whereas laminar flow occurs in slow flows in pipe of relatively small cross-sectional dimensions. The role of viscosity and density in affecting the type of motion is not well-characterized.

According to Reynolds in the laminar flow the pressure drop is linear in the average velocity of the fluid, whereas in turbulent flow he observed that it was approximately proportional to $V^{1.72}$, where V is the average velocity. The actual dependence of the pressure drop on the velocity for turbulent flow in circular pipe is more complicated. The roughness of the interior pipe wall in contact with the fluid affects the pressure drop. He proposed that the change in the nature of the flow occurs when a certain combination of the parameters in the flow crosses a threshold. This combination was named after his name as Reynolds number.

For flow in a circular pipe of diameter 'D' at an average velocity 'V', the Reynolds number 'Re' is defined as follows,

$$Re = \frac{DV\rho}{\mu} \qquad \qquad \ldots (1.13)$$

$$= \frac{DV}{\mu} \qquad \qquad \ldots (1.14)$$

Here, 'μ' is the dynamic viscosity of the fluid, and 'ρ' is the density of the fluid. The ratio '$V\rho/\mu$' is called as kinematic viscosity. For circular tubes, the transition from laminar to turbulent flow occurs over a range of Reynolds numbers from approximately 2,300 to 4,000, regardless of the nature of the fluid or the dimensions of the pipe or the average velocity but is dependent of combination of the parameters known as the Reynolds number that falls in the range. Thus, when the Reynolds number is below 2,300, the flow

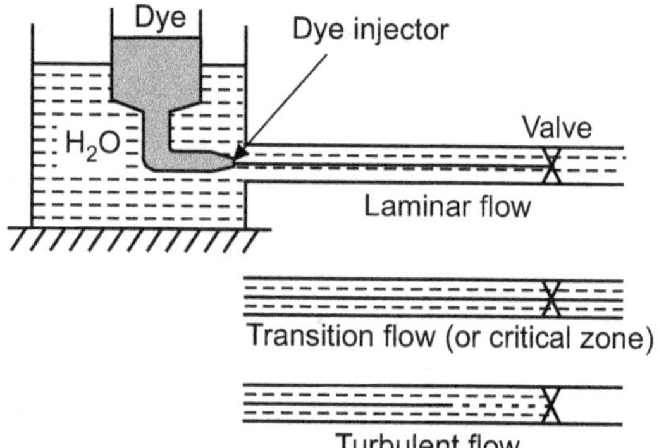

Fig. 1.7: Experimental Set-up of Reynolds Number

is laminar, and when it is above 4,000, the flow is turbulent. In between these two limits, the flow is termed to be transition flow.

Reynolds number can be ascribed a physical significance if multiplied both the numerator and the denominator by the average velocity V as follows.

$$Re = \frac{\rho V^2}{\mu \left(\dfrac{V}{D}\right)} \qquad \qquad \ldots (1.15)$$

In the equation (1.15), denominator represents a characteristic shear stress in the flow as it is the product of the viscosity of the fluid and a characteristic velocity gradient obtained by dividing the average velocity by the diameter of the tube. On the other hand the numerator describes an inertial stress. This is the reason for calling the product '$2\rho V$' a characteristic inertial stress. Thus, the Reynolds number as the ratio of two characteristic stresses in the flow.

$$Re = \frac{\text{Inertial stress}}{\text{Viscous stress}} \qquad \qquad \ldots (1.16)$$

Stress is force per unit area. Therefore, the physical significance of the Reynolds number is expressed as follows.

$$Re = \frac{\text{Inertia force}}{\text{Viscous force}} \qquad \qquad \ldots (1.17)$$

The nature of the flow in a tube, whether laminar or turbulent, depends on the relative importance of the inertia force in comparison with the viscous force. At relatively low values of the Reynolds number, the viscous force is relatively more important, and disturbances in the flow are compensated by viscosity. Thus, it is difficult for disturbances to grow and sustain themselves. On the other hand, at relatively large values of the Reynolds number, the damping of disturbances by viscosity is less effective, and inertia is more important, so that disturbances can perpetuate themselves. Thus, Reynolds number serves as a measure for determining type of flow (i.e. laminar or turbulent). The use of the diameter in the definition of the Reynolds number is an arbitrary choice. The length of the tube in defining the Reynolds number is considered because the typical velocity variation in this flow is across the cross-section of the tube and not along its length. Thus, if we had used the length 'L', the entity 'μ (V/L)' would not be representative of the shear stress in this flow.

Reynolds number for the steady motion of a sphere through a fluid:

When dimensional analysis is performed on the drag experienced by a sphere of diameter 'd_p' moving at a velocity 'V' through a fluid with viscosity 'μ' and density 'ρ', a Reynolds number in this situation is defined as:

$$\text{Re} = \frac{d_p V_p}{\mu} \qquad \qquad \dots (1.18)$$

The drag coefficient, which is a dimensionless drag, depends on this Reynolds number. The flow past a sphere is more involved than that in a tube. At high Reynolds number, a boundary layer, in which viscous effects are important, forms on the sphere, and outside of this boundary layer, viscous effects are relatively unimportant, and the flow is dominated by inertia. The low velocity for simple and ordered flow indicates that Re should be low. Hence, laminar flow takes place when ρ, V and L are small and μ is large. The flow turns out to be turbulent from laminar if the velocity is increased, keeping all other parameters constant. Since Reynolds' number is directly proportional to velocity, the flow should be a linear function of velocity. However, the pressure drop which these types of flow create while flowing in a pipe does not follow the linearity in case of turbulent flow. Thus the relation between pressure drop and velocity is expressed as

$$\Delta P \propto V \text{ for laminar flow}$$

$$\Delta P \propto V^2 \text{ for turbulent flow}$$

1.3 BERNOULLI'S THEOREM AND ITS APPLICATIONS

1.3.1 Bernoulli's Theorem

Bernoulli's theorem is the principle of energy conservation for ideal fluids in steady or streamline flow. This theorem describes relation among the pressure, velocity, and elevation in a moving fluid such as liquid or gas. According to this theorem the compressibility and viscosity (internal friction) are negligible and the flow is steady, or laminar. First derived (1738) by the Swiss mathematician Daniel Bernoulli, the theorem states that 'the total mechanical energy of the flowing fluid comprising the energy associated with fluid pressure, the gravitational potential energy of elevation, and the kinetic energy of fluid remains constant'. In simple terms Bernoulli's theorem can be described as 'within a horizontal flow of fluid, points of higher fluid speed will have less pressure than points of slower fluid speed'.

Incompressible fluids have to speed-up when they reach a narrow constricted section in order to maintain a constant volume flow rate. This is why a narrow nozzle on a hose causes water to speed-up. If the water is speeding-up at a constriction means it is gaining kinetic energy. To give kinetic energy is to do work. So if a portion of fluid is speeding-up, something external to that portion of fluid must be doing work it. For example, consider that water flowing along streamlines from left to right, Fig. 1.8. As the outlined volume of water enters the constricted region it speeds up. The force from pressure P_1 on water pushes to the right and does positive work. The force from pressure P_2 on the fluid pushes to the left and does negative work since it pushes in the opposite direction as the motion of the fluid.

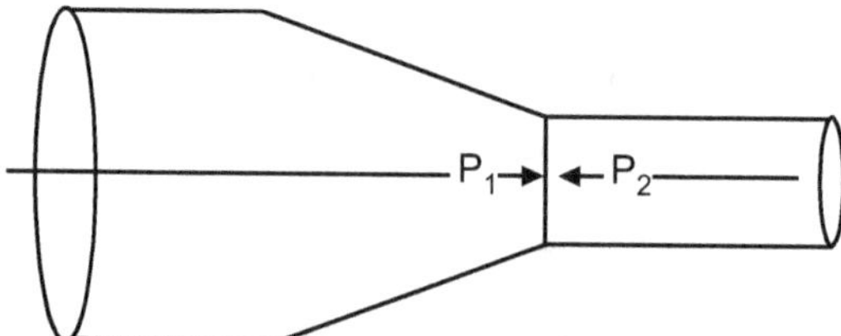

Fig. 1.8: Fluid Speed-up at Constricted End

The pressure on the wider/slower side P_1 has to be larger than the pressure on the narrow/faster side P_2. This inverse relationship between the pressure and speed at a point in a fluid is called Bernoulli's principle.

Bernoulli's Equation:

Bernoulli's equation is a general and mathematical form of Bernoulli's principle that takes into account changes in gravitational potential energy. Bernoulli's equation relates the pressure, speed, and height of any two points (1 and 2) in a steady streamline flowing fluid of density 'ρ'.

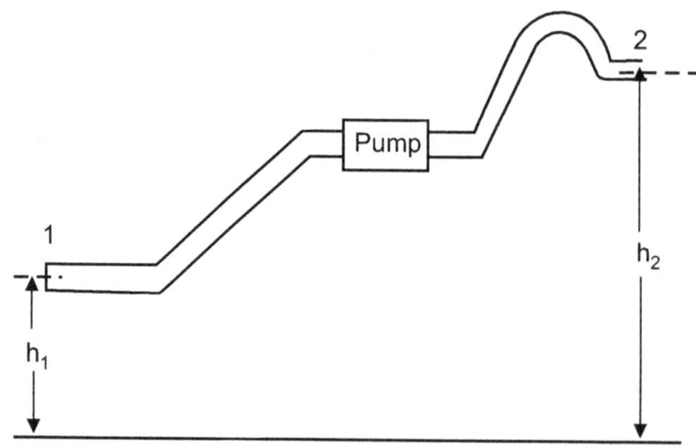

Fig. 1.9: Schematic to Describe Bernoulli's Theorem

Bernoulli's theorem investigates the distribution of pressure in a moving incompressible fluid.

For the instance consider that throughout the system the diameter of the pipe and the temperature is constant. The Fig. 1.9 represents a channel conveying a fluid from point 1 to point 2. The pump provides energy to cause the flow in upward direction. Assume that one pound of fluid enters the channel at point 1. The pressure at this point is P_1 lb/ft^2. If the average velocity of fluid is V_1 lb/sec and specific volume of fluid is V_1 ft^3/lb. The point 1 is at height h_1 above the horizontal bottom plane. The potential energy of a pound of fluid at point 1 is equal to h_1 ft.lb. Since fluid is in motion with velocity V_1, a pound of fluid will have a kinetic energy equal to $V_1^2/2g_c$ ft.lb. This expression is based on average velocity (V) of fluid in the system. In reality the average velocity differs from the mean velocity. The kinetic energy per pound of fluid flowing in channel is given by

$$\frac{1}{w} \int_0^{T_1} \frac{V_1^2}{2g_c} \qquad \text{... (1.19)}$$

where, w is weight of fluid in the system, r_1 is radius of channel and V_L is local velocity at distance r from the axis of channel. As we know, distribution of velocity vary widely within the channel at different localities, the true integral is obtained only when the actual velocity distribution is known. For each case a different velocity distribution curve is obtained. Thus, the kinetic energy in real sense is written as $\dfrac{V^2}{\alpha g_c}$, where α is a correction factor for variations in velocities at different locations in the channel. It was found that for viscous flow $\alpha = 1$ and for turbulent flow $\alpha = 2$.

Since one pound of fluid enters the channel, it enters against pressure P_1 lb/ft^2 and thus work is equal to P_1V_1 ft.lb done on one pound of fluid and is added to the potential energy. The sum of all three energies represents the energy of one pound fluid entering the section of channel. According to principle of conservation of mass whenever the system reaches a steady state, and when one pound fluid enters at point 1, another pound of fluid is displaced at point 2. The energy content of fluid leaving at point 2 can be expressed as

$$E = h_2 + \frac{V_2^2}{2g_c} + P_2V_2^* \qquad \text{... (1.20)}$$

where, V_2 is velocity, P_2 is pressure and V_2^* specific volume of fluid at point 2.

If there is no gain or loss of energy in the system between point 1 and 2 it follows the principle of conservation energy. But it has been postulated that the energy is added by the pump. This energy is 'W' ft.lb/lb of fluid. Some of the energy is converted into heat by friction and dissipated into environment through radiation as system is at constant temperature.

The loss of energy due to friction is 'F' ft.lb/lb of fluid. The total energies of the system under consideration that balances between point 1 and 2 will be

$$h_1 + \frac{V_1^2}{2g_c} + P_1 V_1^* - F + W = h_2 + \frac{V_2^2}{2g_c} + P_2 V_2^* \qquad \dots (1.21)$$

If the density of fluid 'ρ' is expressed as lb/ft³, then

$$V_1^* = \frac{1}{\rho_2} \text{ and } V_2^* = \frac{1}{\rho_2} \qquad \dots (1.22)$$

Then the equation (1.22) becomes,

$$h_1 + \frac{V_1^2}{2g_c} + \frac{P_1}{\rho_1} - F + W = h_2 + \frac{V_2^2}{2g_c} + \frac{P_2}{\rho_2} \qquad \dots (1.23)$$

This expression is based on the consideration of one pound of fluid entering in the system and all energy terms in above equation (1.23) are per pound mass of fluid.

1.3.2 Applications

(i) Bernoulli's equation allows us to estimate the flow rate of fluid through a pipe.

(ii) It allows us to measure the change in velocity and pressure experienced by a fluid running from a pipe of some cross-sectional area into a pipe of a different cross-sectional area. A fluid will have increased velocity and decreased pressure as it flows from a bigger pipe to a smaller pipe. This relationship is especially important in preventing a malfunction in water pipes through maintaining the stable fluid pressure. If the pressure is too high, the pipe explodes causing damage and other problems.

(iii) It can be used to calculate the lift force on an airfoil, if the behaviour of the fluid flow in the vicinity of the foil is known.

(iv) The Pitot tube and static port on an aircraft are used to determine the air speed of the aircraft. Bernoulli's principle is used to calibrate the air speed indicator so that it displays the indicated air speed appropriate to the dynamic pressure.

(v) A De Laval nozzle utilizes Bernoulli's principle to create a force by turning pressure energy generated by the combustion of propellants into velocity.

(vi) The flow speed of a fluid can be measured using a device such as a Venturi meter or an orifice plate, which can be placed into a pipeline to reduce the diameter of the flow. For an incompressible fluid, the reduction in diameter may cause an increase in the fluid flow speed. Bernoulli's principle shows that there must be a decrease in the pressure in the reduced diameter region.

(vii) The maximum possible drain rate for a tank with a hole or tap at the base can be calculated directly from Bernoulli's equation, and is found to be proportional to the square root of the height of the fluid in the tank. Viscosity lowers this drain rate. This is reflected in the discharge coefficient, which is a function of the Reynolds number and the shape of the orifice.

(viii) The Bernoulli grip relies on this principle to create a non-contact adhesive force between a surface and the gripper.

1.4 ENERGY LOSSES

The change in velocity of the fluid in a flow (either in magnitude or direction) induces large scale turbulence due to formation of eddies. So, a portion of energy possessed by the flowing fluid is ultimately dissipated as heat by radiation and is considered to be the loss of energy. Some of the reasons for loss of energy caused by the change in velocity are sudden pipe enlargement, sudden contraction, entrance to a pipe from large vessel, exit from a pipe, obstruction in the flow passage, gradual contraction or enlargement, bends and various pipe fittings etc. These losses of energy are termed as 'minor' losses because the magnitude of these losses is quite small compared to the loss due to friction in long pipes which are distinguished as 'major losses'. The 'minor losses' are confined to a very short length of the passage of the flowing liquid. The analytical expressions representing the loss of energy for above cases are discussed below.

1.4.1 Energy Loss by Sudden Enlargement

Consider a pipe of cross-sectional area A_1 carrying a liquid of specific weight w. It is connected to another pipe of larger cross-sectional area A_2. As there is sudden increase in the cross-sectional area of flow passage the liquid released from smaller pipe is unable to follow the abrupt change in boundary, Fig. 1.10.

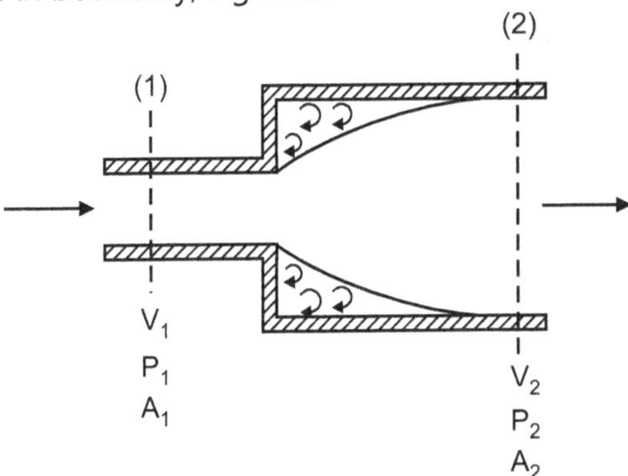

Fig. 1.10: Flow Through Sudden Enlargement in a Pipe

Consequently, the flow separates from the boundary, forming turbulent eddies that results in the loss of energy dissipated as heat by radiation. If P_1, V_1 and P_2, V_2 are the pressures and velocities of flow of liquid in the narrower and wider pipe, respectively, then by continuity equation, the discharge (Q) is,

$$Q = A_1V_1 = A_2V_2 \qquad \qquad .... (1.24)$$

The force acting on the liquid in the controlled volume in the direction of flow is expressed as

$$P_1A_1 + P_1(A_2 - A_1) - P_2A_2 = (P_1 - P_2)A_2 \qquad .... (1.25)$$

Using Newton's second law for the rate of change of momentum and the head loss between two sections '1' and '2' due to sudden enlargement, upon applying Bernoulli's equation we get

$$h_1 = \frac{(V_1 - V_2)^2}{2g} \qquad \qquad ... (1.26)$$

Using continuity equation, equation (1.26) may be expressed as,

$$h_1 = \frac{V_1^2}{2g}\left(1 - \frac{A_1}{A_2}\right)^2 = \frac{V_2^2}{2g}\left(\frac{A_2}{A_1} - 1\right)^2 \qquad ... (1.27)$$

The equations (1.26) and (1.27) is the expression for head loss due to sudden enlargement.

1.4.2 Energy Loss by Sudden Contraction

Consider a pipe carrying certain liquid of specific weight w whose cross-sectional area at a certain-section reduces abruptly from A_1 to A_2 as shown in Fig. 1.11. A sudden contraction in geometry of pipe leads to streamlines between section '1' and '2' curved and the liquid is accelerated. Thus, pressure at the annular face varies in an unknown manner and it cannot be determined. There is no major loss of energy in the region between the section 1 and the accelerating flow in the converging part.

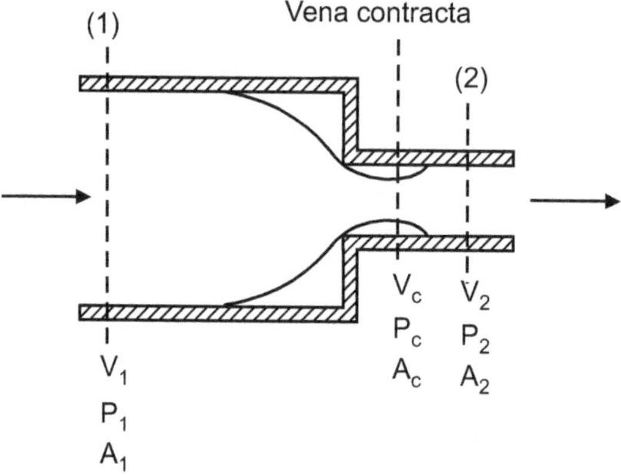

Fig. 1.11: Flow Through Sudden Contraction in a Pipe

As the liquid flows from the wider pipe to narrower pipe, a vena-contracta is formed and is followed by further widening of liquid stream to fill up completely the narrower pipe. In between the vena-contracta and the wall of the pipe, lot of eddies are formed that accounts for considerable dissipation of energy. In this region, the flow pattern is almost similar to that of sudden enlargement.

In general, the loss of head due to sudden contraction is expressed as :

$$\text{Loss of head } (h_L) = 0.5 \times \frac{V_2^2}{2g} \qquad \qquad ... (1.28)$$

1.4.3 Energy Loss at Pipe Entrance

Energy loss at the entrance to the pipe is also called as 'inlet loss'. It occurs, when the liquid enters to the pipe from a large vessel (or tank). The flow pattern is similar to that of sudden contraction. In general, for a sharp-cornered entrance, the loss of head at the entrance is expressed as :

$$\text{Loss } h_L = 0.5 \times \frac{V_2^2}{2g} \qquad \text{... (1.29)}$$

where, V_2 is the mean velocity of flow of liquid in the pipe.

1.4.4 Energy Loss at Pipe Exit

The outlet end of a pipe carrying liquid may be either left free or connected to a large reservoir. The liquid leaving the pipe possesses some kinetic energy corresponding to the velocity of the flow in the pipe which is ultimately dissipated either in the form of free jet or turbulence in the reservoir depending on the outlet condition in the pipe. The loss may be determined by using Eq. (1.30) with the conditions for which $A_2 \rightarrow \infty$. So, the loss of head at the exit of the pipe expressed as

$$\text{Loss } h_L = \frac{V^2}{2g} \qquad \text{... (1.30)}$$

where, V is the mean velocity of flow of liquid in the pipe.

1.4.5 Energy Loss by Obstruction in Flow Passage

The loss of energy due to flow obstruction in a pipe occurs due to the sudden reduction in the cross-sectional area followed by an abrupt enlargement of the stream beyond the obstruction, Fig. 1.12.

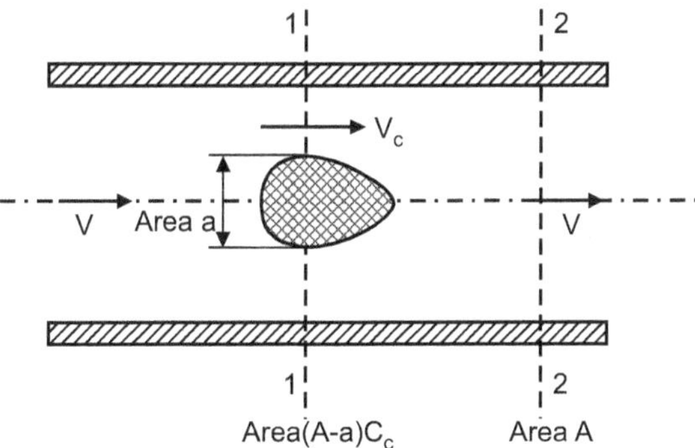

Fig. 1.12: Flow Through a Pipe With Obstruction

Consider a pipe flow (cross-sectional area of the pipe is A) in which an obstruction is placed with maximum cross-sectional area 'a'. As the flow passage is reduced to (A − a), a vena-contracta is formed beyond which the flow becomes uniform after certain distance from vena-contracta. If V_c and V be the velocities at vena-contracta and at section where the flow is uniform, then the loss of head due to obstruction can be deduced as

$$h_L = \frac{V^2}{2g}\left[\frac{A}{C_c\,(A - a)} - 1\right]^2 \qquad \text{... (1.31)}$$

1.5 FLOW MEASUREMENT DEVICES

Flow measurement is the quantification of bulk fluid. Volumetric flow rate is measured in "standard cubic centimeters per minute", a unit acceptable for use with SI. In engineering, the volumetric flow rate (also known as volume flow rate, rate of fluid flow or volume velocity) is the volume of fluid which passes per unit time; usually represented by the symbol Q (sometimes $\dot{V}$). The SI unit is m^3/s. Flow rate can be measured in a variety of ways. Positive-displacement flow meters accumulate a fixed volume of fluid and then count the number of times the volume is filled to measure flow. Other flow measurement methods rely on forces produced by the flowing stream as it overcomes a known constriction, to indirectly calculate flow. Flow may be measured by measuring the velocity of fluid over a known area.

1.5.1 Orifice Meter

The orifice meter is made-up of stainless steel, phosper bronze, nickel and monel. An orifice meter provides a simpler and cheaper arrangement for the measurement of flow through a pipe. Orifice is a thin circular plate with a sharp edged concentric circular hole in it. The main part of an orifice flow meter is a stainless steel orifice plate which is held between flanges of a pipe carrying the fluid whose flow rate is being measured. An orifice plate is fitted between the flanges which are at a certain distance. In order to maintain laminar flow conditions the pipe carrying the fluid is straight. Openings are provided at two places (a) and (b) for attaching a differential pressure sensor (U-tube manometer, a differential pressure gauge) as shown in the Fig. 1.13. The area (A_0) of the orifice is much smaller than the cross-sectional area of the pipe. The flow from an upstream is uniform and adjusts itself in such a manner that it contracts until a section downstream the orifice plate is reached at vena contracta (b) and then expands to fill the passage of the pipe. The vena-contracta length depends on the roughness of the inner wall of the pipe and sharpness of the orifice plate. One of the pressure tapings is provided at a distance equal to diameter of pipe at upstream to the orifice plate where the flow is almost uniform (a) and the other at a distance of half a diameter of pipe to downstream the orifice plate.

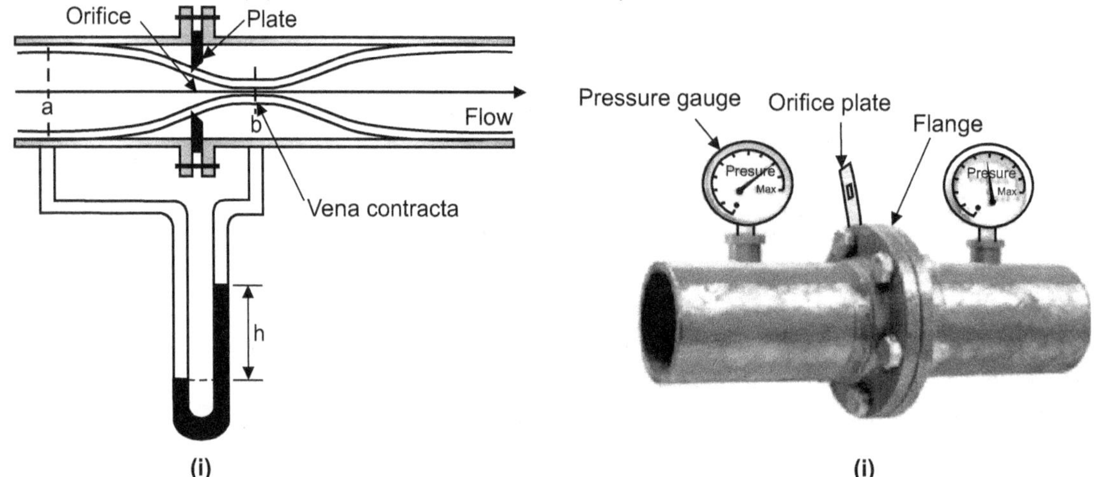

Fig. 1.13: Orifice Meter (I) Schematic (II) Real One Used In Practice

Operation:

In order to know how orifice meter works the details of the fluid movement inside the pipe and orifice plate has to be understood. The fluid having uniform cross-section of flow converges into the orifice plate's opening in its upstream (left side). When the fluid comes out of the orifice plate's opening, its cross-section is minimum and uniform for a particular distance and then the cross-section of the fluid starts diverging in the downstream (right side). At the upstream of the orifice, before the converging of the fluid, the pressure of the fluid (P_1) is at maximum. As the fluid starts converging and enters the orifice opening its pressure drops. Whereas, when the fluid comes out of the orifice opening, its pressure is minimum (P_2) and this minimum pressure remains constant in the minimum cross-sectional area of fluid flow at the downstream. This minimum cross-sectional area of the fluid obtained at downstream from the orifice edge is called vena-contracta. The manometer attached between points (a) and (b) records the pressure difference ($\Delta P = P_1 - P_2$) between these two points which becomes an indication of the flow rate of the fluid through the pipe when calibrated.

Considering the fluid to be ideal and the downstream pressure taping to be at the vena contracta, we can write, by applying Bernoulli's theorem between (a) and (b) as

$$\frac{P_1^*}{\rho g} + \frac{V_1^2}{2g} = \frac{P_2^*}{\rho g} + \frac{V_2^2}{2g} \qquad \ldots (1.32)$$

where, P_1^* and P_2^* are the piezometric pressures at (a) and (b), respectively. From the equation of continuity,

$$V_1 A_1 = V_2 A_2 \qquad \ldots (1.33)$$

where, A_2 is the area of the vena contracta. With the help of equation (1.32), equation (1.33) can be written as,

$$V_2 = \sqrt{\frac{2(P_1^* - P_2^*)}{\rho\left(1 - \dfrac{A_2^2}{A_1^2}\right)}} \qquad \ldots (1.34)$$

Applications:

(i)   The concentric orifice plate is used to measure flow rates of pure fluids.

(ii) The eccentric and segmental orifice plates are used to measure flow rates of fluids containing suspended materials such as solids, oil mixed with water and wet steam.

Advantages:

(i)   It is very cheap and easy method.

(ii) It has predictable characteristics and requires less space.

(iii) It can be used to measure flow rates in large pipes.

Limitations:

(i)   In certain cases it becomes difficult to tap the minimum pressure (P_2) due to roughness of the inner wall of the pipe and sharpness of the orifice plate.

(ii) Pressure recovery at downstream is poor, i.e. overall loss varies from 40% to 90% of the differential pressure.

(iii) The upstream pipe must be straight to obtain laminar flow.

(iv) Chances of clogging the orifice when the suspended fluid flows.

(v)   The orifice plate gets corroded and due to this there may be inaccuracy in determination.

(vi) The orifice plate has low physical strength.

(vii) The coefficient of discharge is low.

1.5.2 Venturi Meter

Venturi meter is a flow measurement instrument or device used to measure discharge through a pipe. It is based on Bernoulli's principle.

Construction:

A venturimeter is essentially a short pipe, Fig. 1.14, consisting of two conical parts with a short portion of uniform cross-section in between. This short portion has the minimum area and is known as the throat. The two conical portions have the same base diameter, but one is having a shorter length with a larger cone angle while the other is having a larger length with a smaller cone angle.

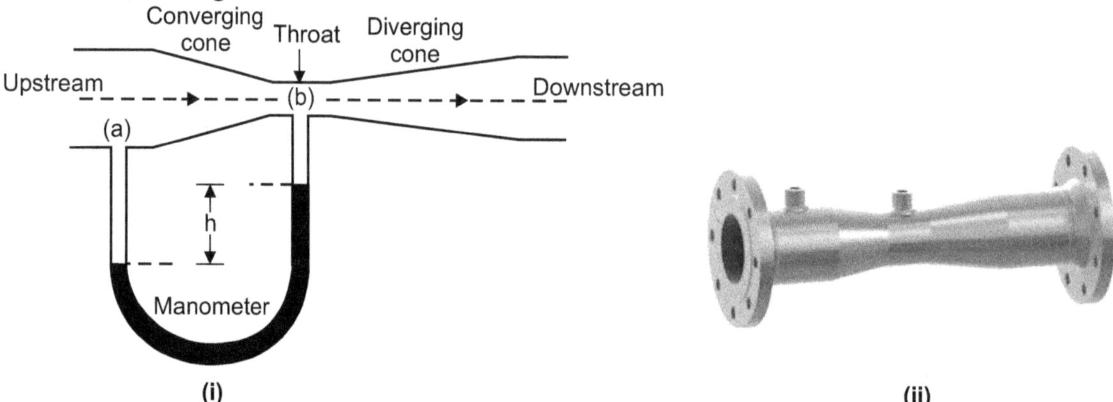

Fig. 1.14: Venturi Meter (I) Schematic (II) Real One Used In Practice

Working:

The variation in the conical portion at upstream and on the downstream ensures a rapid converging passage and a gradual diverging passage in the direction of flow. This is just to avoid the loss of energy due to separation at the throat. During a flow through the converging part, the velocity increases in the direction of flow according to the principle of continuity, while the pressure decreases according to Bernoulli's theorem. The velocity reaches its maximum and pressure reaches its minimum at the throat. Subsequently, a decrease in the velocity and an increase in the pressure take place in course of flow through the divergent part. The Fig. 1.15 shows that a venturimeter is inserted in an inclined pipeline in a vertical plane to measure the flow rate through the pipe. Let us consider a steady, ideal and one dimensional (along the axis of the venturi meter) flow of fluid. Under this situation, the velocity and pressure at any section will be uniform.

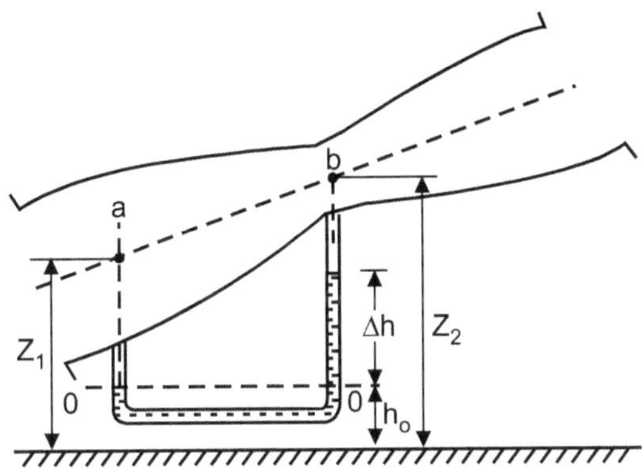

Fig. 1.15: Measurement of Flow by a Venturimeter

Let the velocity and pressure at the inlet (a) are V_1 and P_1, respectively, while those at the throat (b) are V_2 and P_2. Now, applying Bernoulli's equation between (a) and (b), we get

$$\frac{P_1}{\rho g} + \frac{V_1^2}{2g} + z_1 = \frac{P_2}{\rho g} + \frac{V_2^2}{2g} + z_2 \qquad \dots (1.35)$$

where, ρ is the density of fluid flowing through the venturi meter. From continuity,

$$V_1 A_1 = V_2 A_2 \qquad \dots (1.36)$$

where, A_1 and A_2 are the cross-sectional areas of the venturi meter at its throat and inlet respectively.

With the help of equation (1.35), equation (1.36) can be written as

$$+ \frac{V_2^2}{2g} \left(1 - \frac{A_2^2}{A_1^2} \right) = \left(\frac{P_1}{2g} + z_1 \right) - \left(\frac{P_2}{2g} + z_2 \right) \qquad \dots (1.37)$$

$$V_2 = \frac{1}{\sqrt{1 - \frac{A_2^2}{A_1^2}}} \sqrt{2g(h_1^* - h_2^*)} \qquad \dots (1.38)$$

where, h_1^* and h_2^* are the piezometric pressure heads at (a) and (b), respectively, and are defined as

$$h_1^* = \frac{P_2}{\rho g} + z_1 \qquad \dots (1.39$$

$$h_2^* = \frac{P_2}{\rho g} + z_2 \qquad \dots (1.40)$$

Hence, the volume flow rate through the pipe is given by

$$Q = A_2 V_2 = \cfrac{1}{\sqrt{1 - \cfrac{A_2^2}{A_1^2}}} \sqrt{2g(h_1^* - h_2^*)} \qquad \ldots (1.41)$$

If the pressure difference between (a) and (b) is measured by a manometer as shown in Fig. 1.14, we can write

$$P_1 + \rho g\,(z_1 - h_0) = P_2 + \rho g\,(z_2 - h_0 - \Delta h) + h\rho_m g \qquad \ldots\ldots (1.42)$$

$$(P_1 + \rho g z_1) - (P_2 + \rho g z_2) = (\rho_m - \rho)\,g\Delta h \qquad \ldots\ldots (1.43)$$

$$\left(\frac{P_1}{\rho g} + z_1\right) - \left(\frac{P_2}{\rho g} + z_2\right) = \left(\frac{\rho_m}{\rho} - 1\right)\Delta h \qquad \ldots (1.44)$$

$$h_1^* - h_2^* = \left(\frac{\rho_m}{\rho} - 1\right)\Delta h \qquad \ldots (1.45)$$

where, ρ_m is the density of the manometric liquid. The equation (1.45) shows that a manometer always registers a direct reading of the difference in piezometric pressures.

Now, substitution of $h_1^* - h_2^*$ from equation (1.45) in equation (1.44) gives,

$$Q = \frac{A_1 A_2}{\sqrt{A_1^2 A_2^2}} \sqrt{2g\left(\frac{\rho_m}{\rho} - 1\right)\Delta h} \qquad \ldots (1.46)$$

If the pipe along with the venturimeter is horizontal, then $z_1 = z_2$; and hence $h_1^* - h_2^*$ becomes $h_1 - h_2$, where h_1 and h_2 are the static pressure heads.

$$h_1 = \frac{P_1}{\rho g} \qquad \ldots (1.47)$$

$$h_2 = \frac{P_2}{\rho g} \qquad \ldots (1.48)$$

Thus, manometric equation (1.45) becomes,

$$h_1 - h_2 = \left(\frac{\rho_m}{\rho} - 1\right)\Delta h \qquad \ldots (1.49)$$

The final expression of flow rate given by equation (1.46), in terms of manometer deflection Δh, remains the same irrespective of whether the pipe-line along with the venturimeter connection is horizontal or not. The measured values of Δh, the difference in piezometric pressures between (a) and (b), for a real fluid will always be greater than that of an ideal fluid because of frictional losses in addition to the change in momentum. Therefore, equation (1.46) always overestimates the actual flow rate. To compensate for this a multiplying factor (C_d), called the coefficient of discharge, is incorporated in the equation (1.46) as

$$Q_{Actual} = C_d \frac{A_1 A_2}{\sqrt{A_1^2 - A_2^2}} \sqrt{2g\left(\frac{\rho_m}{\rho} - 1\right)\Delta h} \qquad \ldots (1.50)$$

The coefficient of discharge C_d is always less than unity and is defined as;

$$C_d = \frac{\text{Actual rate of discharge}}{\text{Theoretical rate of discharge}} = \frac{Q_{actual}}{Q_{theoretical}} \qquad ... (1.51)$$

Where, the theoretical discharge rate is predicted by the Eq. (1.46) with the measured value of Δh, and the actual rate of discharge is the discharge rate measured in practice. Value of C_d for a venturimeter usually lies between 0.95 to 0.98.

Applications:
   (i)   Venturimeter can be used for the measurement of flow of water, liquids, gases, dirty liquids etc.
   (ii) They are commonly used in water supply industry.

Advantages:
   (i)   It has low head loss of about 10% of differential pressure head.
   (ii) It can measure higher flow rates in pipes having few meters of diameters due to high coefficient of discharge owing to lower loss.
   (iii) It is suitable for use in any position, for example, horizontal, vertical or inclined.
   (iv) Higher sensitivities can be achieved due to smaller size throat which leads to higher pressure differential.

Disadvantages:
   (i)   It has space limitations due to larger size.
   (ii) Due to large size, the cost of venturimeter is higher.
   (iii) Very small diameter of throat results into cavitations of fluid in the throat.
   (iv) It is more susceptible to errors due to burrs or deposits round the downstream (throat) tapping.

1.5.3 Pitot Tube

Pitot tube is a device, invented by Henri Pitot, a French engineer in 18th century, used to measure the fluid flow. The principle of flow measurement by Pitot tube was first used for measuring velocities of water in the river. A right angled large glass tube was used for the purpose. One end of the tube faces the fluid flow while the other end remains open to the atmosphere, Fig. 1.16 (a).

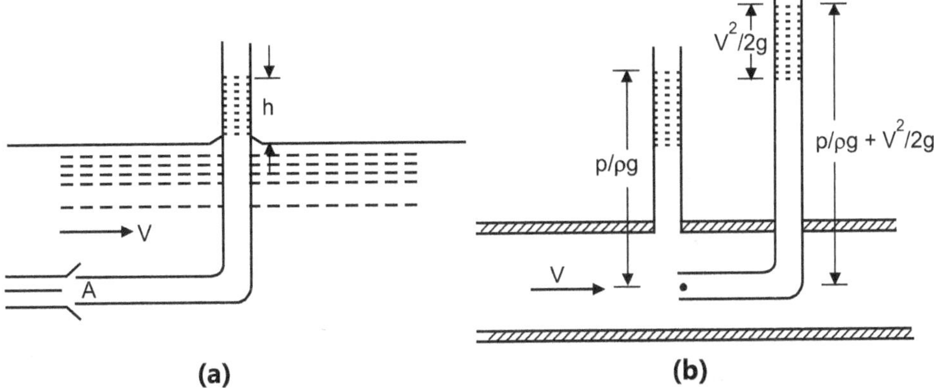

Fig. 1.16: Simple Pitot tube (a) Tube for Measuring the Stagnation Pressure (b) Static and Stagnation Tubes Together

Working:

A pitot tube is a simple round cylinder with one end opened with a small hole and the other end is enclosed. The fluid flowing through the pipe enters the Pitot tube and rest there. There is another chamber within the Pitot tube filled with fluid with static pressure. A diaphragm separates both the chambers. The differential pressure is measured between both the pressures that give the dynamic pressure. The difference in level between the liquid in the tube and the free surface becomes the measure of dynamic pressure. The flow rate is calculated from the square root of the pressure. The flow rate depends on the tube design and the location of the static tap. The Pitot-static probe incorporates the static holes in the tube system to eliminate this parameter.

The liquid flow-up the tube and when equilibrium is attained, the liquid reaches a height above the free surface of the water stream. The measurement of static pressure and the impact pressure is performed through the attachment of proper differential pressure meter that determines flow velocity and thus the flow rate is calculated. Since the static pressure, under this situation, is equal to the hydrostatic pressure due to its depth below the free surface, the difference in level between the liquid in the glass tube and the free surface becomes the measure of dynamic pressure. Therefore, neglecting friction, we can write,

$$P_0 - P \ = \ \frac{\rho V^2}{2} = h\rho g \qquad\qquad\qquad \ldots (1.52)$$

where, P_0, P and V are the stagnation pressure, static pressure and velocity respectively at point A, Fig. 1.16 (a).

For an open stream of liquid with a free surface, this single tube is sufficient to determine the velocity. But for a fluid flowing through a closed duct, the Pitot tube measures only the stagnation pressure and so the static pressure must be measured separately. Measurement of static pressure in this case is made at the boundary of the wall, Fig. 1.16 (b). The axis of the tube measuring the static pressure must be perpendicular to the boundary and free from burrs, so that the boundary is smooth and hence the streamlines adjacent to it are not curved. This is done to sense the static pressure only without any part of the dynamic pressure. A Pitot tube is inserted to sense the stagnation pressure. The end of the Pitot tube, measures the stagnation pressure, and the piezometric tube, measuring the static pressure, may be connected to a suitable differential manometer for the determination of flow velocity and hence the flow rate.

The tubes recording static pressure and the stagnation pressure are combined into one instrument known as Pitot static tube, Fig. 1.17. The tube for sensing the static pressure is known as static tube which surrounds the Pitot tube that measures the stagnation pressure. Two or more holes are drilled radially through the outer wall of the static tube into annular space. The position of these static holes is important. Downstream of the nose of tube, the flow is accelerated somewhat with consequent reduction in static pressure. But in front of the supporting stem, there is a reduction in velocity and increase in pressure. The static holes should therefore be at the position where the two opposing effects are counterbalanced and the reading corresponds to the undisturbed static pressure.

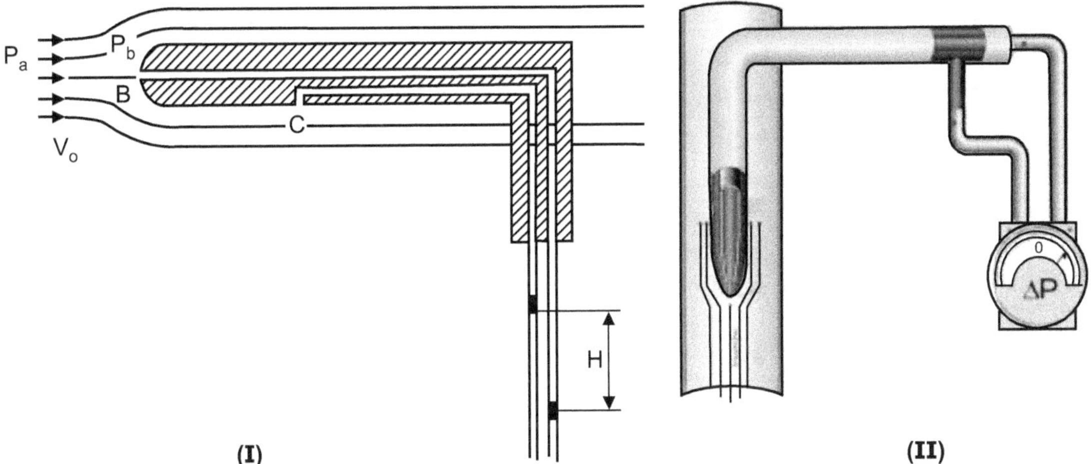

Fig. 1.17: Pitot Static Tube (I) Schematic (II) Real One Used In Practice

The flow velocity is given by $V = C\sqrt{2\left(\dfrac{\Delta P}{\rho}\right)}$　　　　　　　　　... (1.53)

where, Δp is the difference between stagnation and static pressures. The factor C takes care of the non-idealities, due to friction, in converting the dynamic head into pressure head and depends, to a large extent, on the geometry of the Pitot tube. The value of C is usually determined from calibration test of the Pitot tube.

Applications:

(i) It is widely used to measure the airspeed of aircrafts, speedboat speed and for fluid flow measurement in industrial application.

(ii) Pitot tubes are mainly used for gas lines.

(iii) These may be employed where the flowing fluid is not enclosed in a pipe or duct. For example, for measuring the flow of river water, or for measuring air flow in aero plane.

Advantages:

(i) Pitot tube is small and do not contain any moving parts.

(ii) Low permanent pressure loss.

(iii) Loss of head is negligible by insertion of Pitot tube.

(iv) It is very cheap as compared to venturi meter, orifice plate and flow nozzle.

(v) Ease of installation into an existing system.

Disadvantages:

(i) The differential pressures produced are usually low, say of the order of 250 Pa, and so their sensitivity is low.

(ii) Pitot tube requires higher flow velocity in order to produce measurable heads.

(iii) It has small openings which get clogged due to passing solid particles and thus may disrupt normal reading as a result.

(iv) It requires high fluid velocity, of the order 15 m/s to produce a measurable differential pressure.

(v) There is no standardization of pitot tubes. Each Pitot tube is required to be calibrated for each installation.

1.5.4 Rota Meter

A rotameter is a device that measures the volumetric flow rate of fluid in a closed tube. These are the most widely used type of variable-area flow meter. It measures flow rate by allowing the cross-sectional area the fluid travels through to vary, causing a measurable effect.

Construction:

A rotameter consists of a tapered tube, typically made of glass with a 'float' (made either of anodized aluminum, ceramic or plastic), inside that is pushed up by the drag force of the flow and pulled down by gravity. The drag force for a given fluid and float cross-section is a function of square of flow speed. A higher volumetric flow rate through a given area increases flow speed and drag force, so the float is pushed upwards. However, as the inside of the rota meter is cone shaped, the area around the float through which the fluid flows increases, the flow speed and drag force decrease until there is mechanical equilibrium with the float's weight.

Floats are made in many different shapes, with spheres and ellipsoids being the most common. The float may be diagonally grooved and partially colored so that it rotates axially as the fluid passes. This shows if the float is stuck since it will only rotate if it is free. Readings are usually taken at the top of the widest part of the float; the center for an ellipsoid, or the top for a cylinder. The float must not float in the fluid and it has to have a higher density than the fluid; otherwise it will float to the top even if there is no flow. The mechanical nature of the device does not require any electrical power. If the tube is made of metal, the float position is transferred to an external indicator via a magnetic coupling. The measurement can be made remotely from the process or used for automatic control.

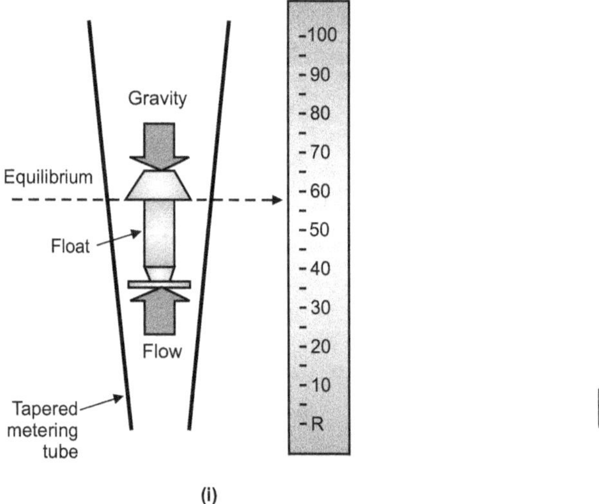

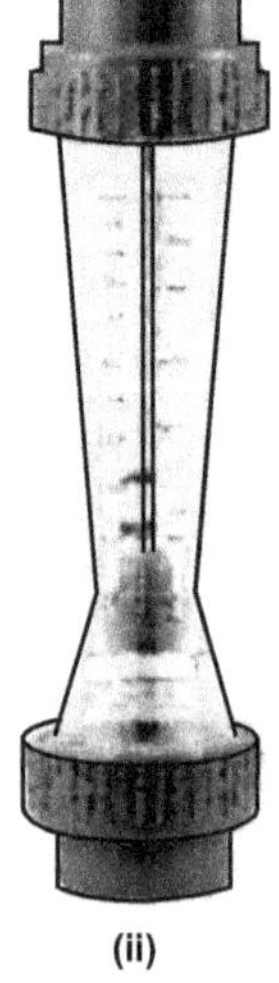

Fig. 1.18: Rota Meter (I) Schematic (II) Real One Used In Practice

Working:

In these devices, the falling and rising action of a float in a tapered tube provides a measure of flow rate. Rota meters are also known as gravity-type flow meters because they are based on the opposition between the downward force of gravity and the upward force of the flowing fluid. When the flow is constant, the float stays in one position that can be related to the volumetric flow rate. That position is indicated on a graduated scale. In order to keep the full force of gravity in effect, this dynamic balancing act requires a vertical measuring tube.

Applications:

(i)   The rotameter is used in process industries to measure fluid flow rates.

(ii) It is used for monitoring gas and water flow in plants or labs.

(iii) It is used for monitoring filtration loading.

Advantages:

(i)   It has good accuracy for low and medium flow rates.

(ii) The pressure loss is nearly constant and small.

(iii) It can be used for corrosive fluids.

(iv) It requires no external power or fuel; it uses only the inherent properties of the fluid, along with gravity.

(v)   A rotameter is a relatively simple device that can be mass manufactured out of cheap materials, allowing for its widespread use and thus cost is low.

(vi) Since the area of the flow passage increases as the float moves-up the tube, the scale is approximately linear.

(vii) Clear glass can be used as this is highly resistant to thermal shock and chemical action.

Disadvantages:

(i)   It is not suitable for opaque fluids as float may not be visible through them.

(ii) Glass tube may be subjected to breakage.

(iii) As this device is based on gravitational force it requires to be installed in vertical position only.

(iv) Calibration scale on rota meter need to be accurate for a given substance at a given temperature.

(v)   A separate rota meter is needed for fluids with different densities and viscosities, or are supplied with multiple scales on the same rota meter.

(vi) Readout uncertainty gets worse near the bottom of the scale.

(vii) Oscillations of the float and parallax may increase the uncertainty of the measurement.

(viii) A transducer may be required for electronically measuring the position of the float.

(ix) Rota meters are not easily adapted for reading automatically.

(x)   Rota meters are not generally manufactured in sizes greater than 6 inches (150 mm).

REVIEW QUESTIONS

1. Define fluid and give its properties. Discuss effect of temperature on viscosity of fluids.
2. State Bernoulli's equation.
3. State the assumptions used in deriving Bernoulli's equation.
4. Write Reynolds equation and describe its terms.
5. Write a short note on different manometers.
6. Write about types of fluid flow.
7. Write short note on laminar flow.
8. Define turbulent flow and write its characteristics.
9. Explain potential energy, kinetic energy and pressure energy.
10. State advantages and limitations of manometers.
11. Differentiate between simple manometer and differential manometer.
12. Write advantages and disadvantages of orifice meter over a Venturi meter.
13. State the limitations of Bernoulli's equation.
14. What is Pitot tube? Discuss its construction, working and applications.
15. What is manometer? How they are classified?
16. Explain the principle of Venturi meter. What are its applications.
17. Why is coefficient of discharge of orifice meter much smaller than that of Venturi meter?
18. What are the limitations of manometers?
19. What is meant by the term Piezometric head?
20. How will you determine the major energy loss?
21. Define major energy loss and minor energy loss in pipes.

Chapter ...2

SIZE REDUCTION

2.0 INTRODUCTION

Pharmaceutical powders are classified as monodispersed (particles of same size) as well as polydispersed (particles of different sizes). Particles of monodispersed type are ideal for pharmaceutical purposes where as polydispersed powders create considerable difficulties in their processing for production of dosage forms. In order to obtain uniform size particles powders are to be reduced in their size by a process called size reduction. Size reduction is defined as a process of reducing large solid unit masses (vegetable or chemical substances) into small unit masses, coarse particles or fine particles. Comminution is the generic term used for size reduction and includes different operations such as crushing, grinding, milling, mincing, and dicing. Size reduction is not enough to obtain monodispersed particles but they are to be further processed by size separation. There are numerous equipments available for size reduction of solids and semisolids to improve performance or to meet specifications. The size-reduction equipments are often developed empirically to handle specific materials. For size reduction knowledge of properties of the material to be processed is essential. The most critical characteristic that enables size reduction is hardness. Size reduction involves techniques to create new surfaces and increase surface area by adding energy proportional to the bonds holding the feed particles together. Other important feature is flow properties because many size-reduction equipments works on continuous mode and often have choke points at which bridging occurs leading to flow interruption. Some of the important applications of size reduction include grinding polymers for recycling, facilitating separation of grain components, boosting the biological availability of medications and producing particles of an appropriate size for a given use. Size reduction may aid other processes such as expression and extraction.

Some of the major applications of size reduction in pharmaceutical field are :

(i) In size reduction of dosage forms such as capsules, insufflations, suppositories and ointments require particle size to be below 60 µm size.

(ii) The therapeutic effectiveness of certain drugs can be increased by reducing the particle size.

(iii) The mixing of solid ingredients is easier if they are reduced to same particle size.

(iv) In case of suspensions particles being finer reduces rate of sedimentation.

(v) The stability of emulsions is increased by decreasing the size of the oil globules.

(vi) Particle size reduction in formulations such as ophthalmics and those meant for external application to the skin could help to reduce irritation of the skin area to which they are applied.

(vii) The rate of drug absorption depends on particle size. The smaller the particle size, quicker and greater will be rate of absorption.

(viii) The physical appearance of semisolids can be improved by reducing its particle size.

Advanced applications of size reduction are:

(i) **Properties of agglomerates:** The breakage behaviour of agglomerates after milling help to investigate effects of the formulation and the mill settings. Both the size of the particles before granulation and the amount of binder used determine the breakage behaviour. These parameters have an influence on the strength of the granule to be milled.

(ii) **Bioavailability enhancement:** The bioavailability of poorly soluble drugs is often intrinsically related to drug particle size. Particle size of pharmaceutical powders for use in inhalation is critical. It dictate areas of the respiratory tract that are to be targeted in order for the product to have the greatest efficacy. Micronisation of solids causes size reduction of a drug substance suitable for an inhalation formulation; it can provide consistent results and is a very cost effective way of achieving small particle sizes.

(iii) **Handling the powder:** Powder handling and processing tends to be problematic because powders exhibit properties similar to both solids and liquids. Normally, they are surrounded by air and the degree of aeration can affect the way the powder behaves. Many common manufacturing problems are attributed to powder flow, including non-uniformity (segregation) in blending, under- or over-dosage, inaccurate filling, obstructions and stoppages. Size reduction help to minimize all those problems.

(iv) **Supercritical fluid technology:** Supercritical fluid technology offers the possibility to produce dry powder formulations suitable for inhalation or needle-free injection. It facilitates controlled particle formation in fine form at near-ambient temperatures and integrates particle formation and solvent removal into a single step.

(v) **Precipitation:** Precipitation with compressed antisolvents is used for generation of monodispersed ultra fine particles. The drug is first dissolved in a solvent, and this solution is mixed with a miscible antisolvent. Mixing processes vary considerably. Precipitation of amorphous material may be favoured at high super saturation when the solubility of the amorphous state exceeded. It utilizes supercritical carbon dioxide as the antisolvent, but the solution jet is deflected by a surface vibrating at an ultrasonic frequency atomizing the jet into much smaller droplets. The advantage is that it can be used for production of organic-solvent free particles, has mild operating temperatures for processing biological materials and is easier for micro-encapsulation of drugs for controlled release of the therapeutic agents.

(vi) Nanotechnology: Wet milling of active drug in the presence of surfactant causes defragmentation. The obtained nanosuspension has increased dissolution rate due to larger surface area exposed, while absence of Ostwald ripening is due to the uniform and narrow particle size range obtained, which eliminates the concentration gradient effect.

2.1 OBJECTIVES

The main objective of size reduction is to produce smaller particles from larger ones. Smaller particles are the desired product either because of their large surface area or because of their shape, size, and number. The energy efficiency of the operation can be related to the new surface formed by the reduction in size. The shape features of particles, both alone and in mixtures, are important for product evaluation after size reduction. In actual processing, using particular equipment does not produce a uniform product, whether the feed is uniformly sized or not. The product normally consists of a mixture of particles, which may contain a wide variety of sizes and even shapes. Some types of equipment are designed to control the magnitude of the largest particles in their products, but the fine sizes are not under such control. In some equipment, fines are minimized, but they cannot be totally eliminated.

In comminuted products, the term "diameter" is generally used to describe the characteristic dimension related to particle size. The shape of an individual particle is conveniently expressed in terms of the sphericity (s), which is independent of particle size. For spherical particles 's' equals unity, while for many crushed materials its value lies between 0.6 and 0.7. There are different types of particle size distributions and no single distribution applies equally well to all comminuted products, particularly in the range of coarser particle sizes. For finer particles, however, the most commonly found distribution follows a log-normal function, which is the most useful among the different types of functions.

Thus, in pharmaceutical practice the objective of this operation is to:

(a) Increase the surface area to enhance the rate of a physical or chemical process.

(b) Perform separation of two constituents in cases where one is dispersed in small isolated pockets.

(c) Meet stringent specifications regarding the sizes of commercial products.

(d) Accomplish intimate mixing of solids in a solid-solid operation since the mixing is more complete if the particle size is small.

(e) Improve dissolution rate, solubility, binding strength and dispersion properties.

(f) Increase the therapeutic effectiveness of certain drugs by reducing the particle size for example, the dose of griseofulvin is reduced to half than that of originally required.

(g) Improve mixing of several solid ingredients.

(h) Improve physical appearance of products.

(i)　Enhance flowability, improve compression and dose uniformity.

(j)　Enhance stability of dispersed system for example, stability of emulsions is increased by decreasing the size of the oil globules.

2.2 MECHANISMS AND LAWS GOVERNING SIZE REDUCTION

The mechanism of size reduction depends upon the nature of the material and each material requires separate treatment. Generally fracture occurs along the lines of weakness. During size reduction fresh surfaces are created or existing cracks and fissures are opened up, wherein the former requires more energy. There may be a tendency that after processing agglomerates of particles are formed. Size reduction is an energy inefficient process because small amount of the energy required in subdividing the particles. In fact, lot of the energy is spent in overcoming friction and inertia of machine parts and the friction between particles and deforming the particles without breaking them. This energy is released as heat.

2.2.1 Laws Governing Size Reduction Process

One of the mechanisms of size reduction called grinding is very inefficient and thus it is important to use energy as efficiently as possible. It is not easy to calculate the minimum energy required for a given size reduction process. Fortunately, there are certain theories which are useful in approximately calculating energy requirement. Although number of theories have been put forth to predict the energy requirements, but none give accurate results.

The theories of size reduction and estimation of energy requirement depend upon the basic assumption that the energy required to produce a change dL in a particle of a typical size dimension L, is a simple power function of L:

$$\frac{dE}{dL} = K\, L^n \qquad\qquad \dots (2.1)$$

Where, dE is differential energy required, dL is change in a typical dimension; L is magnitude of a typical length dimension and K, n, are constants.

Kicks Law:

Kick assumed that the energy required to reduce a material in size was directly proportional to the size reduction ratio dL/L. This implies that n in equation (2.1) is equal to -1.

If,　　　　　　　　　　　　$K = K_K\, f_c$　　　　　　　　　　　　.... (2.2)

Where K_K is called Kick's constant and f_c is called the crushing strength of the material. Thus, we have:

$$\frac{dE}{dL} = K_K\, f_c\, L^{-1} \qquad\qquad \dots (2.3)$$

On integrating equation (2.3) gives:

$$E = K_K\, f_c\, \log_e \frac{L_1}{L_2} \qquad\qquad \dots. (2.4)$$

Equation (2.4) is a statement of Kick's Law. It states that the specific energy required to crush a material, for example, from 10 cm to 5 cm. The same energy is required to crush the same material from 5 mm to 2.5 mm. Thus, in simple terms Kicks law can be stated as energy required to reduce the size of a given quantity of material is constant for the same reduction ratio regardless of the original size.

Rittinger's Law:

Rittinger assumed that the energy required for size reduction is directly proportional to the change in surface area. This leads to a value of −2 for n in equation (2.1) as area is proportional to length squared. If we put:

$$K = K_R \, fc \qquad\qquad .... (2.5)$$

Then,
$$\frac{dE}{dL} = K_R \, f_c \, L^{-2} \qquad\qquad .... (2.6)$$

where, K_R is called Rittinger's constant. On integrating equation (2.6), we obtain:

$$E = K_R \, f_c \left(\frac{1}{L_2} - \frac{1}{L_1} \right) \qquad\qquad ... (2.7)$$

Equation (2.7) is known as Rittinger's Law.

The specific surface of a particle (the surface area per unit mass) is proportional to 1/L. Rittinger's Law states that the energy required to reduce L for a mass of particles from 10 cm to 5 cm would be the same as that required to reduce the same mass of 5 mm particles down to 4.7 mm. This is a very much smaller reduction, in terms of energy per unit mass for the smaller particles, than that predicted by Kick's Law. Thus in simple terms Rittinger's law can be stated as energy used for particulate size reduction is directly proportional to the new surface produced.

Griffith theory : The Griffith theory states that the amount of force to be applied depends on the crack length and focus of stress at the atomic bond of the crack apex.

Bond's law : Bond's law states that energy used to reduce particle size is proportional to the square root of the diameter of the particle produced.

For the grinding of coarse particles wherein the increase in surface area per unit mass is relatively small, Kick's Law is a reasonable approximation. For size reduction of fine powders where large areas of new surfaces are being created better fits the Rittinger's Law.

Size reduction of pharmaceutical products involves reduction mechanism consisting of deforming the material pieces until it breaks or tears. This deformation may be achieved by applying diverse forces. The types of forces commonly used in size reduction process arc compression, impact, attrition or shear and cutting Fig. 2.1. In this operation more than one type of force is usually acts. Table 2.1 summarizes these types of forces and examples of some of the mills commonly used in the pharmaceutical industry.

Table 2.1: Types of Forces Used In Size Reduction

Force	Principle	Example of equipment	Approximate particle size (μm)
Compression	Nutcracker	Roller mill Pestle-Mortar Crushing rolls	50 - 10,000
Impact	Hammer	Hammer mill disintegrator	50 - 8000
Attrition	File	Colloidal mill roller mill	1 - 50
Cutting	Scissors	Scissors shears cutter mill rotary knife cutter	100 - 80,000
Combined impact and attrition	Ball	Ball mill	1 - 2000

2.2.2 Compression

In this mechanism, the material is crushed by application of pressure. Compressive forces are used for coarse crushing of hard materials. Coarse crushing implies reduction to a size of about 3 mm.

2.2.3 Impact

Impact occurs when the material is more or less stationary and is hit by an object moving at high speed or when the moving particle strikes a stationary surface. In both the cases the material is crushed in to smaller pieces. Usually both will take place, since the substance is hit by a moving hammer and the particles formed are then thrown against the casing of the machine. Impact forces can be regarded as general purpose forces and may be associated with coarse, medium and fine grinding of a variety of materials.

2.2.4 Attrition

In attrition, the material is subjected to pressure as in compression, but the surfaces are moving relative to each other, resulting in shear forces which break the particles. Shear or attrition forces are applied in fine pulverization, when the size of products can reach the micrometer range. Sometimes a term referred to as ultra-fine grinding is associated with processes in which the sub-micron range of particles is attained.

2.2.5 Cutting

Cutting reduces the size of solid materials by mechanical action (sharp blade/s) by dividing them into smaller particles. Cutting is used to break down large pieces of material into smaller pieces and definite shape suitable for further processing, such as in the preparation of powders and granules.

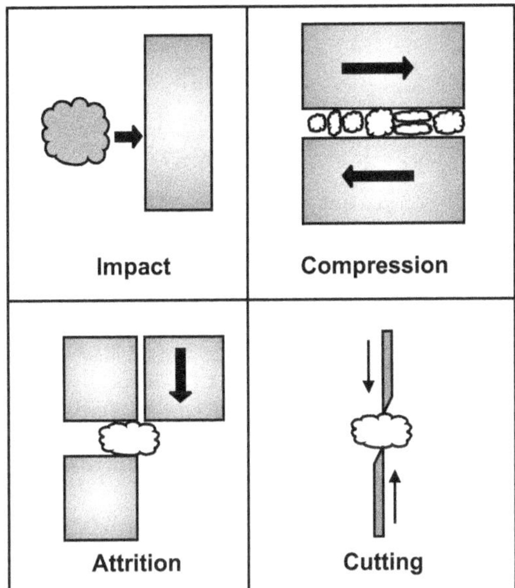

Fig. 2.1: Mechanisms of Size Reduction

2.3 FACTORS AFFECTING SIZE REDUCTION

2.3.1 Hardness

Hardness is a surface property of the material and is frequently confused with strength. It is possible that material is very hard posing a size reduction difficult. If material is brittle then size reduction may present no special problems. An arbitrary scale of hardness has been devised known as Moh's Scale. A series of mineral substances has been given hardness numbers between 1 and 10, ranging from graphite to diamond. Up to 3 are known as soft and can be marked with the fingernail. Hardness above 7 are designated as hard and cannot be marked with a good pen knife blade, while those between 3 and 7 are described as intermediate. In general, the harder the material the more difficult it is to reduce in size.

2.3.2 Toughness

Toughness of a material is generally much more of importance than the hardness. A soft but tough material may present more problems in size reduction than a hard material. For example, tough material like rubber is difficult to break than brittle substance, for example, stick of blackboard chalk. Toughness is encountered in fibrous drugs, and is often related to moisture content. Sometimes material toughness can be reduced by treating them with a liquefied nitrogen at a temperatures lower than −100 to −150 °C. The method has additional advantages that there is a reduction in the decomposition of thermolabile materials, in the loss of volatile materials, in the oxidation of constituents, and in the risk of explosion.

2.3.3 Abrasiveness

Abrasiveness is a property of hard materials (minerals) that limits the mill to be used for size reduction. During the grinding of some very abrasive substances the final powder may be contaminated with more than 0.1 % of metal worn from the grinding mill.

2.3.4 Stickiness

Stickiness of material causes considerable difficulty in size reduction. This type of materials may adhere to the grinding surfaces, or choke the meshes of the sieve. Usually the size reduction equipments produce heat. Gummy or resinous substances may be troublesome to reduce in size as their hardness changes with generation of heat and becomes sticky. Sometimes the addition of inert substances such as kaolin to sulphur may reduce stickiness.

2.3.5 Slipperiness

Slipperiness is the reverse of stickiness. This property also gives rise to size reduction difficulties, since the material acts as a lubricant and lowers the efficiency of the grinding surfaces. While size reduction material slips creating problem in milling.

2.3.6 Softening Temperature

During size reduction process sometimes heat is generated which may cause some substances to soften, and thus the temperature at which this occurs is important. For example, waxy substances such as stearic acid or drugs containing oils or fats may find difficulties in size reduction with reduction in their functionalities. This can be overcome by cooling the mill, either by a water jacket or by passing a stream of cold air through the equipment. Another alternative is to use liquid nitrogen.

2.3.7 Material Structure

Materials used in pharmaceuticals are of wide variety with some are homogeneous but the majority show some special structures.

For example, mineral substances have lines of weakness. Along the lines of weakness these materials splits in to forms like flakes, while vegetable drugs have a cellular structure that often leads to long fibrous particles. Thus, the resulting product at particular operating conditions may vary in their size. The energy required to perform this operation may vary.

2.3.8 Moisture Content

Moisture content of substances influences a number of properties that can affect size reduction. These properties include hardness, toughness or stickiness etc. In general for size reduction materials should be dry or wet and not entirely damp. Usually, less than 5 % moisture is suitable if the substance is to be ground dry or more than 50 % if it is being subjected to wet grinding

2.3.9 Physiological Effect

Some substances are very potent and small amounts of fines generated have an effect on the operator's health. To avoid these fines, mills must be enclosed; in addition exhaust systems should be provided. If possible wet grinding is performed to entirely eliminate the problem.

2.3.10 Purity Required

Some of the size reduction equipments cause wear and tear of the grinding surfaces. Use of these equipments must be avoided whenever high degree of purity of product is needed. Similarly, some of those equipments are so complex that they are unsuitable for cleaning between batches of different materials.

2.3.11 Ratio of Feed Size to Product Ratio

Machines that produce a fine may need to carry out the size reduction in several stages with different equipments. For example, preliminary crushing followed by coarse grinding and then fine grinding. In such cases feed size is needed to be controlled in order to perform reduction efficiently.

2.3.12 Bulk Density

The capacities of most batch mills depend on volume. These mills usually demand solid materials by weight rather than volume. The output of the mill is related to the bulk density of the substance. Higher the bulk density more is the product.

2.4 PRINCIPLES, CONSTRUCTION, WORKING, USES, MERITS AND DEMERITS OF SIZE REDUCTION EQUIPMENTS

From the beginning of time, humans have found it necessary to make little pieces out of big ones. It was a slow, laborious process for many centuries. The first breakthrough was a hammer which worked better than ever, in fact, it's still one of the most widely used tools in size reduction. As we know size reduction requires adding energy to a material to make large pieces smaller, the output depends on energy utilized. Different types of size reduction equipment are available and each has its own mechanism of reduction. The right equipment for the task is the one that can add energy most efficiently for the application. There are many different size reduction equipments available to make little pieces out of big ones. Particle size-reduction equipment includes impact crushers and milling machines such as ball mills, hammer mills, pulverizers and grinders. Materials processed fall into broad categories including abrasive, non-abrasive, wet or dry, sticky and friable. Several factors mentioned earlier helps to select the correct equipment for each unique application. These equipments are classified into three classes according to the nature of the forces applied.

- **(a) Class I:** The size reduction is accomplished by application of continuous pressure and this class includes equipment for coarse crushing.

- **(b) Class II:** The reduction is effected by blow or impact. An example of impact is breaking of a brittle lumpy material by throwing against a wall when the material breaks into pieces due to sudden release of force.

- **(c) Class III:** In the third type shearing forces are applied by grinding or abrasion and this class gives fine grinding.

   There is no sharp demarcation line between first two classes since some mills use a combination of these forces for size reduction. Thus a broad classification could be a crushing, impact and grinding mills.

The materials to be reduced in their size must be thoroughly dried to avoid accumulation in the mill. The necessary care must be employed to avoid possible jamming with wet material and to prevent agglomeration of the particles after size reduction. Crystalline inorganic and organic medicinal compounds which are isolated by normal precipitation and crystallization methods must be thoroughly dried. Vegetable drugs, due to their wide variation in physical state, may require an initial reduction to small pieces. Materials like camphor and spermaceti, the particles of which tend to cohere as quickly as they are produced, need wetting with alcohol before size reduction to avoid this difficulty. On the small-scale initial size reduction of vegetable drugs may be done by slicing, rasping or contusion. Slicing or cutting may be done both transversely and longitudinally so that the tissues may be laid open as completely as possible for quicker drying of the material. Rasping or grating can be done with a nutmeg grater and is mainly used for soaps and waxes that are normally required in coarse state. Bruising is accomplished by beating the drug in heavy motor using pestles whose shape and material of construction vary. They are made of iron, marble, porcelain, glass, steel etc. The bottom surfaces of the mortar and pestle may be shallow or round. Shallow mortars give more grinding effect and are more efficient for size reduction of dry materials and for preparation of fine emulsions.

2.4.1　Hammer Mill

A hammer mill is an essential machine in the pharmaceutical and food processing industries. It can be used to crush, pulverize, shred, grind and reduce material to suitable sizes. In a hammer mill, swinging hammer heads are attached to a rotor that rotates at high speed inside a hard casing.

Principle:

The working principle of hammer mill is simple to understand. The principle is illustrated in Fig. 2.2(a). It only requires choosing an appropriate motor, crushing hammers/knives and material to be crushed. It operates on the principle of impact between rapidly moving hammers mounted on rotor and the stationary powder bed. The material is crushed and pulverized between the hammers and the casing and remains in the mill until it is fine enough to pass through a sieve which forms the bottom of the casing. Both brittle and fibrous materials can be handled in hammer mills, though with fibrous material, projecting sections on the casing may be used to give a cutting action.

Construction:

Hammer mill has five main parts. Fully assembled pharmaceutical hammer mill is showed in Fig. 2.2(b). Normally, the number of parts may vary depending on the complexity of the machine design. Every part in the hammer mill plays an integral role in the overall working of hammer mills. However, the milling process mainly takes place in the crushing chamber. It consists of a stout steel casing in which a central shaft is enclosed to which four or more swinging hammers are attached. When the shaft is rotated by motor the hammers swing out to a radial position. On the lower part of the casing a sieve of desired size is fitted which can be easily replaced according to the particle size required. The material is crushed and pulverized between the hammers and the casing and remains in the mill until it is fine enough to pass through a sieve. Some mills consist of projecting sections on the casing used to give a cutting action if fibrous materials are to be processed. The hammer mills are available in various size, designs and shapes. In pharmaceutical industry they are used for grinding dry materials, wet filter cakes, ointments and slurries etc.

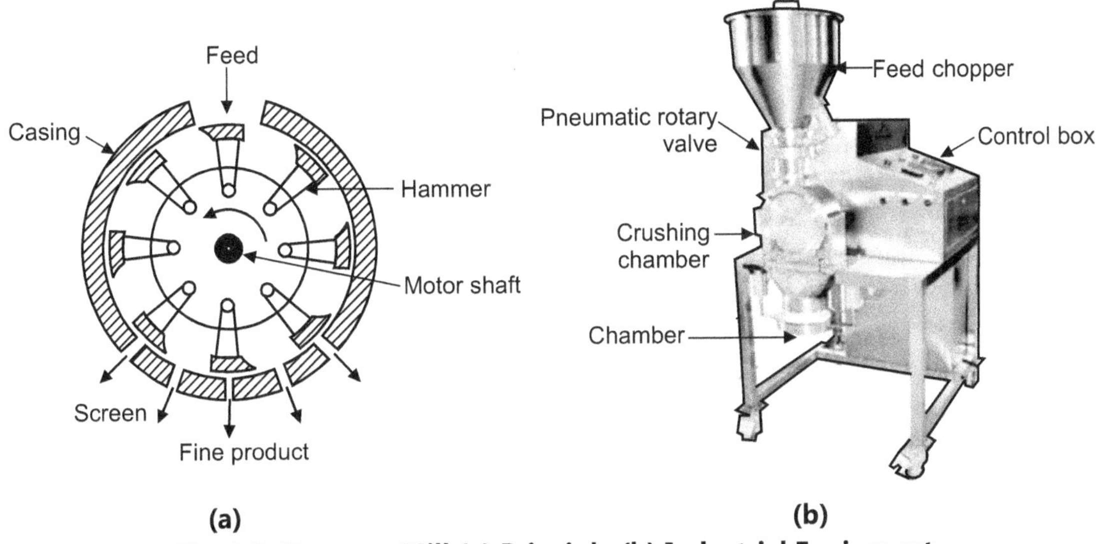

Fig. 2.2: Hammer Mill (a) Principle (b) Industrial Equipment

Working:

Feeding mechanism refers to the process by which particles enter the crushing chamber. Depending on the design of the hammer in mill machine, it may use either gravity or a metered feeding system. Metered feeding systems are used when product uniformity is a major concern as they eliminate all possible variables that may cause output product inconsistencies. A good example in this case is the pneumatic rotary valve found between the feeding hopper and the crushing chamber. In the gravity feeding system, the milling machines solely depend on the gravitational force that helps to feed particles into the crushing chamber.

Users can switch ON/OFF the machine from the control box. Operator may control the feeding system or motor speed. Some pharmaceutical milling machines come with a display panel where users can monitor all processes. This mill operates at a high speed that may vary from 2,500 to 60,000 r.p.m. In most cases, hammers are mounted on horizontal shafts where they may rotate either clockwise or anti-clockwise. This may depend on the direction of the rotor rotation. A rotor is the rotating shaft coupled to an electric motor. The hammers come in different styles and shapes. Hammer mill's crushing tools may be coupled directly to a motor or driven by a belt. As opposed to direct connection, the belts can cushion the motor from shock and allows for accurate speed adjustment. The output of a pharmaceutical hammer mill varies broadly. Normally, the size of the particles depends on the sieve variation. These hammer mills may have over 12 different types of sieve meshes. Pharmaceutical materials that enter the systems are reduced to very small particle due to the rotating hammers.

The basic working steps are as follows:

(i) Introducing material through the feed hopper: Materials with suitable physical properties that have been cut to the right size are selected. Depending on the design of the hammer mill it will move into the crushing chamber either by gravity or controlled/metered process.

(ii) In the crushing chamber: The ganged hammers or chopping knives hit the material severally. These components rotate at high speed reducing materials to a desired size. Only particles whose diameter conforms to that of the sieve size passes through sieves. Otherwise, the hammers continue to hit these materials until they are reduced to the required size. Basically, within this chamber, the material is hit by a repeated combination of knives/hammer impact and collision with the wall of the milling chamber. Moreover, collision between particles plays an instrumental role in this size reduction process. It is adviced for not to open the crushing chamber when the machine is operating.

(iii) Outlet of the milling chamber: The outlet of the milling chamber has perforated metal sieves (bar gates). Depending on the size and design of the metal sieve, it allows the required size of particles to pass through while retaining coarse material. The material that passes through is basically the finished product called output.

Factors determining output and capacity of hammer mill:

Basically, there are three aspects that determine the particle size of a hammer mill. These include hammer or cutting knife configuration, shaft speed and sieve size. In most cases reducing large particles into small size may result in a fine or coarse finish. To obtain a fine particles key aspects such as size, a fast rotating rotor speed, small sieve size and large or/and more crushing knives/hammers are preferred. For coarse finished output key aspects are few or/and small crushing hammers/knives, slow rotor speed and large sieve. The overall capacity of hammer mills depends on many critical aspects that include characteristics of materials to be crushed, nature or type of the crushing hammers or knives, number of rows of crushing hammers or knives and feed size.

Merits:

(i)   It is rapid in action, and is capable of grinding many different types of materials.

(ii) They are easy to install and operate, the operation is continuous.

(iii) There is little contamination of the product with metal abraded from the mill as no surface move against each other.

(iv) The particle size of the material can be easily controlled by changing the speed of the rotor, hammer type, shape and size of the sieve.

Demerits:

(i)   The high speed of operation causes generation of heat that may affect thermolabile materials or drugs containing gum, fat or resin. The mill may be water-cooled to reduce this heat damage.

(ii) The rate of feed must be controlled carefully as the mill may be choked, resulting in decreased efficiency or even damage.

(iii) Because of the high speed of operation, the hammer mill is susceptible to damage by foreign objects such as stones or metal in the feed. Magnets may be used to remove iron, but the feed must be checked visually for any other contamination.

Uses:

(i)   Fibrous materials can be handled in hammer mills by cutting edges.

(ii)   Brittle material is best fractured by impact of blunt hammers.

(iii) It is capable of producing intermediate grades of powders of almost all substances.

(iv)   Powdering of barks, leaves, roots, crystals and filter cakes.

(v)   Useful for granulation where the damp mass is cut in to granules by the hammers.

2.4.2 Ball Mill

The general idea behind the ball mill is an ancient one that it was used for grinding flint for pottery. A pharmaceutical ball mill is a type of grinder used to grind and blend materials while manufacturing various dosage forms. The size reduction is done by impact as the balls drop from near the top of the shell. Ball mills are used primarily for single stage fine grinding, regrinding, and as the second stage in two stage grinding circuits. According to the need ball mill can be either for wet or dry designs. Ball mills have been designed in standard sizes of the final products between 0.074 mm and 0.4 mm in diameter.

Principle:

The size reduction in ball mill is a result of fragmentation mechanisms (impact and attrition) as the balls drop from near the top of the shell. Mixing of feed is achieved by the high energy impact of balls. The energy levels of balls are as high as 12 times the gravitational acceleration. Rotation of base plate provides the centrifugal force to the grinding balls and independent rotation of shell to make the balls hit the inner wall of the shell. Since the shell is rotating in alternate (one forward cycle and one reverse cycle) directions a considerable part of grinding take place in addition to homogenous mixing. The operating principle of the ball mill consists of following steps. In a continuously operating ball mill, feed material is fed through the central hole into the drum (shell) and moves there along with grinding media (balls).

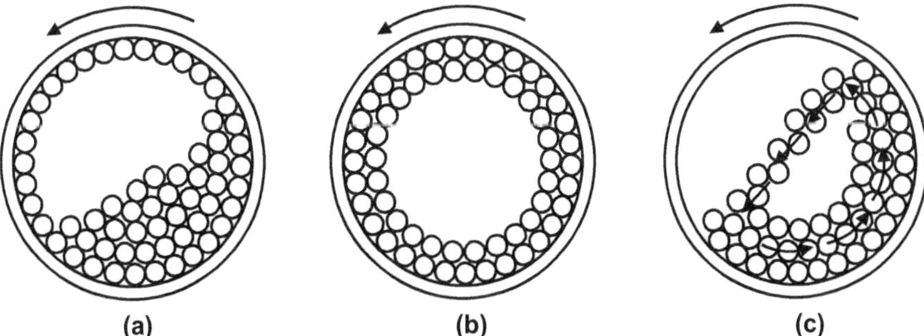

(a)   (b)   (c)

Fig. 2.3: Cascade Operation in Ball Mill (a) Low Speed (b) High Speed (c) Correct Speed

The material to be ground is fed from hopper at a 60° angle and the product is discharged through a 30° angle. As the shell rotates the balls are lifted up on the rising side of the shell and cascade down (or drop down on to the feed) from near the top of the shell. The material grinding occurs during impact of falling grinding balls and abrasion of the particles between the balls. The discharge of ground material is performed through the central hole in the discharge cap (mills with center unloading the milled product) or through the grid (mills with unloading the milled product through the grid). In ball mill depending on the rotational speed following possible modes of the grinding media motion could be achieved.

(a) **Low speed:** Speed mode with a rolling of grinding balls without flight.

(b) **Mixed mode (Cascade mode motion):** Speed mode with a partial rolling and a partial flight of grinding balls.

(c) **High speed:** Speed mode with circular motion of balls with no fall.

In ball milling the speed of the rotation is more important. At a low speed, Fig. 2.3(a), the mass of the ball slides or rolls over each other with inefficient output. At a high speed, Fig. 2.3(b), the balls are thrown out to the walls by centrifugal force. Since at this speed there is absence of any impact or attrition no grinding occurs. Compression by the ball against the shell wall is not enough for comminution. But at $2/3^{rd}$ of the speed (50 to 80% of the critical speed), Fig. 2.3(c), the centrifugal speed force just occurs with the result that the balls are carried almost to the top of the mill and then fall to the bottom. By this way the maximum size reduction is effected by the impact of particles between the balls and by attrition between the balls. After the suitable time the material is taken out and passed through a sieve to get powder of the required size. Ball mills are very effective for grinding smooth, aqueous or oily dispersions by wet grinding since it gives particles of 10 microns or less.

Construction:

The basic parts of ball mill are a shell, balls and motor Fig. 2.4. A ball mill is also known as pebble mill or tumbling mill. It consists of a hollow cylindrical shell (drum) containing balls mounted on a metallic frame such that it can be rotated along its longitudinal axis. The axis of the shell may be either horizontal or at a small angle to the horizontal. It is partially filled with balls. The grinding media is the balls, which may be made of chrome steel, stainless steel or ceramic. The balls which could be of different diameter occupy 30 - 50% of the mill volume and its size depends on the feed and mill size. The large balls tend to break down the coarse feed materials and the smaller balls help to form the fine product by reducing void spaces between the balls. Usually the grinding media balls weight is kept constant. The ball size depends on the feed and the diameter of the mill. The inner surface of the cylindrical shell is usually lined with an abrasion-resistant material such as manganese steel or rubber. Less wear takes place in rubber lined mills. The metallic cylinder which is coated with different materials is helpful in the mechanism of attrition. The length of the mill is approximately equal to or slightly greater than its diameter.

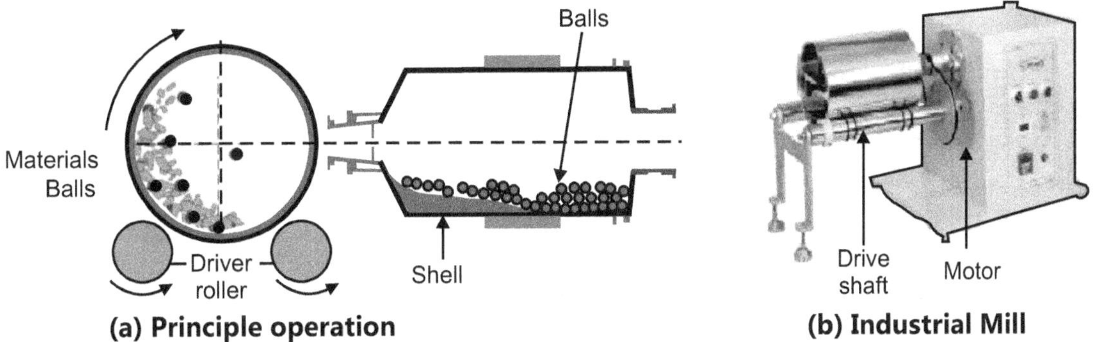

(a) Principle operation　　　　　　　　　**(b) Industrial Mill**

Fig. 2.4: Pharmaceutical Ball Mill

An internal cascading effect reduces the material to a fine powder. Industrial ball mills can operate continuously to fed at one end and discharged at the other. Large to medium ball mills are mechanically rotated on their axis, but small ones normally consist of a cylindrical capped container that sits on two drive shafts. High quality ball mills are potentially expensive and can grind mixture particles to as small as 0.0001 mm, enormously increasing surface area and reaction rates.

Factors determining efficiency of ball mill:

The degree of milling in a ball mill is influenced by;

(i)　Residence time of the material in the mill chamber.

(ii)　The size, density and number of the balls.

(iii) The nature (hardness) of the balls and material to be grinded.

(iv) Feed rate and feed level in the vessel.

(v)　Rotation speed of the cylinder.

Working:

Several types of ball mill exist. They differ to an extent in their operating principle. They also differ in their maximum capacity of the milling shell, ranging from 0.010 liters for planetary ball mill, mixer mill or vibration ball mill to several 100 liters for horizontal rolling ball mills. The steps involved in the working process of ball mill are as follows:

(i)　**Initial stage:** The powder particles are get flattened by the collision of the balls. It leads it changes in the shapes of individual particles or cluster of particles being impacted repeatedly by the milling balls with high kinetic energy.

(ii)　**Intermediate stage:** Significant changes occur in comparison with those in the initial stage.

(iii) **Final stage:** Reduction in particle size takes place. The microstructure of the particle also appears to be more homogenous in microscopic scale than those at the initial and intermediate stages.

(iv) **Completion stage:** The powder particles possess an extremely deformed metastable structure.

Types of ball mill:

There are various types of ball mills used for different applications amongst which first two are commonly used in pharmaceutical practice. These includes Pebble ball mill, Vibrating ball mill, Drum ball mills, Jet-mills, Bead-mills, Horizontal rotary ball mills,

(i) Pebble ball mill: Pebble mills are sometimes called as jar mill or pot mill which works on the principle of attrition and impact. The grinding is effected by placing the substance in the cylindrical vessel or jar vessels that are lined by the porcelain or other hard substance containing pebbles or balls. The cylindrical vessel revolves horizontally on their long axis and the tumbling of the pebbles over one another and against the sides of the cylinder produce pulverization with a minimum loss of material.

(ii) Vibrating ball mill: Vibrating ball mill also works on the principle of attrition and impact. It consists of mill shell containing a charge of balls similar to that of ball mills. In this case the shell vibrates due to some frequency rather than rotated.

Uses:

  (i) Small capacity ball mills are used for the final grinding of drugs or for grinding suspensions.

  (ii) The high capacity ball mills are used for milling ores prior to manufacture of pharmaceutical chemicals.

  (iii) Ball mills are an efficient tool for grinding many brittle and sticky materials into fine powder.

  (iv) The hard and abrasive as well as wet and dry materials can be grinded in the ball mills for pharmaceutical purpose.

  (v) Powders for ophthalmic and parenteral products can be reduced in size.

  (vi) Ball mill is used for the milling of pigments and insecticides for industrial purpose.

  (vii) Ball mills are also used in manufacture of black powder.

  (viii) Blending of explosives is an example of an application for rubber balls.

  (ix) For systems with multiple components, ball milling has been shown to be effective in increasing solid-state chemical reactivity.

  (x) Ball milling has been shown effective for production of amorphous materials.

Merits:

  (i) It produces very fine powder (particle size less than or equal to 10 microns).

  (ii) It is suitable for milling toxic materials because of its design as a completely enclosed form.

  (iii) It is used in milling highly abrasive materials.

  (iv) Strong adaptability to the fluctuation of the physical property of the materials such as granularity, water content and hardness.

  (v) Ball mill has a big crushing ratio and high production capacity.

   (vi) It has simple design, ease of examination and change of abraded spare parts.

  (vii) Reliable operation, simple maintenance and management.

 (viii) It can be used for continuous operation, if sieve or classifier is attached to the mill.

   (ix) It is capable of grinding a large variety of materials of different characters and different degree of hardness.

    (x) It is suitable for wet as well as dry grinding processes.

   (xi) The cost of installation, power and grinding medium is low.

  (xii) It is suitable for both batch and continuous operation.

 (xiii) Suitable for grinding material with high hardness.

 (xiv) The shape of the final products is circular.

  (xv) No contamination in the powder with ceramic ball.

 (xvi) The capacity and fineness can be adjusted by adjusting the diameter of the ball.

Demerits:

    (i) Contamination of product may occur as a result of wear and tear of the balls and partially from the casing.

   (ii) High machine noise level especially if the hollow cylinder is mode of metal, but much less if rubber is used.

  (iii) It has relatively long milling time due to low rotary speed and thus has low working efficiency.

  (iv) It is difficult to clean the machine after use.

   (v) High production cost and high unit electricity consumption.

  (vi) Heavy equipment so very high one time capital investment.

 (vii) Some raw materials may become damaged by steel balls.

 (vii) Not suitable for sensitive and flammable substances.

2.4.3 Fluid Energy Mill

Fluid energy mill is also known as pulverizer, micronizer or jet mill. It is used for fine grinding and for close particle size control. The reduction of the particles takes place by the attrition and impact mechanism by the air or inert gas introduced through the nozzles presents in the chamber. This mill is mainly used to grind heat sensitive materials to the fine powder.

Principle:

It operates on the principle of impact and attrition. The inlet and outlets are attached with classifier which prevents the particles to pass until they become sufficiently fine, Fig. 2.5(a). It helps in determination of particle size and shape. The speed of air/inert gas is directly related with efficiency. Solids introduced into the stream through inlet result in high degree of turbulence, impact and attritional forces to occur between the particles. This erratic motion between the feed and air result in breakdown of particles. This mill involves no heat generation and hence used to grind heat sensitive materials.

Construction:

The main basic parts present in the fluidized energy mill are inlet, nozzles, classifier and hollow toroid (Loop). Through inlet the solid material is introduced into the chamber made of stainless steel. The air or the inert gas is introduced through nozzles into the chamber at the bottom of the loop. The cyclone separator called classifier is attached at the top from which the fine particles are collected. The loop of a pipe has a diameter of 20 to 200 mm depending on the overall height of the loop which may be up to about 2 meters. The high pressure of fluid exerts a high velocity circulation in the loop in a very turbulent manner. A classifier is incorporated in the system, so that particles are retained in loop until sufficiently fine.

Fluidized energy mills are available in other subclasses. They have no moving parts and are primarily distinguished from one another by the configuration and/or shape of their chambers, nozzles and classifiers. They include tangential jet, loop/oval, opposed jet, opposed jet with dynamic classifiers, fluidized bed, moving target, fixed target and high pressure homogenizers.

Working:

The feed introduced in to fluid energy mill is pre-treated to reduce the particles size to the order of 100 meshes. This enables the process to yield a product as small as 5 micrometers or less. Despite this, mills capable of output up to 40 kg/h are also available. Air or inert gas is injected as a high pressure jet through nozzles at the bottom of the loop.

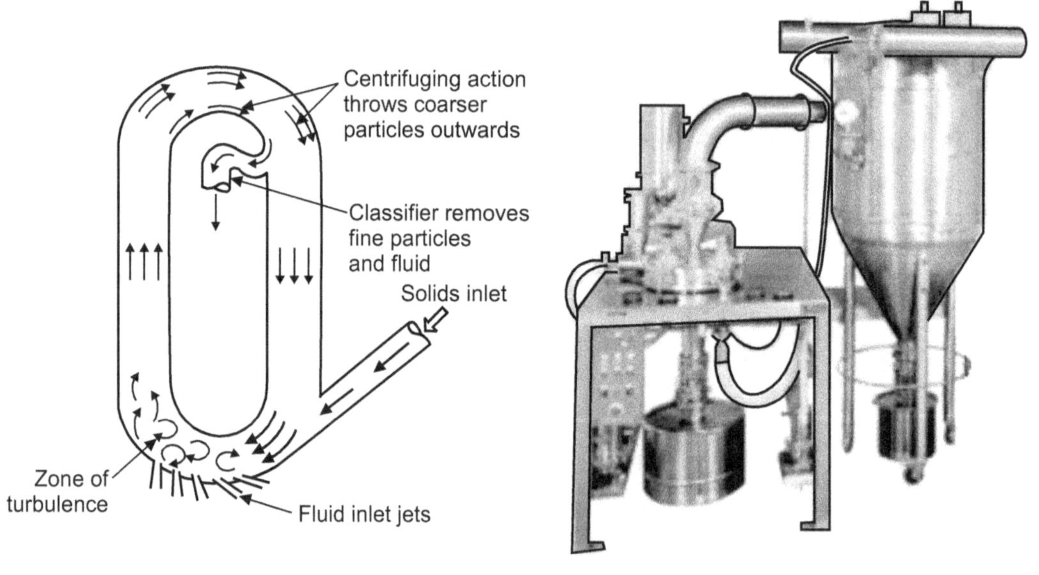

(a) Schematic   **(b) Industrial mill**

Fig. 2.5: Fluid Energy Mill

The powder particles in the mill are accelerated to high velocity by gas pressure. The kinetic energy of the air and the resulting turbulence due to high pressure causes inter particle collision and attrition due to particle-wall contact resulting in particle size reduction up to 5 μm. Size-reduction in this mill also depends on the energy supplied by a compressed air that enters the grinding chamber at high speed. The fluidized effect carries particles to a classifier zone where the larger particles are retained until they become sufficiently fine. Fine particles are collected through a classifier.

Types of fluid energy mills:

There are two main classes of pulverizers (fluid energy mills)

(i) Air Swept Pulverizer: In this mill the particles along with air are fed into the mill inlet. Air swept pulverizers uses air to transport particles to the pulverizing section of the apparatus. The beater plates support the hammers and distribute the particles around the periphery of the grinding chamber. The hammers grind the solid against the liner of the grinding chamber. The beater plates rotate between 1600 and 7000 rpm to reduce the size of the incoming particles. The classifier plate separates the fine product and exit through the discharge outlet. The larger material is back feed to the mill inlet through the recycle housing.

(ii) Air Impact Pulverizer: In air impact pulverizers superheated steam or compressed air produces the force that reduces the size of large particles. It results in the smashing of the particles into smaller particles. This pulverizer uses high speed air to pulverize the particles.

The products from both air swept and air impact pulverizers produces particles which do not require further sieving or classifying.

Factors determining efficiency of fluid energy mills:

   (i)   The speed of air/inert gas.

   (ii) Feed rate and size.

   (iii) The configuration of the mill.

   (iv) Design of the classifier.

   (v) The position of the nozzle.

   (vi) The impact between the feed and air.

Uses:

   (i)   Fluid energy mill is used when fine powders are required, for example, antibiotics, sulphonamides and vitamins.

   (ii) Suitable for laboratories where small samples are needed.

   (iii) The mill is used to grind heat sensitive material to fine powder.

   (iv) The major advantage is fine grinding of pigments, kaolin, zircon, titanium and calcium, alumina, ceramic frit, powder insecticides such as DDT, diatomaceous earth, feldspar, fluorspar, graphite, gypsum, iron ore, iron oxide, iron powder, limestone, polymers, rare earth ores carbon, talc etc.

   (v) It is the choice of mill when higher degree of drug purity is required

Merits:

(i) The particle size of the product is smaller than produced by any other method.

(ii) Expansion of gases at the nozzles leads to cooling, counteracting the frictional heat thus protecting heat-sensitive materials.

(iii) There is little or no abrasion of the mill and so no contamination of the product.

(iv) To protect sensitive drugs from oxidative degradation this mill has facility to use inert gases.

(v) Presence of classifier permits control of particle size and particle size distribution.

(vi) Suitable for size reduction of materials capable of generating a static charge.

(vii) The process is suitable for friable, abrasive or crystalline materials.

(viii) Air needed is freely available.

(ix) Homogeneous blend of large range of sizes available.

(x) The equipment is easily sterilized.

(xi) At the end of milling product particle size between 2 and 10 µm is obtained.

Demerits:

(i) This mill is energy consuming and the energy consumed per ton of milled product is high.

(ii) High head space is required.

(iii) Coarse feed size is not suitable.

(iv) The fed device may be clogged with the clump materials.

(v) Special feeding devices should be provided for the feeding of the materials.

(vi) The use of compressed air leads to generation of static electricity.

(vii) Material recovered in the collection bags is difficult or impossible to remove by the normal blow back procedures.

(viii) Tendency of forming aggregates or agglomerates after milling.

(ix) Generation of amorphous content due to high energy impact.

(x) Formation of unwanted ultra-fine particles.

2.4.4 Edge Runner Mill

The edge runner mill is also called as roller stone mill and is mechanized form of mortar and pestle-type compression comminution. It crushes the materials into fine powders by the rotating stones. The edge runner mill consists of two large rotating grinding wheels or stones turning slowly in a large bowl. In this mill material can be crushed or ground in a continuous operation.

Principle:

The edge runner mill mainly works on the attrition and impaction by which the crushing or grinding of the powder material takes place. The principle of size reduction by this mill are crushing due to heavy weight of the stones or metal and shearing force. Movement of stones or metal causes size reduction. The Edge-runner mill has the pastel equivalent mounted horizontally and rotating against a bed of powders.

Construction:

The basic parts of this mill consist of two heavy rollers and a bed made of stones or granite which is used for the grinding of the materials, Fig. 2.6. The rollers are mounted on the central horizontal shaft and move around the bed in a shallow circular pan.

Working:

The material to be milled is fed into the centre of the pan and is worked outwards by the action of the wheels. Scrapers are employed in scraping the material constantly from the bottom of the wheel vessel after which it is fed to the wheel where it gets crushed to powders. The material is ground for a definite period and then it is passed through the sieves to get the powder of the required size. An electric motor in the basement provides power for the mill to start the device as used in flour mills. This mill is used for crushing or grinding various materials without the danger of clogging or jamming of the machine by accumulation of the ore with greater efficiency and in high comparative quantities. The crushed powder is discharged through outlet at the bottom.

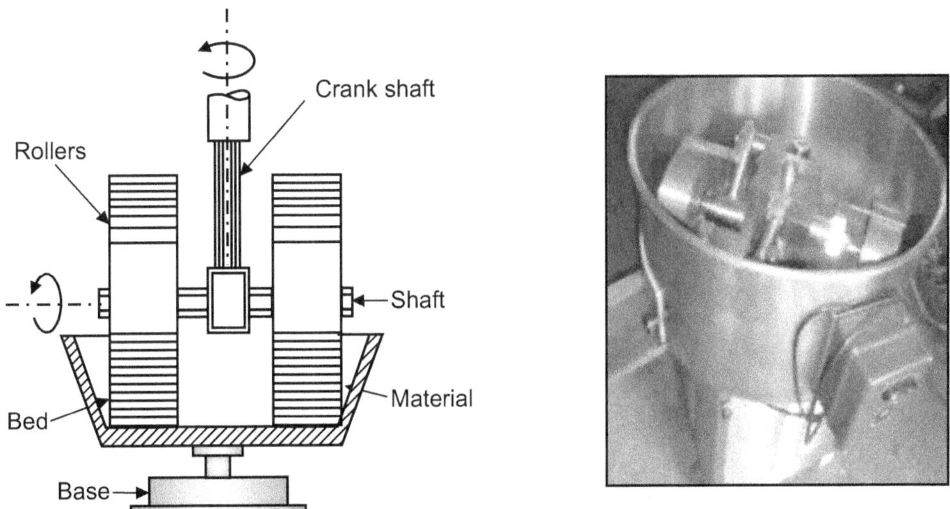

Fig. 2.6: Edge Runner Mill (a) Schematic (b) Industrial Mill Used In Practice

Uses:

(i)   This mill is used for grinding most of the drugs to very fine powder.

(ii) It is used to crush or grind all types of the drugs.

(iii) It is most preferred for size reduction of non-sticky materials

Merits:

(i)   Very fine particle sized materials can be obtained by this edge runner mill.

(ii) It has simple design.

(iii) The major advantage of this mill is that it requires less attention during operation.

(iv) The combinations of various elements in this machine makes it to operate with greater efficiency.

(v) Utilizes less power, and does not require frequent clean-up and particular adjustment.

Demerits:

(i)   It requires more floor space than the other commonly used mills.

(ii) It is not suitable for sticky materials.

(iii) This mill produce lot of noise pollution.

2.4.5 End Runner Mill

End-runner mill similar to edge runner mill is a mechanized form of mortar and pestle type size reduction equipment. A heavy weight pestle rotates due to the friction of material present between mortar and pestle upon rotation of mortar driven by motor at the base.

Principle:

The principle of size reduction applied in these mills are crushing due to heavy weight of the stones or metal pestle and shearing force as a result of movement of these stones or metal. In the end-runner mill, a weighted pestle is turned by the friction of material passing beneath it as the mortar rotates under powder to be processed.

Construction:

End-runner mills are the mechanized forms of mortar and pestle-type compression comminution. This milling equipment consists of pestle made of either stone or metal, connected by a shaft, Fig. 2.7. The pastel rotates at its axis in a shallow steel or porcelain mortar. The pestle is mostly dumb-bell shaped. The mortar is fixed to a flanged plate at the bottom. It also consists of scrappers at the centre and alongside of the circular pan. The pestle is mounted horizontally and rotating against a bed of powders.

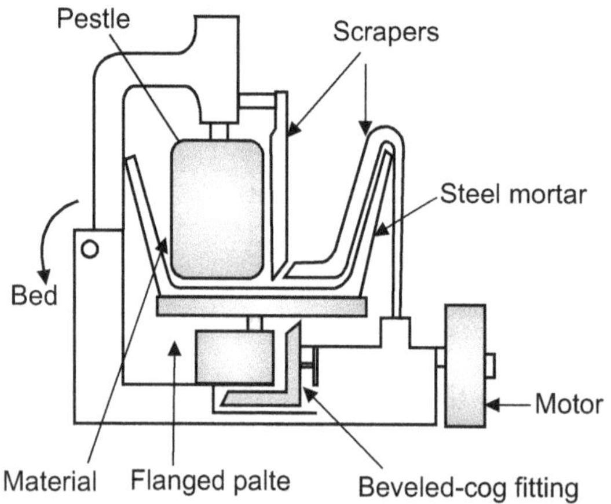

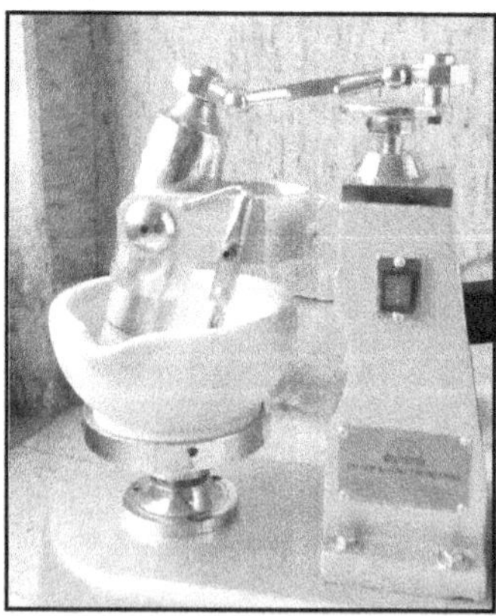

Fig. 2.7: End Runner Mill (a) Schematic (b) Mill Used in Practice

Working:

The material to be milled is fed into the centre of the circular mechanical mortar (pan) and is worked outwards by the action of the wheels and mill is operated. The pestle rotates against a bed of powders. Mortar revolves at high speed and causes the pestle to revolve. Scrapers are employed in scraping the material constantly from the bottom of the wheel and are feed back to the wheel were it gets crushed further. Finally, pestle is raised from the mortar manually or automatically to facilitate emptying and cleaning.

Uses:

(i)   It is used to reduce fibrous crude drugs to a fine size.

(ii) It used for grinding semisolid preparations such as ointments and pastes to fine size.

(iii) It is used for uniform distribution of the contents in viscous dispersion medium.

(iv) It can be used for both wet and dry grinding of crude drugs.

Merits:

(i)   It has simple design and thus cleaning and maintenance is easy.

(ii) It utilizes less electrical power.

(iii) It produces fine and sometimes very fine particles.

(iv) Requires less attention during the milling operation.

(v)   It has no problem of chocking or clogging as it has no sieves for size separation.

Demerits:

(i)   It runs only on batch operation.

(ii) It is not suitable for milling sticky materials.

(iii) Unsuitable for drugs which are hard and unbroken or in slightly broken condition.

(iv) Machine noise causes lot of noise pollution.

(v)   It requires scrapper adjustment intermittently.

REVIEW QUESTIONS

1.   What is size reduction? What are objectives of size reduction?

2.   Write pharmaceutical applications of size reduction.

3.   What is Kick's law? What is its significance in size reduction?

4.   Discuss energy calculation theories involved in size reduction.

5.   What is Rittinger's Law? What is its significance in size reduction?

6.   What is Griffith theory and Bond's law?

7.   Discuss mechanisms involved in size reduction of material.

8. Discuss factors affecting size reduction.

9. Classify size reduction equipments based on nature of forces applied.

10. Describe principle, construction, working, uses, merits and demerits of hammer mill.

11. What are factors that determine output and capacity of hammer mill?

12. Describe principle, construction, working, uses, merits and demerits of ball mill.

13. What is cascading effect and critical speed in ball mill operation? Write about its significance.

14. Describe principles, construction, working, uses, merits and demerits of ball mill.

15. Write note on types of ball mills.

16. Discuss principle, construction, working, uses, merits and demerits of fluid energy mill.

17. Write about various types of fluid energy mills.

18. Describe principles, construction, working, uses, merits and demerits of fluid energy mill,

19. Discuss principle, construction, working, uses, merits and demerits of edge runner mill.

20. Discuss principle, construction, working, uses, merits and demerits of end runner mill,

21. Differentiate between edge runner mill and end runner mill.

☙ ☙ ☙

Chapter ... **3**

SIZE SEPARATION

Large pieces of material are usually estimated visually but difficulties arise only when powders are to be estimated. The aim of any estimation, including particle size separation, is either analytical or preparative. Size separation is a unit operation that involves the separation of a mixture of various size particles into two or more portions by means of sieveing surfaces. Size separation is performed by processes known as sieving, sifting, segregation etc. Size separation is a method of classifying particles into fractions based on size. Granular mixtures separate according to particle size when shaken, with large particles rising; a phenomenon termed the 'Brazil-nut effect'. It is well known fact that differences in particle density affect size separation in mixtures of granular particles.

Particles of many kinds and various sizes have played an important role in development and production of dosage forms. If particles are spherical or cubical, it would be easy to characterize them. Unfortunately, most of the particles or granules in pharmaceuticals are of irregular size and shape. Therefore, various methods and techniques have been developed to characterize such particles. Particle size analysis is important in studying particle behaviour in a medium during industrial applications. Particle size analysis in various processes involves many concepts and techniques; however, this chapter is focused on the methods of particle size separation utilizing mechanical techniques.

3.1 OBJECTIVES

Particles of many kinds and various sizes play an important role in performing specific function in development and use of dosage forms. If particles are spherical or cubical, it is easy to characterize them. Unfortunately, most of the particles employed in pharmaceuticals are of irregular size and shape. Therefore, it is desirable to develop methods and techniques to characterize particles of irregular size and shape, and this is the main objective of particle size separation. Apart from this other objectives of size separation are:

(i) Size separation is useful in grading powders or granules. Any solid materials after size reduction never give particles of the same size but contain particles of varying sizes. The size-reduced particles are then passed through sieves with the objective to get fractions of narrow size range.

(ii) To control size variations in the materials. During tablet granulation the granules should be within narrow size range, otherwise, weight variation will take place during tablet punching.

(iii) To classify materials in to different sizes for the desired purpose.

(iv) To enhance performance (topical powders), efficacy (powders for inhalation) and stability of dosage forms (suspensions).

(v) To judge uniformity in a mixing materials.

(vi) To avoid variations in the bulk properties of materials.

(vii) To specify the quality parameter of a intermediate and finished dosage forms.

3.2 APPLICATIONS

Particle size separation is important in studying particle behaviour in a medium as in many analytical sciences and industrial applications. Size separation has following major applications in pharmacy:

(i) Size separation has significance in formulating uniform dosage forms with respect to drug content.

(ii) It can be used to obtain granules of required size.

(iii) It helps to ensure good flowability.

(iv) It can also be useful in separating undesirable size solids from desired ones.

(v) It has applications in determination of particle size and their distribution in the given samples.

(vi) It can also be used to investigate efficiency and validate size reduction equipments.

(vii) It is used to obtain monosized powders/particles which undergo least size segregation.

3.3 OFFICIAL STANDARDS FOR POWDER SIZE

Standards for powders used in pharmaceuticals are reported in the British Pharmacopoeia (B.P.) which states that "the degree of coarseness or fineness of a powder is differentiated and expressed by the size of the mesh of the sieve through which the powder is able to pass". The B.P. specifies five grades of powder and the number of the sieve through which all the particles must pass, Table 3.1.

Table 3.1: Standards for Powders given B.P.

Grade of powder	Sieve number through which all particles must pass
Coarse	10
Moderately coarse	22
Moderately fine	44
Fine	85
Very fine	120

The B.P. specifies a use of smaller size of sieve for the coarser powders but states that not more than 40 % shall pass through. The relevant grades of powder and sieve number are presented in the Table 3.2. Thus, the coarse powder is that wherein all the particles which pass through a No. 10 sieve and not more than 40 % through a No. 44 sieve. This is usually referred as a 10/44 powder.

The B.P. states that when a powder is described by a number, all particles must pass through the specified sieve and when a vegetable drug is being ground and sifted, none must be rejected. This classification is must if the character of a vegetable drug is compared with a chemical substance.

Table 3.2: Classification of Powders as per B.P.

Grade of powder	Sieve number through which all particles must pass	Sieve number through which not more than 40 % of particles pass
Coarse	10	44
Moderately coarse	22	60
Moderately fine	44	85
Fine	85	Not specified
Very fine	120	Not specified

The chemical materials are generally homogeneous. If a certain quantity of a powder is required, an excess may be ground so as to get a sufficient amount of the desired size range by sieving, and the oversize particles may be discarded. As we know vegetable drugs consists of a variety of tissues of different degrees of hardness that softer tissues are ground first and oversize mass is obtained by sifting contain a higher proportion of the harder tissues. In many cases, constituents are not distributed uniformly through vegetable tissues. For example, digitalis contains glycosides concentrated in the mid-rib and veins of the plant. Hence, if tailings are discarded while grinding and sifting the drug, it is likely that a high proportion of the active constituents may be lost.

The British Pharmaceutical Codex has given a further grade of powder known as ultra-fine powder. For these powders it is required that the maximum dimension of at least 90 % of the particles must be not greater than 5 μm and none must be greater than 50 μm. Determination of particle size for this grade is carried out by a microscopic method.

3.4 SIEVES

A sieve, also called sifter, is a device for separating desired elements from unwanted material or for characterizing the particle size distribution of a sample. This is a device typically made-up of using a woven sieve such as a mesh or net or metal. The word "sift" is derived from "sieve". A sieve has very small holes. The sieving process is comparatively inexpensive, simple in concept and easy to use. Coarse particles are separated or broken-up by grinding against one-another and sieve openings. Sieves are the most commonly used devices for particle size analysis. Depending upon the types of particles to be separated, sieves with different types of holes are used. Sieving plays an important role in pharmaceutical and food industries where they (often vibrating) are used to prevent the contamination of the product by foreign bodies. The design of the industrial sieve is of primary importance. Each sieve has a specific number that denotes the number of meshes in a length of 2.54 cm ($\approx$1 inch).

3.4.1 Construction of Sieves

Based upon application specially constructed sieves are used. Various types of sieves includes electroformed sieves, perforated plate sieves, sonic sifters, air jet sieves, wet wash sieves etc. Generally pharmaceutical sieves are made up of stainless steel, brass, bronze etc. and are not coated with any material to avoid wear and tear as well as contamination in the products. Sieves should be non-reactive and resistant to corrosion. The most common choice of material for sieves is iron because it is cheap. Iron has limitation for its use when there is possibility of corrosion and contamination. This can be avoided by coating iron surfaces with galvanizing agent. Stainless steel, brass and phosphorus bronze due to their corrosion resistant, good strength and non-contaminating qualities are preferred as an alternative to iron. Even non-metals such as nylon and terylene are used if contamination is to be avoided. Sieves with different type of holes viz. size and shapes made in plates as perforations can be used as separating devices. Sieves made-up of woven cloth are used if fine powders are to be separated. This cloth can be made of cotton, nylon or silk.

3.4.2 Types of Sieves

Pharmaceutical sieves are extensively used for size separations from 300 mm down to around 38 μm. The efficiency of sieving decreases rapidly with fineness. Dry sieving is used for material above 5 mm in size and wet sieving is common in use down to 250 μm but is possible to about 40 μm. In its simplest form, a sieve is a surface having many apertures (holes), usually with uniform dimensions. Particles presented to that surface will either pass through or be retained, according to whether the particles are smaller or larger than the dimension of the apertures. There are numerous different types of industrial sieves available, Fig. 3.1. Some of the most common are vibrating sieves, static sieves, trommels, roller sieves, flip-flow sieves, circular sieves, linear sieves etc.

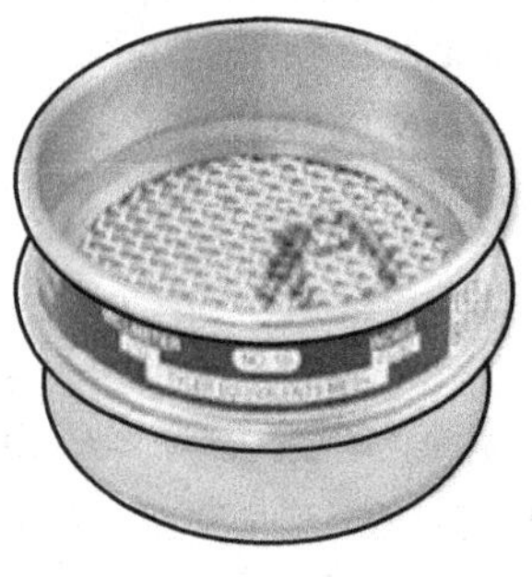
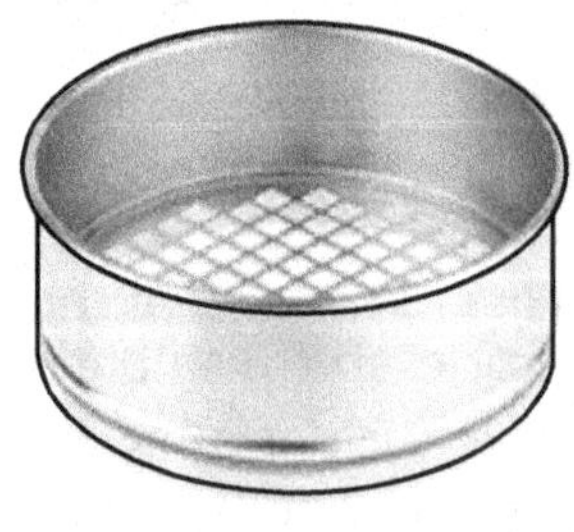
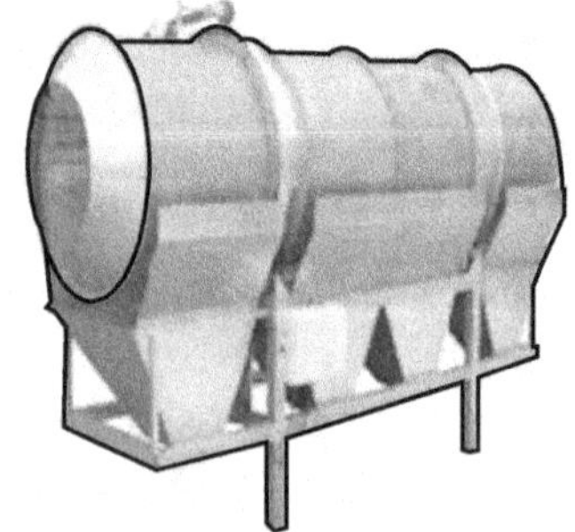

(a) Wire Sieve	**(b) Perforated Sieve**	**(c) Horizontal Sieve**

Fig. 3.1: Types of Sieves

(i) Vibrating Sieves:

The commonest sieve type in industrial applications is the vibrating sieve. There are many subtypes of vibrating sieves in use for coarse- and fine-sieving applications. Vibrating sieves have a rectangular sieving surface with feed and oversize discharge at opposite ends. They are used in a variety of sizing, grading, scalping, dewatering, wet sieving, and washing applications. Sieves are vibrated in order to throw particles off the sieving surface so that they can again be presented to the sieve and to convey the particles along the sieve. Vibrating motion is generally produced by vibrating mechanisms based on eccentric rotating masses with amplitude of 1.5–5 mm and operating in a range of 700–1000 r.p.m. The right type of vibration also induces stratification of the feed material, which allows the finer particles to work through the layer of particles to the sieve surface while causing larger particles to rise to the top. Vibrating sieves of most types can be manufactured with more than one sieve deck. On multiple-deck systems, the feed is introduced to the top coarse sieve, the undersize falling through to the lower sieve decks, thus producing a range of sized fractions from a single sieve.

(ii) Inclined or circular motion sieves:

This type of vibrating sieve is widely used for sizing applications. A vertical circular or elliptical vibration is induced mechanically by the rotation of unbalanced weights or flywheels attached usually to a single drive shaft. The amplitude of throw can be adjusted by adding or removing weight elements bolted to the flywheels. The rotation direction can be contra flow or in-flow. Contra flow slows the material flow more and permits more efficient separation, whereas in-flow permits a greater throughput. Single-shaft sieves must be installed on a slope, usually between 15° and 28° angle to permit flow of material along the sieve.

(iii) Static sieves:

Very coarse material is usually sieved on an inclined sieve called grizzly sieve. Grizzlies are characterized by parallel steel bars or rails set at a fixed distance apart and installed in line with the flow of ore. The gap between grizzly bars is usually greater than 50 mm and can be as large as 300 mm, with feed top size as large as 1 m. The most common use of grizzlies in mineral processing is for sizing the feed to primary and secondary crushers.

(iv) Horizontal low-head or linear vibrating sieves:

These sieves have a horizontal or near-horizontal sieving surface and therefore need less headroom than inclined sieves. Horizontal sieves must be vibrated with a linear or an elliptical vibration. The accuracy of particle sizing on horizontal sieves is superior to that on inclined sieves; however, because gravity does not assist the transport of material along the sieve, they have lower capacity than inclined sieves. Horizontal sieves are used in sizing applications where sieving efficiency is critical and as drain-and-rinse sieves in heavy medium circuits.

(v) Banana or multislope sieves:

These sieves become widely used in high-tonnage sizing applications where both efficiency and capacity are important. Banana sieves typically have a variable slope of around 40–30° at the feed end of the sieve, reducing to around 0–15° at the discharge end in increments of 3.5–5°. The steep sections of the sieve cause the feed material to flow rapidly at the feed end of the sieve. The resulting thin bed of particles stratifies more quickly and therefore has a faster sieving rate for the very fine material than would be possible on a slower moving thick bed. Toward the discharge end of the sieve, the slope decreases to slow down the remaining material, enabling more efficient sieving of the near-size material. The capacity of banana sieves is significantly greater and is reported to be up to three or four times that of conventional vibrating sieves.

(vi) Rotary scrubbers:

These sieves are cost-effective washing units that are an integral part of a material handling system to upgrade a wide variety of primary crushed hard rock and ore, including iron ore. A rotary scrubber is a cylindrical drum with internal lifters, typically supported by trunnion rollers at either end. These are high-capacity, high-retention time machines primarily used to remove water-soluble clays, deleterious materials, and coatings from a wide variety of hard rock and ore. Rotary scrubber designs include the solid shell and combination scrubber sieves and are available in a variety of diameters and lengths. Drive transmission choices include chain and sprocket, gear and pinion, or pedestal mount hydraulic motor.

(vii) Test Sieves

Test sieves are measuring devices used to determine the size and size distribution of particles in a material sample using wire mesh of different openings to separate particles of different sizes. Test sieves come in different materials such as brass, stainless steel, or brass frames with stainless steel mesh. Diameters include 3", 8", and 12" with mesh sizes ranging from 4 mm to 38 microns. When stacked on a sieve shaker, the top test sieve has the largest mesh size and the bottom one the smallest mesh size. The sieve stack consists of pan at the bottom and covers at the top.

3.4.3 Calibration of Sieves

Sieves used for sieving are to be cleaned regularly. The frequent use can cause changes in mesh openings but much of the damage sustained to working sieves occurs during cleaning. Often, the operator hurries to clear the mesh of residual particles by strongly tapping the frame. This tapping can distort the mesh. Operators also use brushes to remove residual particles after use. This process often distorts sections of the sieve mesh. These alterations of the sieve may change the quality of products in terms of size hence sieves are calibrated intermittently.

3.4.4 Standards for Sieves

Sieving is the separation of fine material from coarse material by means of a meshed or perforated surface. The technique was used since early Egyptian days as a way to size grains. These early sieves were made of woven reeds and grasses. Today the sieve test is the technique used most often for analyzing particle-size distribution. Although at first look the sieving process appears to be elementary, in practice, there is a science and art involved in producing reliable and consistent results. To better understand sieving, there are several areas of sieve specifications that should to be explained and some of them are given Table 3.3. Sieves used in pharmaceuticals must comply with the standards given in Pharmacopoeia, Table 3.4.

Table 3.3: I.P. Standards for Sieves

1.	Sieve (mesh) Number	The sieve number is number of meshes in length of 2.54 cm in each transverse direction parallel to the wires. Mesh is arranged in multiple configurations. Mesh can be a square pattern, long-slotted rectangular pattern, circular pattern, or diamond pattern.
2.	Nominal size of aperture	This term is the distance between the wires. It represents the length of side of a square aperture. The relation between nominal size of aperture and size in mm or micrometer is given in I.P.
3.	Nominal diameter of the wire	The diameter of wires used to make sieves gives strength to avoid distortion in the meshes. A wire with specific diameter is used for particular sieve.
4.	Approximate percent sieving area	This standard expresses the area of meshes in percent to total area of sieve. The approximate sieving area range from 35 to 40% of sieve area. This area is suitable to give enough strength to sieve while sieving. It depends on diameter of wire.
5.	Aperture tolerance average percent	During making or while use some variations in the aperture size takes place. This variation is expressed as aperture tolerance average percent. It is small for coarse sieves while greater for small size sieves.

Table 3.4: Specifications for Wire and Aperture Size of Sieves as Per I.P.

Sieve No.	Nominal aperture size (mm)	Nominal wire diameter (mm)	Standard wire gauge	Approximate screen area (%)	Average aperture tolerance (%)
6	3.812	1.422	17.0	44	3.2
8	2.057	1.118	18.5	42	3.3
10	1.676	0.864	20.5	44	3.3
22	0.699	0.457	26.0	36	4.0
25	0.599	0.417	27.0	35	4.2
30	0.500	0.345	29.0	35	4.4
36	0.422	0.284	31.5	36	4.9
44	0.353	0.224	34.5	38	4.8
60	0.251	0.173	37.0	35	5.3
85	0.178	0.122	40.0	35	5.9
100	0.152	0.102	42.0	35	6.2
200	0.076	0.051	47.0	36	8.2

Table 3.5 presents the different international sieve standards and the corresponding sieve types. There are several sieve aperture progression ratios commonly available depending on the different international standards. In the USA, a progression ratio of $2^{1/2}$ is used. This ratio corresponds to successive particle groups of 2 : 1 particle surface ratio. The progression rate of $2^{1/3}$ ($10^{0.1}$) has been adopted by the French which corresponds to successive particle groups of 2:1 particle volume ratio. The progression ratios of $10^{0.1}$ and $10^{0.05}$ are recommended for narrow size distributions.

Table 3.5: International Sieve Standards

Country	Standard	Sieve type
Great Britain	BS 410	Woven wire
USA	ASTM E11	Woven wire
	ASTM E161-607	Micromesh (electroformed)
Germany	DIN 4188	Woven wire
	DIN 4187	Perforated plate
France	AFNOR NFX 11-501	Woven wire
International	ISO R565 1972(E)	Woven wire, Perforated plate

3.5 MECHANISMS OF SIZE SEPARATION

Size separation is useful since particles are sorted into categories solely on the basis of size, independently of other properties such as density, surface, etc. It can be used to classify dry or wet powders and generates narrowly classified fractions. While doing this mechanical sieving equipments used works on the principle of agitation, brushing and centrifugal force.

3.5.1 Agitation Method

A single sieve or sieves in a set may be agitated in different ways.

(i) Oscillation: In this case the sieve is mounted in inclined frame or rack that oscillates back and forth. This is most common and simple mechanism in which material rolls on the surface of sieve and sometimes forms a ball. This movement is achieved by ordinary eccentric movement of the rotating motor shaft.

(ii) Vibration: Sieves in this mechanism are mechanically or electrically vibrated at high speed allowing powder material to pass through. Vibration are either sinusoidal or gyratory. Sinusoidal vibration occurs at an angled plane relative to the horizontal. The vibration in a wave pattern are determined by frequency and amplitude. This motion can causes sieves to move-up and down or left to right.

(iii) Gyration: The sieves are kept on rubber mounting which is attached to rotary eccentric flywheel. This produces a movement of desired amplitude with required intensity to induce motion in the material. Rotary motion allows particles to spin and pass through the meshes. Gyratory vibration occurs at near level plane at low angles in a reciprocating side-to-side motion.

3.5.2 Brushing Method

Material to be processed for size separation using sieving is passed through sieves by use of brushes in different directions. For motion in circular sieves brush is rotated at centre of sieve while in horizontal cylindrical sieves it rotates around its longitudinal axis. Brush helps to keep the meshes clean. This method is suitable for wet, greasy and sticky materials.

3.5.3 Centrifugal Method

In this method vertical cylindrical type mechanical sieve is used. It consists of high speed rotor inside the cylinder that throws particles on the sieve by centrifugal force. A current of air generated due to movement of rotor causes particle separation. To aid particle separation further an air jet can be fixed in the cylinder.

Other mechanisms of particle separation are gravitational force, density and electrostatic force. Gravity is a physical interaction in the sense that when the material is thrown from the sieve causes it to fall to a lower level. Gravity also pulls the particles through the sieve media. The density of the material relates to material stratification. The classification in this case is based upon weight of material. Electrostatic force can be applied to sieve when particles are extremely dry or wet that help to sieving.

3.6 PRINCIPLE, CONSTRUCTION, WORKING, USES, MERITS AND DEMERITS

There are different techniques used in particle size separation. The most common mechanical techniques for particle size separation relevant to pharmaceutical sciences and industrial applications are: sieving, sedimentation (gravitational or centrifugal), elutriation, electrostatic precipitation, thermal precipitation, hydrodynamic chromatography and impaction. Some of the major equipments are briefly presented below.

3.6.1 Sieve Shaker

Sieving is most widely used technique in pharmaceutical industry for particle size analysis. The particles are classified based on their size, independent of any other particle characteristics such as density and surface properties. Micromesh sieves are used to classify particles of size range 5 - 20 μm, while particles of size range 20 -125 μm are classified in the standard woven wire sieves. Coarse particles (>125 μm) are classified in punched plate sieves. Punched plate sieves are commonly used in industrial applications where the openings are circular or rectangular. The sieves can take different configurations.

Principle:

The principle of sieve shaker is based upon vibration, agitation or gyration. Efficiency of sieving by sieve shaker depends on the particles size distribution, sieve load, the method of sieve shaking, the dimension and shape of the particle, and the ratio of open area of sieve to total area. The sieving operation can be affected by the friability and cohesiveness of the powder. During sieving the sample is subjected to horizontal or vertical movement in accordance with the chosen method. This causes a relative movement between the particles and the sieve. Depending on size the individual particles either pass through the sieve mesh or are retained on the sieve surface. The likelihood of a particle passing through the sieve mesh is determined by the ratio of the particle size to the sieve openings, the orientation of the particle and the number of encounters between the particle and the mesh openings. Thus sieving depends on the sieve movement and the sieving time.

Construction:

The sieve shaker consists basically of a cradle for holding the sieves, a power unit and a base. The cradle consists of a platform fastened to the lower ends of two vertical support rods, Fig. 3.2. The upper ends of which are shock mounted to a horizontal support that is free to pivot about its mounting. A sieve holder, a retaining ring and nuts on the vertical support rods hold the top bar firmly against the nest of sieves. The standard sieves of different sieve numbers are used.

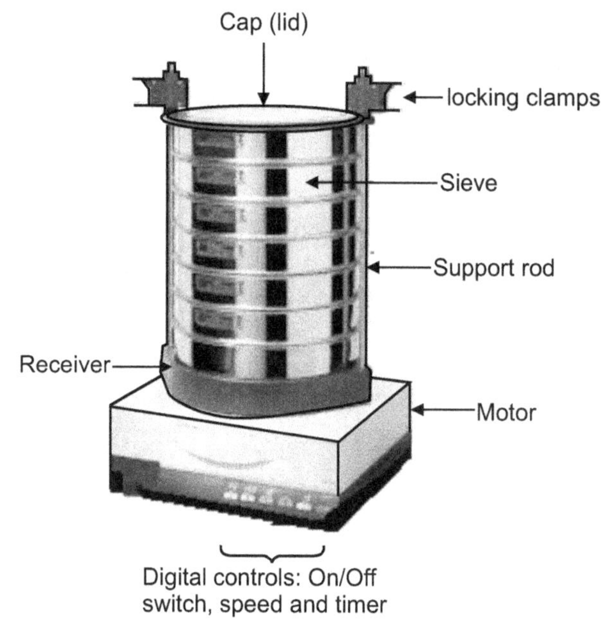

Fig. 3.2: Sieve Shaker

Working:

The sieving by sieve shaker is conducted using up to 11 sieves stacked with progressively larger aperture openings towards the top. The sample is placed on the top sieve. A closed pan (receiver) is placed at the bottom. There are several methods for shaking the sieves by mechanical or ultrasonic means. The residues in each sieve are recorded and expressed in percentage as cumulative values against the nominal sieve aperture values. The common methods of sieving are machine, wet, hand and air-jet sieving. Wet-sieving is recommended for material originally suspended in a liquid and is necessary for powders which form aggregates when dry-sieved. In such sieving the stack of sieves is filled with liquid and the sample is fed to the top sieve. Sieving is accomplished by rinsing, vibration, reciprocating action, vacuum, ultrasonication or a combination of these.

(a) Manual and mechanical sieving:

Today, manual sieving is only used where no electricity supply is available, for example, for rapid on-site random checking for oversize and undersize. It is only used for orientation purposes. In contrast, sieve analyses in the laboratory and for quality assurance are carried out with sieve shakers. Modern sieve shakers are characterized by the fact that their mechanical parameters, such as sieving time and amplitude or speed, are carried out with exact reproducibility. In the laboratory a differentiation is made between horizontal sieve shakers and throw-action sieve shakers.

(b) Throw-action sieving:

Throw-action sieve shakers are also known as vibratory sieve shakers. An electromagnetic drive sets a spring-mass system in motion and transfers the oscillations to the sieve stack. The sample is subjected to a 3-dimensional movement and is distributed uniformly across the whole area of the sieve, Fig. 3.3. The amplitude can normally be set continuously in the range from 0-2 mm or 0-3 mm. Modern instruments enable the required amplitude to be entered digitally. During the sieving process, a built-in measuring system and control unit performs a continuous comparison between the set and actual amplitude values. This provides the optimal preconditions for reproducible sieving parameters. Digital accuracy for the sieving time and the interval function is a matter of course.

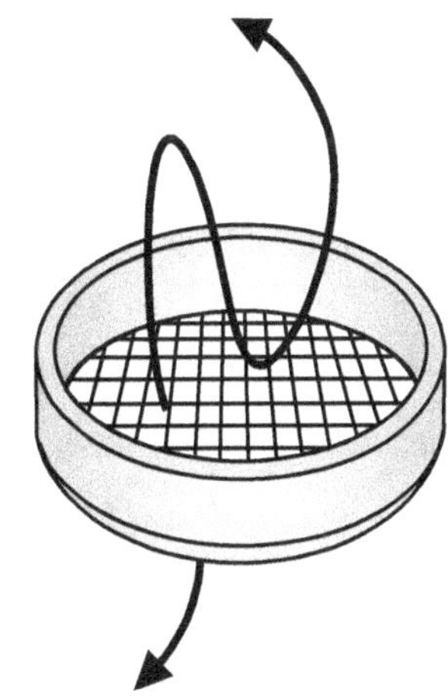

Fig. 3.3: In Throw-Action Sieving the Sample is Subjected to a 3-Dimensional Movement

(c) Horizontal sieving:

In a horizontal sieve shaker the sieves move in horizontal circles in one plane, Fig. 3.4. Horizontal sieve shakers are preferably used for needle-shaped, flat, long or fibrous samples, as their horizontal orientation means that only a few disorientated particles enter the mesh and the sieve is not blocked so quickly.

The AS 400 control permits the use of test sieves with a diameter up to 400 mm. The large sieving area makes it possible to sieve large amounts of sample, for example as encountered in the particle size analysis of coarse granules and aggregates. In addition, in the fine particle size range and for obtaining single fractions, ultrasonic and air-jet sieving is used for special applications.

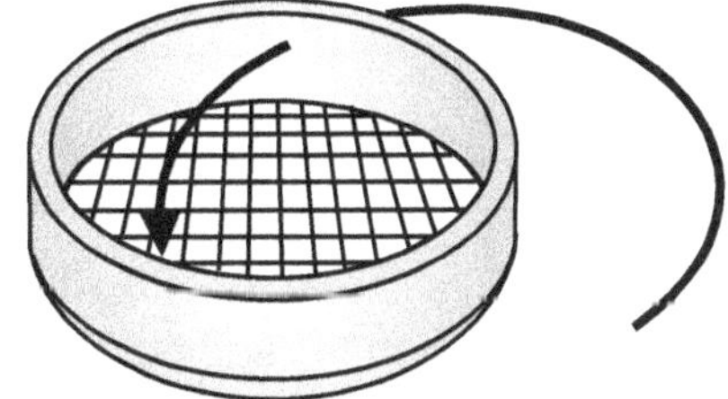

Fig. 3.4: In Horizontal Sieving the Sample Moves in Horizontal Circles

(d) Sieve set sieving:

Sieve set sieving is the process in which a set of several sieves is used together with a collector pan. The tests sieves are arranged in a stack with the largest mesh openings at the top of the stack. The sample is placed on the top sieve and allowed to pass through in lower sieves.

(e) Dry and wet sieving:

Most sieving processes are carried out on dry materials. However, there are many applications in which wet sieving cannot be avoided, for example, suspension or when a very fine sample that tends to agglomerate has to be sieved. As in dry sieving, a sieve stack is assembled on a sieve shaker. The sieving process is additionally supported by water from a spray nozzle located above the uppermost sieve. The sample is placed on the uppermost sieve in the form of a suspension. Rinsing is carried out until the sieving liquid leaving the sieve stack outlet is no longer turbid with solid particles. In wet sieving, the sieving liquid must not alter the physical or chemical properties of the sample.

Optimal sieving time and amplitude or speed:

The settings for the sieving time and the optimal amplitude or speed depend on the material to be sieved. National and international standards, internal regulations and standards normally provide detailed information about product-specific sieve analyses and their associated sieving parameters. The instruction manual for the sieve shaker should also provide guidelines for this. If this basic information does not exist then the sieving time and amplitude or speed must be determined experimentally. This is done by first selecting a relatively short sieving time (for example, 5 min) and carrying out sieving at various amplitudes or speeds to determine at which values the largest amount of sample passes through the sieves (optimal sieving quality).

Sieving Aids:

Sieving aids are used for very fine samples that tend to adhere together. They are used to make the sample sievable. A differentiation is made between mechanical sieving aids (for example, rubber cubes, brushes, balls, chains) for eliminating molecular adhesive forces, and additives (for example, talcum, Aerosil) for greasy, sticky and oil-containing products. Antistatic sprays reduce electrostatic charges whereas surfactants reduce the surface tension in wet sieving.

A complete sieving process includes the following steps which should be performed in a precise careful manner.

(a) Sampling.

(b) Sample division (if required).

(c) Selection of suitable test sieves.

(d) Selection of sieving parameters.

(e) Actual sieve analysis.

(f)　Recovery of sample material.

(g)　Data evaluation.

(h)　Cleaning and drying the test sieves.

Merits:

(i)　Sieve shaker is simple to operate.

(ii)　It separates samples rapidly.

(iii)　It is suitable only for particle size up to 50 μm.

(iv)　Requires less area for its installation.

(v)　Results of particle sizing are accurate and reproducible.

(vi)　Cost of the instrument is lower than other methods.

Demerits:

(i)　For materials finer than 100 mesh, dry sieving can be significantly less accurate.

(ii)　Sieve analysis assumes that all particle will be round (spherical) or nearly so but in reality it is not the fact.

(iii)　For elongated and flat particles a sieve analysis does not yield reliable mass-based results.

(iv)　Not suitable for particles smaller than 50 μm.

(v)　There is a possibility of further reduction in size, which can cause errors.

(vi)　Sieves could be clogged and distorted if not properly handled and maintained.

Applications:

(i)　Sieve shaker is used for particle size analysis of variety of materials.

(ii)　It is suitable for coarse material down to 150 μm.

(iii)　It can be used for wet sieve analysis where the material analyzed is not affected by the liquid - except to disperse it.

3.6.2 Cyclone Separator

Cyclone separators provide a method of removing particulate matter from air or other gas streams at low cost and low maintenance. This separator is mainly used for the separation of solids from the liquids. It mainly consists of tangential inlet to feed the materials inside the chamber. It has solid and fluid outlets which separate fluid through one side and solids through the other side.

Principle:

In the cyclone separator the centrifugal force is used to separate solids from the fluids (liquid or gas/air). The separation depends on the particle size as well as on the density of the particles. Hence depending on the fluid velocity the cyclone separator can be used to separate all types of the particles. Especially it is used to remove only coarse particles and allows fine particles to be carried through with the fluid. It simply transforms the inertia force of a gas particle to a centrifugal force by means of a vortex generated in the cyclone body.

In a cyclone, the air containing particulate material is forced along the tangential axis. A helical flow pattern is set up within the chamber. The centrifugal force causes the particles to migrate to the outside of the chamber. Here they fall down to the bottom of the cyclone by gravity. The collected particulates are allowed to exit out an underflow pipe while the gas phase reverses its axial direction of flow and exits out through the vortex finder (gas outlet tube). The air moves-up the center of the cyclone and reaches the top.

Construction:

Cyclone separators are a bit complicated in design with better particle removal efficiency. Cyclones are basically centrifugal separators. It consists of a cylindrical vessel referred to as the barrel with the conical base, Fig. 3.5. The upper part of the vessel is fitted with a tangential inlet and a fluid outlet and at the base it is fitted with the solid outlet. Cyclones have no moving parts and are available in many shapes and sizes.

For example, cyclone separators of 1 to 2 cm diameter is used for particle size analysis and upto 5 m diameter is used after wet scrubbers, but the basic separation principle remains the same.

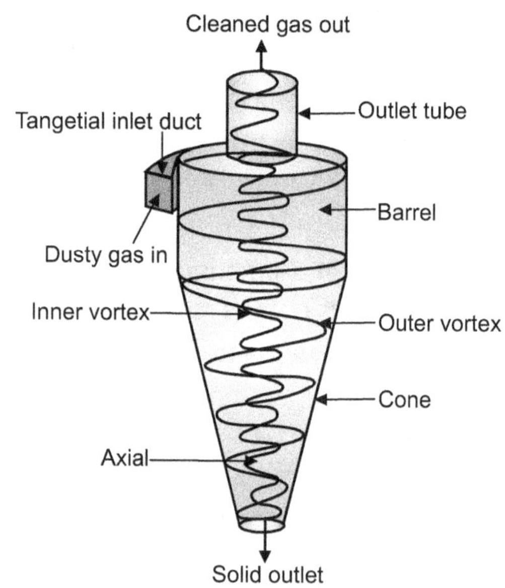

Fig. 3.5: A Schematic of Cyclone Separator

Working:

In the suspensions of a solid-gas usually air is introduced tangentially at a very high velocity so that rotary movement takes place within the vessel. The fluid (gas) is removed from the central outlet at the top. The rotatory flow within the cyclone separator causes the particles to be acted on by centrifugal force. The solids are thrown out to the walls forming an outer vortex, thereafter it falls to the conical base and discharged out through solids outlet. The increasing air velocity in the outer vortex results in a centrifugal force on the particles separating them from the air stream. When the air reaches the bottom of the cone, it begins to flow radially inwards and out at the top as clean air/gas while the particulates fall into the dust collection chamber at the bottom of the cyclone.

The collection efficiency of cyclones varies as a function of density, particle size and cyclone design. Cyclone efficiency generally increases with increase in particle size and/or density, inlet duct velocity, cyclone body length, number of gas revolutions in the cyclone, ratio of cyclone body diameter to gas exit diameter, inlet dust loading, smoothness of the cyclone inner wall etc. Similarly, cyclone efficiency may decrease with increases in the parameters such as gas viscosity, cyclone body diameter, gas exit diameter, gas inlet duct area, gas density, leakage of air into the dust outlet etc.

Merits:

   (i) Cyclone separator requires low capital investment.

   (ii) It has high efficiency for 5 - 200 μm particles.

   (iii) It produces high volume flow rate.

   (iv) A lack of moving parts reduces wear and tear.

   (v) It can be operated on continuous or batch process.

   (vi) It requires virtually no downtime for maintenance or recovery.

   (vii) It has versatile applications.

   (viii) It is small in size relative to other separation equipment.

   (ix) It can be operated at a wide range of temperatures and pressures.

Demerits:

   (i) It shows reduced efficiency when overloaded than its capacity.

   (ii) It finds difficulty in obtaining good separation of substances with similar densities.

   (iii) It cannot handle viscous flow.

   (iv) The extremely high velocities cause abrasive wear.

   (v) Clogging of the dust outlet is common in reverse flow cyclones.

Applications:

A cyclone separator is most often used to separate "heavies" from a liquid mixture originating at a centrifugal pump or some other continuous source of pressurized liquid. A cyclone separator is most likely to be the right choice for processes where "lights" are the greater part of the mixture and where the "heavies" settle fairly easily. These may be used to separate solids from water.

   (i) Cyclone separator is used to separate the suspensions of a solid in a gas or air. It can be used with the liquids suspensions of solids.

   (ii) It is used in the production of active pharmaceutical ingredients (API) through drying systems such as spray or fluid bed drying.

   (iii) It can also be used for separation of particles based upon size, specific gravity, porosity and concentration from solids, liquids and gases.

   (iv) In pharmaceutical industry it is mostly used for separation of fines from coarse granules.

   (v) In tablet compression cyclone is used to extract waste powder before it reaches the central extraction system.

   (vi) It can be used in air-handling systems to produce particle free clean air.

   (vii) It is used in oil industry to separate oil from water or vice versa.

3.6.3 Air Separator

An air separator is usually a mechanical device with large metal box containing a blower, heating or cooling elements and filter racks or chambers, sound attenuators, and dampers. Air separators are usually connected to a duct of a ventilation system that distributes the air and fine particles.

Principle:

The air separator works on the same principle of cyclone separator. The cyclone separators sometimes are not efficient in separating powders that contain very fine size particles. In such situations an additional provision is made that combines current of air with the centrifugal force. This causes fines to separate along with air and coarse particles to thrown away by centrifugal force which is collected at the bottom.

Construction:

It consists of vertical metal cylindrical vessel with conical base at the bottom, Fig. 3.6. The feed inlet is fitted tangentially at the upper part of vessel. The outlet for collected solids is at the base of conical portion where as fluid outlet is at the centre of the top portion. The fluid outlet pipe extends down below inlet section to avoid air short-circuiting directly from the inlet into the outlet. The rotating disc and rotating blades are fitted on shaft is placed at the center of the vessel. It has two separate outlets at bottom for finer and coarser/heavy particles.

Working:

The feed enters through the inlet tangentially in the upper part of vessel. Feed falls on the rotating blades. The rotating blades produce an air jet in the direction indicated in Fig. 3.6. The fine particles are blown away on the walls by centrifugal force generated with the air jet and are collected at the bottom. The coarser particles due to their large mass travel less distance from the centre of the separator and falls in the coarse particle collection zone which is collected at its discharge.

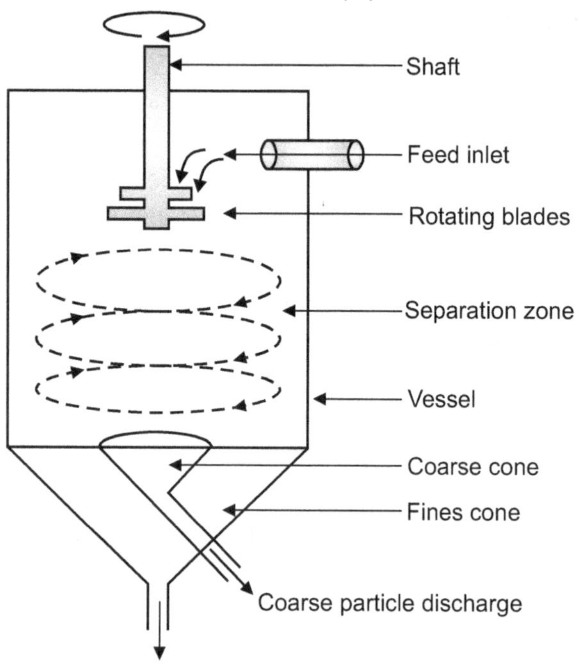

Fig. 3.6: Air Separator

Merits:

(i) It is easy to install.

(ii) The rotor speed as well as air flow is adjustable.

(iii) It has high product output.

(iv) It is easy to clean and maintain.

(v) It is superior to sieving method in terms of output and quality of products.

(vi) It is used in batch as well as continues mode.

Demerits:

(i)   If particles are too fine (<5 µm) its efficiency decreases.

(ii) It is not suitable for wet and sticky materials.

Applications:

(i)   It is used as dust collectors in many processes to either recover valuable granular solid or powder from process streams.

(ii) It can be used to separate sub micron size particles those cannot be handled by sieving.

(iii) It is often used as an air pollution control device to maintain or improve air quality in pharmaceutical production areas.

(iv) It can be used as mist collectors to remove particulate matter in the form of fine liquid droplets from the air to improve or maintain the quality of air in the workplace environment.

(v) It can be used to remove granular solid pollutants from exhaust gases prior to venting to the atmosphere.

(vi) It can be used for the collection of metal working fluids, and coolant or oil mists.

3.6.4 Bag Filter

The bag filter is a mechanical device used in quality of air in pharmaceutical production and other allied areas. In pharmaceutical production very potent drugs such as hormones, vitamins, antibiotics etc generates lot of dust during processing which may be life threatening to the operators. These processes include screening, blending, mixing, drying, granulating, tableting, compression, packaging etc. It causes air pollution and chemical hazards. In order to avoid these unwanted situations the air is needed to be maintained clean. This is achieved by use of filter bags. A fabric filter is a dust collection device made using a woven or non-woven filter bag that filters and collects the dust in process gas. When the filter cloth is made into a cylindrical-shaped bag and suspended, it is referred to as a bag house or a fabric filter.

Principle:

The purpose of filter bag to collect dust is based upon the principle of filtration. The dust layer adheres to and is deposited on the surface of the filter bag and the interior of the filter cloth (the primary dust layer) filters and collects the dust contained in the process gas. The fabric provides surface for dust particles to get accumulated. The accumulation or collection takes place by inertial or electrostatic interaction, interception and Brownian movement. Together these mechanism results in formation of the dust cake on fabric surface.

Construction:

This equipment consists of a big metal vessel (bag house) with series of fabric bags in compartments, Fig. 3.7. The bags are made-up of woven cotton, wool, membranes, sintered metal fibers or ceramic cartridges. The selection is based upon the operating temperature and pressure and stability of filter medium to these conditions. Filter bags are suspended in invert position in the vessel. The length of bags varies from 2 to 10 m with a diameter up to 40 cm. The open ends of the bags are attached to the manifold. The number of bags in a vessel varies from 100 to 1000 or more depending on bag house. In the bottom portion hopper is provided to collect dust held by the filter.

Working:

The processing gas enters through the inlet pipe that strikes the baffle plate. This striking causes large particles to fall down due to gravity in the hopper at the bottom. Carrier gas then flows in upward direction and leaves through the bags leaving behind fine particulate matter on its interior surface. Normally the filtration velocity of the process gas passing through a filter cloth is about 0.3-2 m/min, and the pressure loss is 1-2 kPa. As the dust layer collected on the surface of the filter cloth becomes thicker, the pressure loss of the filter cloth increases, so the collected dust is intermittently removed. Removing the dust layer is carried out by mechanical shaking, reverse pressure, or pulse jet. In most cases the dust collection efficiency of fabric filters is 99% or higher, and the dust concentration at the outlet is less than 10 mg/m^3. In order to achieve better efficiency filter bags are cleaned, maintained and changed intermittently.

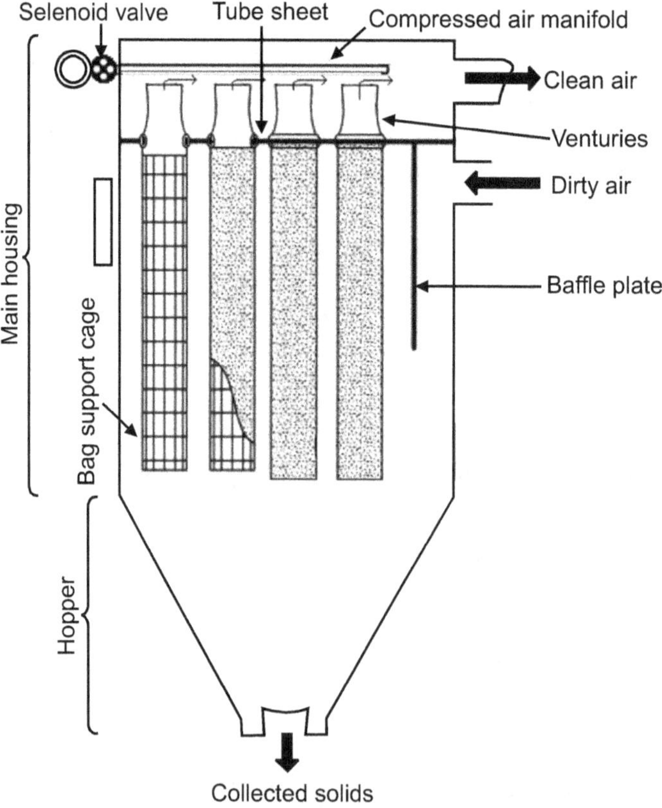

Fig. 3.7: Filter Bag

Merits:

(i) Filter bag is best method amongst all for removing fines from the air.

(ii) Electricity consumption is low.

(iii) It help to maintain and protect healthy environment.

(iv) They are simple in construction and operation.

(v) It has versatility and effective design.

(vi) It help to reduce housekeeping and better product quality.

(vii) Filter bags has effective design according to American Ventilation System Standards

(viii) High quality filter bags has trouble free operation.

(ix) It has robust construction.

Demerits:

(i) It has limitations for its operation due to high gas temperature and high humidity.

(ii) The maintenance cost is high as fabric used is costly.

(iii) The characteristics of fabric change with operating parameters.

(iv) Comparatively it is large in size.

(v) Condensation of vapours and presence of hygroscopic material reduces its efficiency.

Applications:

(i) Bag filters are used in industries to separate dust particles from the air.

(ii) These are used to clean the air in working areas.

(iii) They are extensively used in large industries that produce different kind of dust such as metals, cement, chalk and lime, ceramics, flour and foundries.

(iv) It is most commonly used in fluidized bed dryer.

3.6.5 Elutriation Tank

An elutriator is a simple device which can separate particles into two or more groups. Elutriation depends on the movement of a fluid against the direction of sedimentation of the particles. Elutriation is based on particle size, shape and density. The air elutriator is mainly used for particles smaller than 1 µm. The smaller or lighter particles rise to the top (overflow) because their terminal sedimentation velocities are lower than the velocity of the rising fluid. The terminal velocity of any particle in any medium can be calculated using Stokes' law if the particle's Reynolds number is below 0.2. In elutriator particles separation is based upon densities. The heavier particles settle due to gravitational force.

Principle:

In the process of elutriation, particles falling in a rising fluid can be classified into two sizes. When the fluid in a sorting column is rising with a certain velocity, the particles having terminal velocities higher than this velocity settle at the bottom of the sorting column and the particles with lower terminal velocities are lifted to the top of the sorting column and are carried away to the next tube. Terminal velocities of the particles falling in a fluid can be calculated using the Stokes' law equation for Reynolds number.

$$R_e \;=\; \frac{2r \times V_m \times (\rho - \rho_o)}{\eta} \qquad\qquad \text{... (3.1)}$$

$$V_m \;=\; \frac{2r^2 \times g \times (\rho - \rho_o)}{9\eta} \qquad\qquad \text{... (3.2)}$$

Where, ρ = specific gravity of the particle, ρ_o specific gravity of the fluid medium, r is radius of the particle, η = viscosity of the medium, V_m = terminal velocity of the particle and g = gravitational acceleration.

In the elutriation, when the volumetric flow rate of rising fluid is constant, the velocity of the rising fluid in the columns depends on their diameters. The narrow diameter column gives high velocity and the one with wide diameter gives low fluid velocity. Higher velocities of the rising medium allow coarser particles to settle while lower velocities allow finer particles to settle. Various size classes of particles can be obtained when the sample is separated in columns of increasing diameters connected in series. Upper size limit of the particles follows Stokes' law.

Construction:

For the gravitational system, the apparatus consists simply of a vertical column with an inlet near the bottom for the suspension, an outlet at the base for coarse particles, and an overflow near the top for fluid, Fig. 3.8. One column will give a single separation into two fractions, but it must be remembered that this will not give a clear cut separation, since there is a velocity gradient across the tube, resulting in the separation of particles of different sizes according to the distance from the wall. If more than one fraction is required, a number of tubes of increasing area of cross-section can be connected in series, Fig. 3.9.

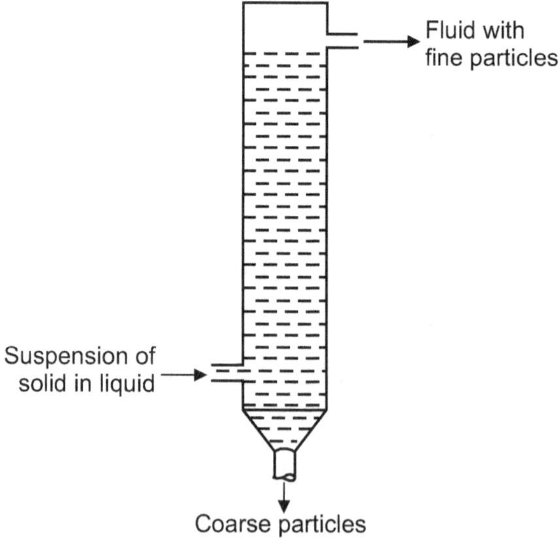

Fig. 3.8: A Schematic of Simple Elutriator

With the same overall flow-rate, the velocity will decrease in succeeding tubes as the area of cross-section increases, giving a number of fractions.

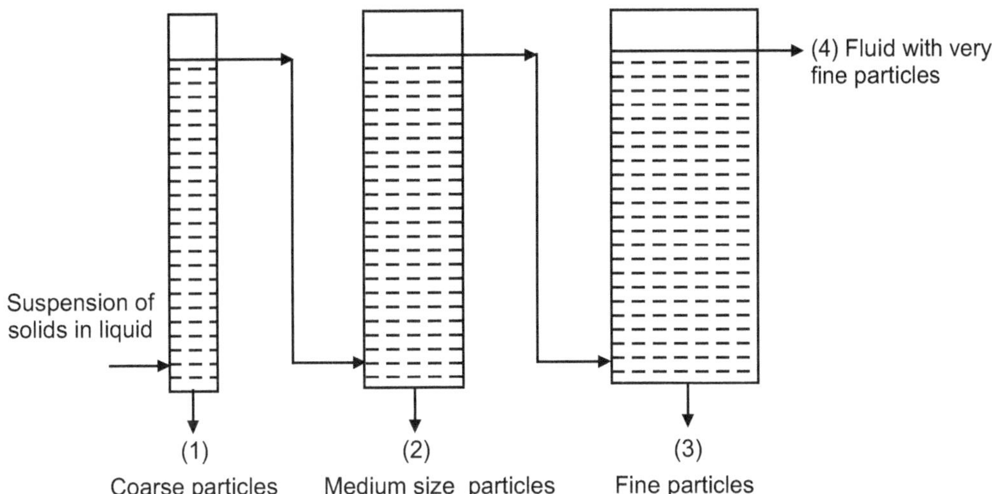

Fig. 3.9: Multi-Stage Elutriator: (1) to (4) is fractions of decreasing particle size

Working:

The material whose particles are to be separated is first levigated and the paste is transferred to elutriation tank. A large amount of water is added to tank so as to make independent particle settling. The contents in the tank are stirred to obtain uniform particle distribution. If left aside undisturbed coarse particles settle at the bottom where as small size particles remain suspended in liquid. These fines can be transferred to next elutriator in connection wherein similar process of separation takes place to obtain further fractions of fines.

Merits:

(i)   The process is continuous.

(ii) The separation is quicker than with sedimentation.

(iii) It has feasibility to add many columns based upon fractions required.

(iv) It needs no skilled operators.

(v)   It is a fast process than sedimentation.

Demerits:

(i)   The suspension has to be dilute; which may sometimes be undesirable.

(ii) It separates particles based on their sedimentation property but not on specific features (for example, surface or shape).

(iii) It cannot separate different types of particles which have similar sedimentation properties.

Applications:

(i)   Both simple and multiple elutriators are used for similar purposes following a size reduction process, with the object of separating oversize particles, which may be returned for further grinding, used for other purposes, or discarded according to the circumstances.

(ii) With liquids, it can be used to separate insoluble solids, such as kaolin or chalk, which are often subjected to wet grinding followed by sedimentation or elutriation with water.

(iii) With gases, it can be applicable to finer solids that would separate too slowly in liquids, to water-soluble substances, or where dry processing is required.

REVIEW QUESTIONS

1.   What is size separation? What are its objectives?
2.   Explain various applications of size separation.
3.   Comment on various official standards for powder size.
4.   Classify powder according to B.P.
5.   What are pharmaceutical sieves? Write about its construction.
6.   Discuss various types of pharmaceutical sieves.
7.   What is significance of calibration of sieves?
8.   Discuss various standards applied to sieves as per I.P.
9.   Discuss various I.P. specifications for wire and aperture size of sieves.
10.   What are various international standards for sieves?
11.   Elaborate on mechanisms of size separation.
12.   Discuss principle, construction, working, uses, merits and demerits of sieve shaker used in pharmaceutical production.
13.   Discuss various sieving mechanisms involved in size separation.
14.   What is sieving time, sieving amplitude and sieving aid?
15.   Enlist and explain various steps involved in sieving process.
16.   Discuss principle, construction working, uses, merits and demerits of cyclone separator.
17.   Discuss principle, construction working, uses, merits and demerits of air separator.
18.   Discuss principle, construction working, uses, merits and demerits of bag filter.
19.   Discuss principle, construction working, uses, merits and demerits of elutriation tank.
20.   How terminal velocities of particle settling are calculated in elutriation tank?
21.   What is significance of multi-stage elutriator?

✍ ✍ ✍

Chapter ... **4**

HEAT TRANSFER

4.0 INTRODUCTION

Heat is a form of energy. As we know matter is made-up of atoms and molecules, atoms in molecules are always in motion represented by translation, rotation and vibration. This motion leads to generation of heat energy. The more the motion of atoms in molecules more is the generation of heat. This heat can only be transferred from a region of higher temperature to a region of lower temperature. Heat is transferred by conduction, convection, and radiation. Conduction is the main method by which heat is transferred through solids. In solids no appreciable displacement of matter occurs. The flow of heat in non-metals is due to transfer of vibrational energy from one molecule to another and, in the case of metals, by the movement of free electrons. In convection, energy is transferred from or to a region by the motion of fluids. The heat flow is caused by buoyancy forces (caused by difference in temperature) induced by variations in the density of the fluid. All substances above absolute zero radiate heat in the form of electromagnetic waves. The radiation may be transmitted, reflected, or absorbed by matter; the fraction absorbed being transformed into heat. Thus, it is known that energy is transferred between systems either as heat or as work. The energy transfer that results across a finite temperature difference is heat transfer and the rest of the energy transfer interactions can be brought under one or other type of work transfer. Heat transfer involves first and the second law of thermodynamics.

4.1 OBJECTIVES

We know that across a finite temperature difference present between a system and its surrounding, heat transfer depends upon the mode of heat transfer for example, conduction, convection or radiation. The amount of heat (q) that transfers depends on several parameters such as the system and surrounding temperatures, their shape, relative movement or flow and thermo-physical properties such as specific heat, thermal conductivity, viscosity, and emissivity. These parameters can be used in understanding the principle and mechanisms involved in heat transfer process which can be further exploited for rapid and economical manufacturing of pharmaceutical API, intermediates and finished dosage forms.

The objectives of heat transfer are given below:

(i)   Formulate basic equation for heat transfer problems.

(ii) Calculate heat transfer between objects with simple geometries.

(iii) Evaluate the impact of initial and boundary conditions on the solutions of a particular heat transfer issue.

(iv) Recognize basic heat transfer mechanism and apply appropriate methods for quantification.

(v) Evaluate the relative contributions of different modes of heat transfer.

(vi) Perform an energy balance to determine temperature and heat flux.

(vii) Apply heat transfer principles to design and size to evaluate performance of heat exchangers.

4.2 APPLICATIONS OF HEAT TRANSFER

(i) **Evaporation:** Heat is supplied in order to convert a liquid into a vapour.

(ii) **Distillation:** Heat is supplied to the liquid mixture for separation of individual vapour component.

(iii) **Drying:** For drying the wet granules and other solids.

(iv) **Crystallization:** Saturated solution is heated to bring out super saturation, which promotes crystallization of drugs.

(v) **Sterilization:** Autoclaves are used with steam as a heating medium.

(vi) **Food processing industries:** The principles of heat transfer are widely used in food processing industries for pasteurization, refrigeration, chilling, and freezing and refrigerative evaporation.

(vii) **Chemical process industries:** Heat transfer methods find a variety of applications in the chemical process industries. Heating and cooling of batch tanks will allow the user to calculate the time it takes to heat up and then cool a batch vessel or tank.

(viii) **Manufacturing of bulk drugs and dosage forms:** Principles of heat transfer is of significance in manufacturing of various bulk drugs, excipients and dosage form.

4.3 FOURIER'S LAW

The law of heat conduction is also known as Fourier's law. It states that "the time rate of heat transfer through a material is proportional to the negative gradient in the temperature and to the area."

The Fourier's equation of heat conduction is expressed as equation (4.1)

$$Q = -k \times A \frac{dT}{dx} \qquad \qquad \ldots (4.1)$$

Where, Q is the heat flow rate by conduction (W), k is the thermal conductivity of body material (W/m.K), A is the cross-sectional area normal to direction of heat flow (m^2) and $\frac{dt}{dx}$ is the temperature gradient (K/m).

The negative sign in Fourier's equation indicates that the heat flow is in the direction of negative gradient temperature and that serves to make heat flow positive. Thermal conductivity is one of the transport properties. Other properties includes viscosity associated with the transport of momentum and diffusion coefficient associated with the transport of mass. Thermal conductivity provides an indication of the rate at which heat energy is transferred through a medium by conduction process.

The assumptions of Fourier equation includes steady state heat conduction, one directional heat flow, isothermal bounding surfaces with constant and uniform temperatures at the two faces, isotropic and homogeneous material and thermal conductivity constant, constant temperature gradient and linear temperature profile and no internal heat generation.

The unique features of Fourier equation are that this equation is valid for all matter solid, liquid or gas. The vector expression indicates that the heat flow rate is normal to an isotherm and is in the direction of decreasing temperature. It cannot be derived from first principle and helps to define the transport property 'k'.

Thermal resistance is reciprocal of the thermal conductance and is associated with the conduction of heat. Consider a plane wall of thickness L and average thermal conductivity k. The two surfaces of the wall are maintained at constant temperatures of T_1 and T_2. For one-dimensional steady heat conduction through the wall, we have T_x. Then Fourier's law of heat conduction for the wall with two surfaces is expressed as:

$$Q_{wall} = - kA \frac{T_2 - T_1}{L} \qquad \text{... (4.2)}$$

$$= - \frac{T_2 - T_1}{L} \qquad \text{... (4.3)}$$

Where, Q_{wall} is the heat flux through the plane (W), k is the materials conductivity (W/m.K), L is the plane thickness (m) and A is the plane area (m^2). Thermal resistance is a heat property and is a measurement of a temperature difference by which an object or material resists a heat flow. The thermal resistance (R_t) for conduction in a plane wall is defined as:

$$R_t = \frac{L}{kA} \qquad \text{... (4.4)}$$

Where, k is the materials conductivity (W/m.K), L is the plane thickness (m) and A is the plane area (m^2).

4.4 MECHANISMS OF HEAT TRANSFER

Heat transfer mechanisms are simply ways by which thermal energy is transferred between objects. It is based on the basic principle that kinetic energy tries to be at equilibrium or at equal energy states. There are three different ways for heat transfer to occur namely conduction, convection, and radiant heat. There is one more related phenomenon that transfers latent heat called evapotranspiration.

4.4.1 Conduction

Conduction heat transfer is energy transport due to molecular motion and interaction. Conduction heat transfer through solids is due to molecular vibration. Fourier determined that Q/A, the heat transfer per unit area (W/m^2) is proportional to the temperature gradient dT/dx . The constant of proportionality is called the material thermal conductivity k.

$$\frac{Q}{A} = - k\frac{dT}{dx} \qquad \qquad \dots (4.5)$$

Table 4.1: Thermal Conductivities of Common Materials

Material	Thermal Conductivities (W/m K)
Copper	400
Aluminum	240
Cast iron	80
Water	0.61
Air	0.026

In conduction the molecules simply gives their energy to adjacent molecules until equilibrium is reached. Conduction models do not deal with the movement of particles within the material. The thermal conductivity k depends on the material, for example, the various materials used in engines have the thermal conductivities (W/m K) as given in Table 4.1. The thermal conductivity also depends somewhat on the temperature of the material.

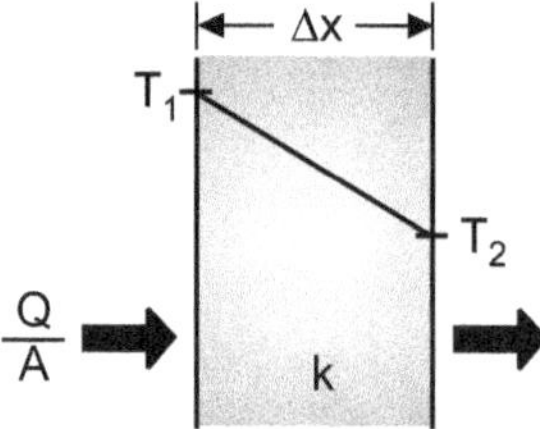

Fig. 4.1: Conduction through Piston Cylinder Wall

For a cast iron 0.012 m cylinder block at steady state, Fig. 4.1, and at T_1 = 100 °C and T_2 = 300 °C heat transfer is given by equation (4.6)

$$\frac{Q}{A} = - k\frac{dT}{dx} = \frac{- k\,(T_1 - T_2)}{\Delta x} \qquad \qquad \dots (4.6)$$

$$= \frac{- 80\,(100 - 300)}{0.012}$$

$$= 1.3 \text{ MW/m}^2$$

4.4.2 Convection

Convection heat transfer is energy transport due to bulk fluid motion. This type of heat transfer through gases and liquids from a solid boundary results from the fluid motion along the surface. Newton determined that the heat transfer/area (Q/A), is proportional to the fluid solid temperature difference (T_s – T_f). The temperature difference usually occurs across a thin layer of fluid adjacent to the solid surface. This thin fluid layer is called a boundary layer. The constant of proportionality is called the heat transfer coefficient (h).

$$\frac{Q}{A} \propto T_s - T_f \qquad\qquad \text{... (4.7)}$$

$$\frac{Q}{A} = h\,(T_s - T_f) \qquad\qquad \text{... (4.8)}$$

The movement of the thermal energy in convection is due to movement of hot fluid. Usually this motion occurs as a result of differences in density. Warmer particles are less dense, so particles with higher temperature will move to regions where the temperature is cooler and the particles with lower temperature will move to areas of higher temperature. Thus, the fluid will remain in motion until equilibrium is reached. The heat transfer coefficient depends on the type of fluid and the fluid velocity. The heat flux depending on the area of interest is the local or area averaged. The various types of convective heat transfer are usually categorized into the following areas:

Table 4.2: Convective Heat Transfer Coefficients

Convection type	Description	Heat Transfer Coefficients (h) (W/m^2K)
Natural convection	Fluid motion is induced by density differences	10 (gas) and 100 (liquid)
Forced convection	Fluid motion is induced by pressure differences from a fan or pump	100 (gas) and 1000 (liquid)
Boiling	Fluid motion is induced by a change of phase from liquid to vapour	20,000
Condensation	Fluid motion is induced by a change of phase from vapour to liquid	20,000

For a cylinder block, Fig. 4.2, with a forced convection (h) of 1000, surface temperature of 100 °C, and a coolant temperature of 80 °C, the local heat transfer rate is calculated as:

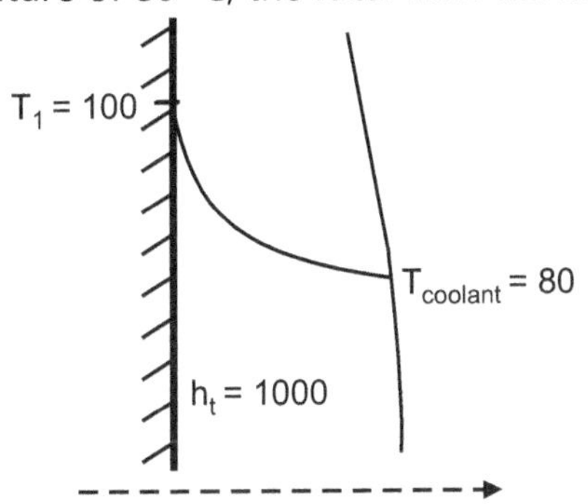

Fig. 4.2: Convection Heat Transfer

$$\frac{Q}{A} = 1000\,(100 - 80)$$

$$= 20000 \; W/m^2$$

4.4.3 Radiation

Radiation heat transfer is energy transport due to emission of electromagnetic waves or photons from a surface or volume, Fig. 4.3. All moving charged particles emit electromagnetic radiation. This emitted wave will travel until it hits another particle. The particle that receives this radiation will receive it as kinetic energy. Particles will receive and emit radiation even after everything is at the same temperature, but it is not noticed due to the fact that the material is at equilibrium at this point. The radiation does not require a heat transfer medium, and can occur in a vacuum.

The heat transfer by radiation is proportional to the fourth power of the absolute material temperature. The proportionality constant is the Stefan-Boltzmann constant $\approx 5.67 \times 10^{-8}\,\text{W/m}^2\,\text{K}^4$. The radiation heat transfer also depends on the material property emissivity (e) of the material.

$$\frac{Q}{A} = \varepsilon \times \sigma \times T^4 \qquad\qquad \dots (4.9)$$

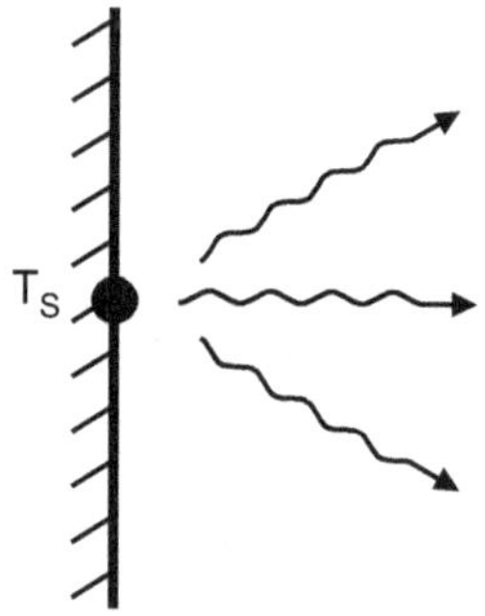

Fig. 4.3: Radiation Through Piston Cylinder Wall

For a surface with an emissivity of e = 0.8 and T = 373 K (100 °C), the radiation heat transfer is

$$\frac{Q}{A} = 0.8 \times 5.67 \times 10^{-8} \times (373)^4$$

$$= 878\ \text{W/m}^2$$

For moderate (less than 100 °C) temperature differences, it should be noted that the radiation and natural convection heat transfer are about the same.

4.4.4 Evapotranspiration

Evapotranspiration is the energy carried by phase changes, like evaporation or sublimation. Water takes a fair amount of energy to change phase, so this process recognizes that water vapour has a fair amount of energy associated with it. This type of energy transfer mechanism is often not listed among the different types of transfer mechanism as it's harder to understand.

4.5 HEAT EXCHANGERS

A heat exchanger is a device that allows heat from a fluid (a liquid or a gas) to pass to a second fluid (another liquid or gas) with the two fluids at different temperatures and in thermal contact. In heat exchangers, there are usually no external heat and work interactions. Heat exchangers are classified according to transfer processes, number of fluids, and degree of surface compactness, construction features, flow arrangements, and heat transfer mechanisms.

Applications:

    (i) Heating or cooling of a fluid stream.

    (ii) Evaporation or condensation of single- or multicomponent fluid streams.

    (iii) To recover or reject heat.

    (iv) Sterilize, pasteurize, fractionate, distill, concentrate, crystallize, or control process fluids.

    (v) Chemical and petrochemical plants .

    (vi) Air conditioning systems.

    (vii) Power production.

    (viii) Waste heat recovery.

    (ix) Automobile radiator.

    (x) Central heating system.

    (xi) Electronic parts.

Classification of heat exchangers:

In general, based on the relative flow direction of the two fluid streams heat exchangers are classified into two general classes as follows.

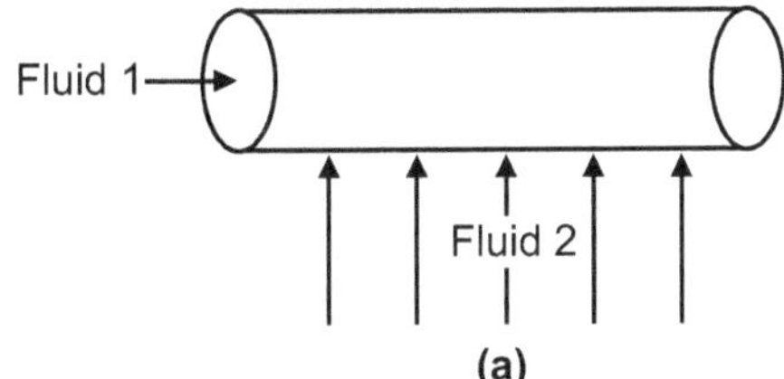

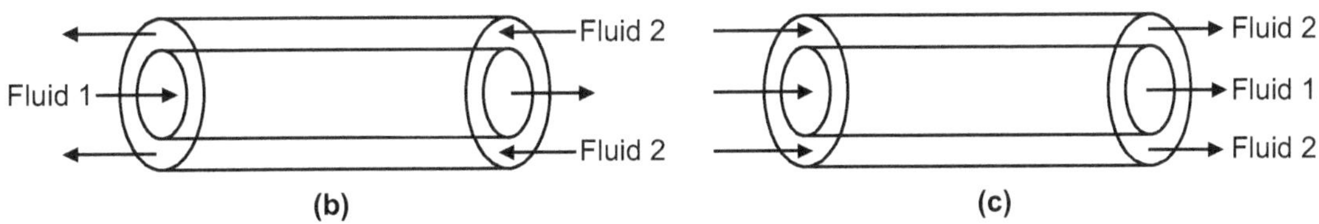

Fig. 4.4: Orientation of Fluid Stream in Heat Exchanger (a) Cross Flow (b) Co-current Flow (c) Parallel Flow

    (i) Cross flow exchangers: Both the fluid streams cross each other in space at right angle, Fig. 4.4(a).

    (ii) Parallel flow exchangers: Both the fluid streams move in parallel direction in space. For example, shell and tube heat exchanger. If the fluid flows in the parallel direction, two situations may arise.

       (a) Fluids flow in same direction.

       (b) Fluids flow in opposites direction.

When the fluid flow is in same direction it is called as "Parallel-flow" heat exchangers and when it is in the opposite direction called as "Co-current flow" heat exchangers, Fig. 4.4.

4.5.1 Shell and Tube Heat Exchanger

The shell and tube heat exchangers are the most commonly used heat exchangers in the chemical process industries. This type of heat exchanger consists of a bundle of tubes properly secured at the ends in tube sheets. The metal sheets have holes into which the tubes are fixed up to have leak proof joints. The entire tube bundle is placed inside a closed shell in such a way that it forms two immiscible zones for hot and cold fluids. One fluid flows through the tubes whereas the other fluid flows around the outside of the tubes within the space between the tube sheets and is enclosed by the outer shell. The proper fluid distribution of the shell side fluid is achieved by placing baffles normal to the tube bundle. Baffle creates turbulence in the shell side fluid and enhances the transfer coefficients for the shell side flow.

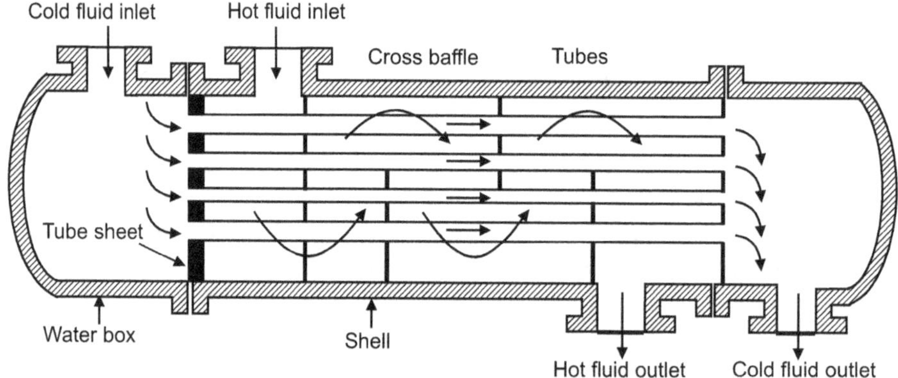

Fig. 4.5: One-Shell Pass, One Tube Pass Heat Exchanger (1-1 Exchanger)

The tube heat exchanger, Fig. 4.5, have one shell and one tube pass since both the shell and tube side fluid make a single traverse through the heat exchanger. Thus, this type of heat exchangers is designated as 1-1 exchanger. If the tube fluid passes twice it is designated as 1-2 exchangers. Similarly, if heat exchanger has 2 shell pass and 4 tube pass, it is designated as 2-4 exchangers. The number of pass in tube side is done by the pass partition plate. A pass partition plate is shown in Fig. 4.6. The shell side pass can be created by a flat plate as shown in Fig. 4.7.

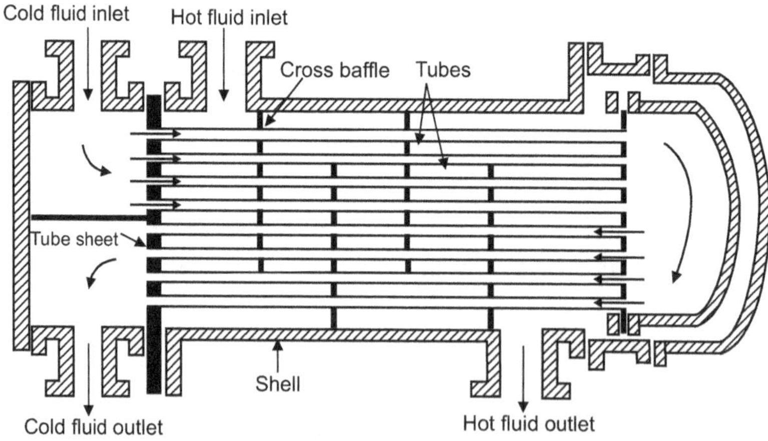

Fig. 4.6: 1-2 Exchanger Showing Pass Partition Plate

In reality, this type of shell and tube heat exchanger is used in the process industry and is quite complex and is improved in design for thermal expansion stresses, tube fouling due to contaminated fluids, ease of assembling and disassembling, size, weight etc. The area available for flow of the tube side fluid is inversely proportional to the number of passes. Thus, on increasing the number of pass the area reduces and as a result the velocity of fluid in the tube increases and henceforth the Reynolds number also increases. It results in increased heat transfer coefficient but it is at the cost of high pressure drop. Generally, even numbers of tube passes are preferred for the multi-pass heat exchangers.

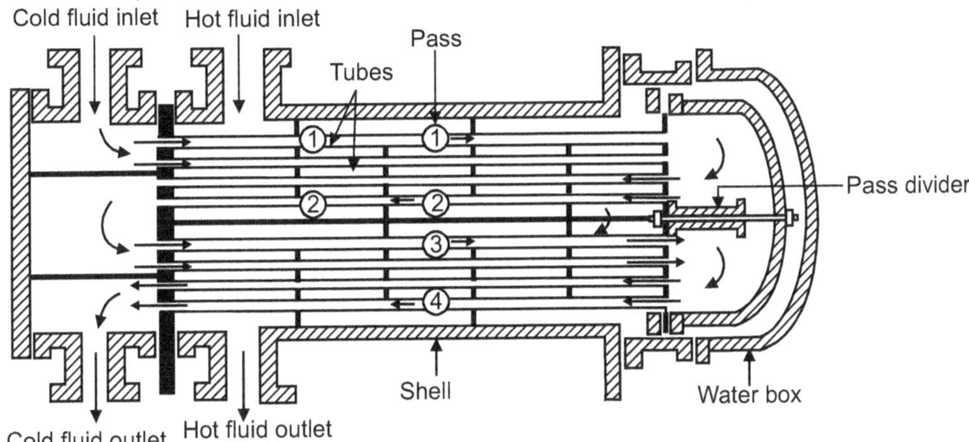

Fig. 4.7: 2-4 Exchanger Showing Shell and Tube Passes

The commonly used method of classifying heat exchangers is indirect contact type or direct contact type heat exchangers.

(A) Indirect contact type heat exchangers: In many heat exchangers, the fluids are separated by a heat transfer surface, and ideally they do not mix or leak. Such exchangers are referred to as direct transfer type.

    (i)   Direct transfer type

    (ii) Storage type

    (iii) Fluidized bed type

(B) Direct contact type: Exchangers in which there is intermittent heat exchange between the hot and cold fluids via thermal energy storage and release through the exchanger surface are referred to as indirect transfer type.

    (i)   Immiscible fluids

    (ii) Gas-liquid

    (iii) Liquid-vapour

4.5.2 Indirect-Contact Heat Exchangers

In an indirect-contact heat exchanger, the fluid streams remain separate and the heat transfers continuously through dividing wall or into and out of a wall. There is no direct contact between thermally interacting fluids. This type of heat exchanger is also called as surface heat exchanger. These type of heat exchangers can be classified into direct-transfer type, storage type, and fluidized-bed type heat exchangers as described below.

(a) Direct-transfer type exchangers:

In this type, heat transfers continuously from the hot fluid to the cold fluid through a dividing wall, Fig. 4.8. Although a simultaneous flow of two fluids is required in the exchanger, there is no direct mixing of the these fluids because each fluid flows in separate fluid passages. In general, there are no moving parts in most such heat exchangers. This type of exchanger is designated as a recuperative heat exchanger or simply as a recuperator. Recuperator is a form of heat exchanger in which heating air is waste gases.

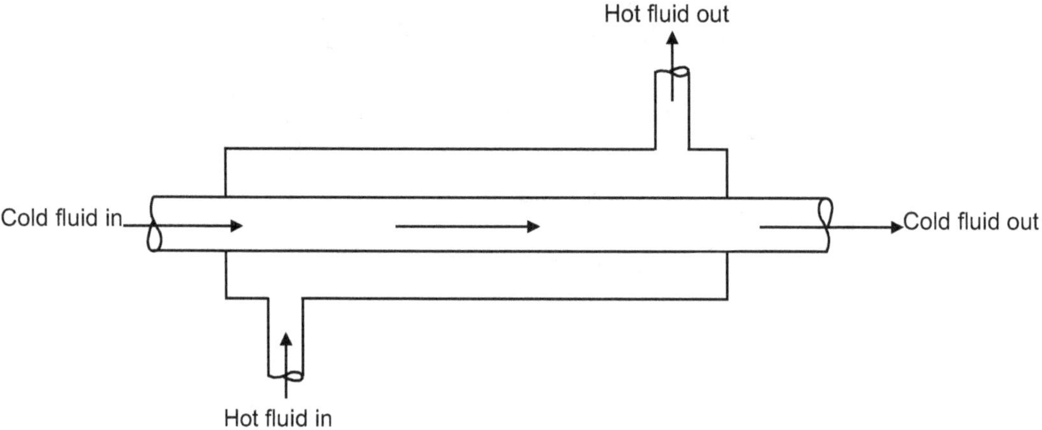

Fig. 4.8: Direct-Transfer Type Exchangers

Some examples of direct transfer type heat exchangers are tubular, plate-type, and extended surface exchangers. The term recuperator is not commonly used in the process industry for shell-and-tube and plate heat exchangers, but they are considered as recuperators. Recuperators are further sub-classified as prime surface exchangers and extended-surface exchangers. Prime surface exchangers do not use fins or extended surfaces on any fluid side. Plain tubular exchangers, shell-and-tube exchangers with plain tubes, and plate exchangers are good examples of prime surface exchangers.

(b) Storage type exchangers:

In storage type exchanger, Fig. 4.9, both the fluids flow alternatively through the same flow passages and thus the heat transfer is intermittent. The heat transfer surface is generally cellular in structure and is referred to as a matrix or it is a permeable solid material, referred to as a packed bed. When hot gas flows over the heat transfer surface the thermal energy from the hot gas is stored in the matrix wall, and thus the hot gas is cooled during the matrix heating period. As cold gas flows through the same passages later, the matrix wall gives up thermal energy, which is absorbed by the cold fluid. Thus, heat is not transferred continuously through the wall as in a direct-transfer type exchanger, but the corresponding thermal energy is alternately stored and released by the matrix wall. This storage type heat exchanger is also referred to as a regenerative heat exchanger, or simply as a regenerator.

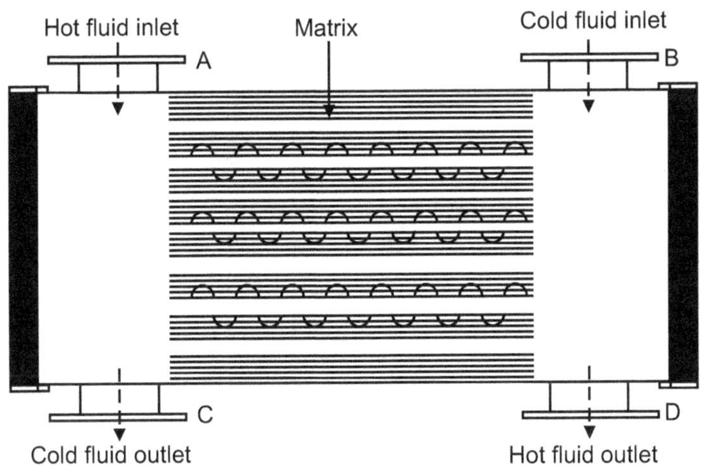

Fig. 4.9: Storage Type Heat Exchanger

To operate continuously and within a desired temperature range, the gases, headers, or matrices are switched periodically so that the same passage is used for hot and cold gases. The actual time required for hot gas to flow through a cold regenerator matrix is called the hot period or hot blow. Whereas time required for cold gas to flow through the hot regenerator matrix is called the cold period or cold blow. It is not necessary to have hot- and cold-gas flow periods of equal duration. There is some unavoidable carryover of a small fraction of the fluid remained in the passage to the other fluid stream after switching of the fluids; this known as carryover leakage. If the hot and cold fluids are at different pressures, the leakage is from the high-pressure fluid to the low-pressure fluid past the radial, peripheral, and axial seals, or across the valves, referred as pressure leakage. These leakages being unavoidable, regenerators are used exclusively in gas-to-gas heat and mass transfer applications with sensible heat transfer. In some applications regenerators may transfer about 5% moisture from humid air to dry air.

(c) Fluidized-bed heat exchangers:

In a fluidized-bed heat exchanger, one side of a two-fluid exchanger is immersed in a bed of finely divided solid material, as shown in Fig. 4.10. If the upward fluid velocity on the bed side is low, the solid particles will remain fixed in position in the bed and the fluid will flow through the interstices of the bed. If the upward fluid velocity is high, the solid particles will be carried away with the fluid. At a "proper" value of the fluid velocity, the upward drag force is slightly higher than the weight of the bed particles. This causes the solid particles to float with dilation of bed behave as a liquid and is referred to as a fluidized condition. In this condition, the fluid pressure drop through the bed remains almost constant, independent of the flow rate, and a strong mixing of the solid particles occurs. This causes uniform temperature in the whole bed with an apparent thermal conductivity of the solid particles as infinity.

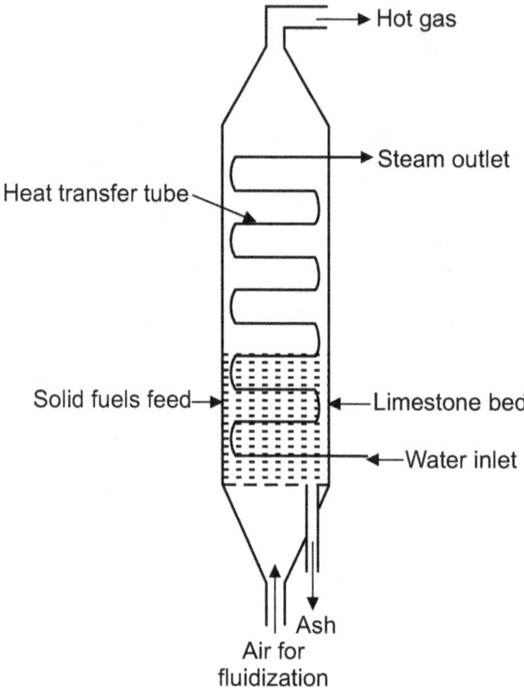

Fig. 4.10: Fluidized-Bed Heat Exchangers

Very high heat transfer coefficients are achieved on the fluidized side compared to particle-free or dilute-phase particle gas. Chemical reaction is common on the fluidized side in many process applications, and combustion takes place in coal combustion fluidized beds. The common applications of the fluidized-bed heat exchanger are drying, mixing, adsorption, reactor engineering, coal combustion, and waste heat recovery. Initial temperature difference between the inlet temperature of the hot fluid and the fluidized bed is reduced by to fluidization and thus the exchanger effectiveness is lowered.

4.5.3 Direct-Contact Heat Exchangers

In a direct-contact exchanger, two fluid streams come into direct contact, exchange heat, and are then separated. Common applications of a direct-contact exchanger involve mass and heat transfer, such as in evaporative cooling and rectification. The enthalpy of phase change in such an exchanger represents a significant portion of the total energy transfer. The phase change generally enhances the heat transfer rate. Direct-contact heat exchangers have very high heat transfer rates, the exchanger construction is relatively inexpensive, and the fouling problem is generally non-existent due to the absence of a heat transfer surface between the two fluids. These exchangers are classified as follows.

(a) Immiscible Fluid Exchangers:

(i) Liquid-liquid exchanger: In this type, two immiscible fluid streams are brought into direct contact. These fluids may be single-phase fluids, or they may involve condensation or vaporization. For example, condensation of organic vapours and oil vapours with water or air.

(ii) Gas–liquid exchangers:

In this type, one fluid is a gas (usually air) and the other a low-pressure liquid (commonly, water) and is readily separable after the energy exchange. In either cooling of liquid (water) or humidification of gas (air) applications, liquid partially evaporates and the vapour is carried away with the gas. In these exchangers, more than 90% of the energy transfer is by virtue of mass transfer due to the evaporation of the liquid and convective heat transfer is a minor mechanism. For example, water cooling tower with forced- or natural-draft airflow, air-conditioning spray chamber, spray drier, spray tower, and spray pond.

(b) Liquid–Vapour Exchangers:

In this type, steam is partially or fully condensed using cooling water, or water is heated with waste steam through direct contact in the exchanger. Non-condensables and residual steam and hot water are the outlet streams. For example, de-superheaters and open feed water heaters (de-aeraters) in power plants.

4.6 HEAT INTERCHANGERS

Most of the chemical and pharmaceutical industries uses a variety of heat transfer equipments. The materials to be heated may be liquids, gases or solids. The heating media is a hot fluid or condensed steam. In pharmacy, operations involved in heat transfer includes preparation of starch paste for granulation, crystallization, evaporation, distillation etc.

In industrial processes, heat energy is transferred by various methods. The heat exchangers are the devices used for transferring heat from one fluid (hot gas or steam) to another fluid (liquid) through a metal wall. Heat interchangers are the devices used for transferring heat from one liquid to another or from one gas to another gas through a metal wall. This classification is vague and may time used interchangeably.

In a heat interchanger, when heat is transferred the film coefficients on both sides of the tube are of the same order of magnitude. In order to increase the overall coefficient, along with increase in the coefficient on one side the fluid velocity on both sides is also increased to enhance both the coefficients. The fluid velocity and heat transfer coefficient could be achieved by placing baffles outside the tubes. The baffle arrangement increases the path length and decrease the cross-section of the path of the second fluid. Thus, provision of baffles increases the velocity of the liquid outside the tubes and also makes it to flow at right angles to the tubes. It leads to additional turbulence which reduces the resistance for heat transfer outside the tubes.

4.6.1 Baffles

Baffles are circular discs of metal with one side cut away. These discs are perforated through which tubes are fitted. In order to avoid or at least minimize the leakage, the clearance is kept small between the baffles, shell and tubes. The baffles are supported on metal rods and are fastened between the tube sheets by set-screws. Baffles are used to create turbulence in the shell side fluid by changing the flow pattern parallel or cross flow to the tube bundles and thus increases the shell side heat transfer coefficient. It also has a function to support the tube all along its length otherwise the tube may bend. Moreover, these baffles may have horizontal or vertical cuts (segmental baffle) as shown in Fig. 4.11.

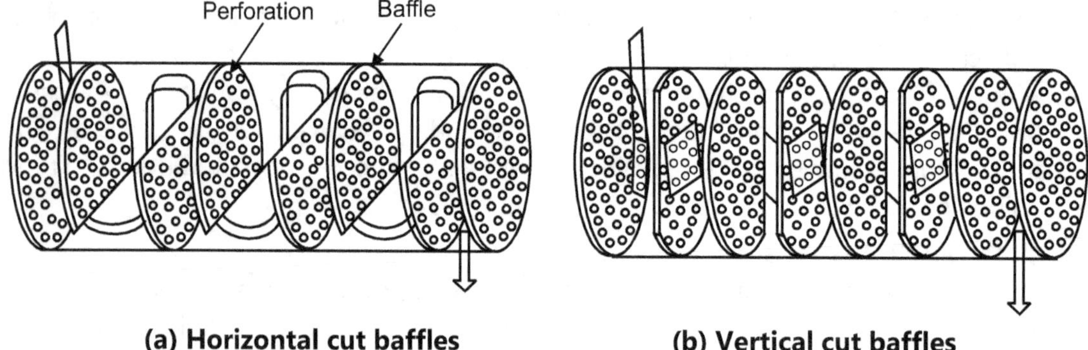

(a) Horizontal cut baffles   **(b) Vertical cut baffles**

Fig. 4.11: Baffles

The cut portion of the baffle is called as baffle window. It provides the area for flow of the shell fluid. The baffle window area ranges from 15% to 50%. At 20% cut segmental baffle means that the area of the cut-out portion is 20% of the area of the baffle. The spacing between the baffles has significance in terms of pressure drop and heat transfer coefficient. A larger spacing reduces the shell side pressure drop, decreases turbulence and heat transfer coefficient. A smaller spacing increases the turbulence and heat transfer coefficient but the pressure drop may increase significantly, thus the advantage attained due to the higher heat transfer coefficient may be nullified. Thus, baffle spacing is selected based on the allowable shell side pressure drop and the desired heat transfer coefficient. Generally, the minimum spacing of segmental baffles is $1/5^{th}$ of the shell diameter.

4.6.2 Liquid-to-Liquid Interchanger

The liquid-to-liquid heat interchanger is a single pass equipment wherein the fluid to be heated is passed only once through the tubes before it gets discharged. Thus, the heat transfer in this case is not efficient. The basic construction includes few modifications and its working remains approximately same.

Working:

Baffles are placed outside the tubes. The presence of baffles increases the velocity of liquid outside the tubes. Baffles make the liquid flow more or less right angles to the tubes, which creates more turbulence. This helps in reducing the resistance to heat transfer outside the tubes. The construction of a liquid-to-liquid heat interchanger illustrates the principle of introducing the baffles into the equipment.

Construction:

The construction of a liquid-to-liquid heat interchanger is shown in Fig. 4.12. It consists of baffles, tube sheets, spacer rods and the tubes. The most important parts in any heat interchanger are the baffles. Appropriate size of tube sheets is used for the fabrication. Guide rods are fixed to the tube sheets and tighten by means of screws. As mentioned before baffles are placed at right places with the support of guide rods. The baffles are separated with proper spacing using short sections of the same tubing. Tubes are inserted through the perforations in baffles where as ends of tubes are expanded into the tube sheets. This whole assembly is enclosed in a shell for introducing the heating fluid. The outlet for the heating fluid is at top of one end of interchanger. On both the sides of the tubes, distribution chambers are provided. At the top of left-side chamber an inlet for fluid to be heated is provided. The outlet for the heated fluid is provided near to the right-side distribution chamber.

Working:

The hot fluid (heating medium) is pumped from the left-side top of the shell. The fluid flows outside the tubes and moves down directly to the bottom. Then, it changes the direction and rises again. This process is continued till it leaves the heater. Baffles increase the velocity of the liquid outside the tubes. Baffles also allow the fluid to flow more or less right angles to the tube, which creates more turbulence. This help in reducing the resistance to heat transfer outside the tubes. Baffles lengthen the path and decrease the cross-section of path of the cold fluid. The baffles get heated and provide greater surface area for heat transfer. Simultaneously, during the flow, the tubes also get heated. As a result, the film coefficient inside the tube also increases. The liquid to be heated is pumped through the inlet provided on left-side distribution chamber. The liquid passes through the tubes and gets heated. The flow of liquid is single-pass. The heated liquid is collected from the right-hand side distribution chamber.

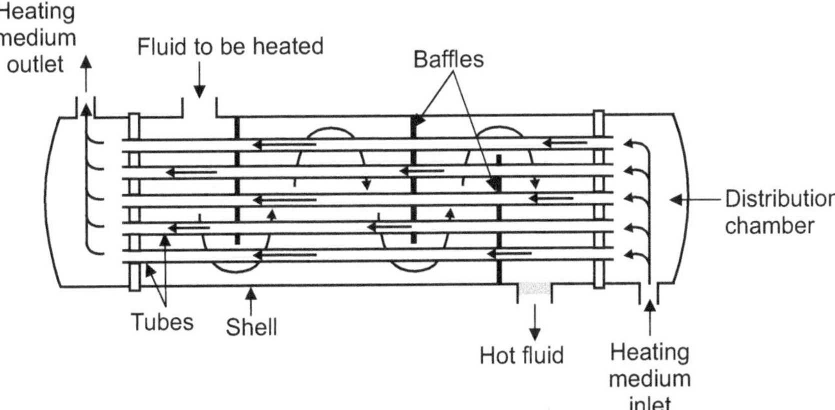

Fig. 4.12: Construction of Liquid-to-Liquid Heat Interchanger

Advantages:

In a liquid-to-liquid interchanger, heat transfer is rapid as the liquid.

(i)   passes at high velocity outside the tubes and,

(ii)   flows more or less at right angles to the tubes.

4.6.3 Double Pipe Heat Interchangers

Double pipe heat interchangers are efficient equipments for the heat transfer as they have few pipes (tubes) per pass.

Construction:

The double-pipe heat interchanger uses two pipes arranged as one inserted into the other, Fig. 4.13. The inner pipe is used for the pumping of cold fluid to be heated whereas the outer acts as a jacket for the circulation of the hot fluid. The components of this interchanger are inter-connected within the shell. As mentioned earlier the number of pipe sections is limited and in addition the length of the pipe is also less. The glass tube, standard iron pipe and graphite materials are used for construction. The metal pipes are assembled with return bends. Few pipes are connected in parallel and stacked vertically and may have longitudinal fins on its outer surface. Outer pipe size varies from 2 to 14 inch with inner tubes varying from 0.75 to 2 inch in size. Some have longitudinal fins on the outside of the inner tube. Counter-current flow in these interchangers is advantageous when very close temperature approaches are required.

Working:

The heating medium (hot liquid) is pumped into the outer jacket and is circulated through the annular spaces between them and carried from one part to the next part and finally it leaves the jacket at bottom on right side. During movement of fluid the pipes get heated and thus hot fluid loses its temperature. The fluid to be heated is pumped into the inner tube through the inlet provided at right side. The liquid gets heated-up and flows through the bent tubes into the part of the pipe. The liquid further gets heated during flow and finally discharges through the exits point on the left side.

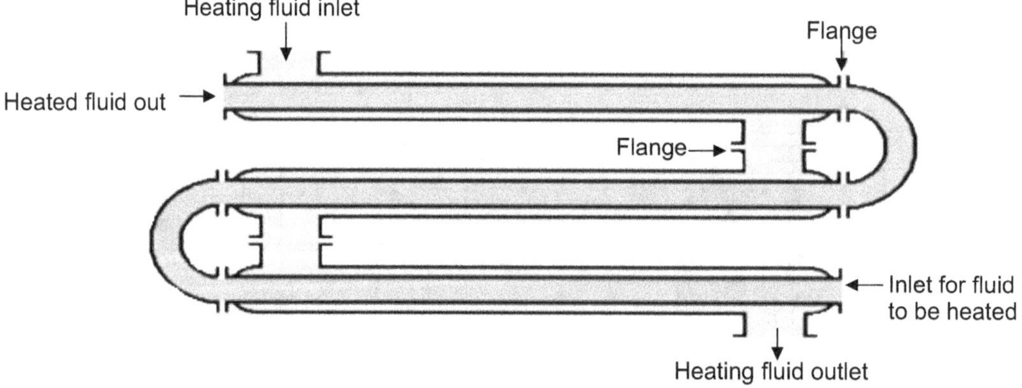

Fig. 4.13: Double Pipe Heat Interchangers

Uses:

(i)   Double pipe heat interchanger is useful when not more than 0.9 to 1.4 m^2 of surface is required.

(ii)   It is best suited when the volume of liquid inside tubes is less and obtain desired velocity and the size of the tube.

(iii) Since, one liquid flows through the inside of the pipe and the second liquid flows through the annular space between the pipes, these are primarily used for low flow rates, high temperature drops and high pressure applications.

4.6.4 Scraped Surface Exchangers

In some of the heat interchangers the drag forces due to flow of viscous liquid a quite thick viscous sub-layer or due to turbulent conditions in the core, liquid exhibits no pressure loss with excessive pumping costs. This problem is solved by physically removing the layers of fluid at the heat transfer surfaces and mixing them with the bulk fluid in the heat exchanger. In this way, if the fluid is being heated, heat is conveyed directly from the wall to the bulk liquid. The technique is particularly attractive for heat sensitive liquids used in pharmaceutical products, because it has low interface temperature between the liquid and heat transfer surface for a given overall temperature driving force.

These types of exchangers have a rotating element with spring loaded scraper blades, Fig. 4.14, to scrape the inner heating surface to effectively remove liquid from it. The blades move against the heat transfer surface under the influence of the rotational forces. Simultaneously, as liquid layers are removed any fouling substance deposited on the surface is also removed. This ensures no contamination of the processed liquid with no change in product qualities. The number of scraper blades may vary but as the number of blades is increased the capital cost rises. A large number of blades are not necessary, since the time interval between successive scrapes is relatively short. The choice of the number of blades is an empirically based compromise between capital cost, acceptable speed of rotation and liquid viscosity. Rotating parts in these exchangers makes the maintenance costlier.

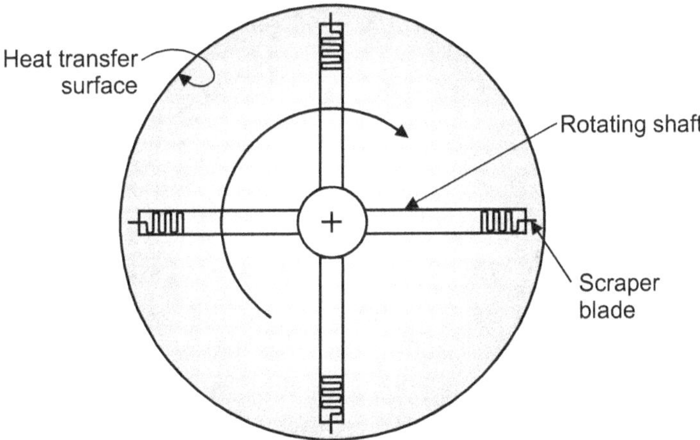

Fig. 4.14: The Scraped Surface Heat Exchanger

Some exchangers have blades that do not actually touch the surface over which they pass, but move in close proximity to it. Such designs may be termed as "wiped surface" heat exchangers, and may be preferred, where the wear of components cannot be tolerated from a view point of mechanical or contamination effects. Scraped surface heat exchangers can either run full of liquid or the liquid may enter the exchanger as a peripheral stream. The design of this heat exchanger is complex and is made usually based on empirically determined parameters derived from experience. Scraped surface heat exchangers are, in general, used only for special applications.

4.6.5 Finned Tube Exchanger

In a heat exchanger while heating the air outside the tubes with steam inside the tubes, the steam side coefficient will be very high and the air side coefficient will be extremely low. While heat transfer, as the overall coefficient approximates that of the lower side (the air side coefficient), the only remedy to increase q is to increase the area term on the air side without putting more tubes in the heater. As we know, metals generally have high thermal conductivity, the temperature of the metal surface rapidly approximates that of steam. If metal fins are attached on the outside of the tubes such that there is good contact between the surface of the tube and base of the fin, heat transfer surface area is increased. A wide variety of fins are used as shown in Fig. 4.15. Rectangular discs of metal may be pressed on to the tube at right angles to them. Spiral fins may be attached to the tubes. Transverse and longitudinal fins are other forms. Use of finned tubes greatly reduces the size of the apparatus. In cases where the heat transfer coefficients on the two sides are close, the question where fins are to be attached is entirely one of economics in design. There are certain cases where fins are used on the inner as well as on the outside of the tubes.

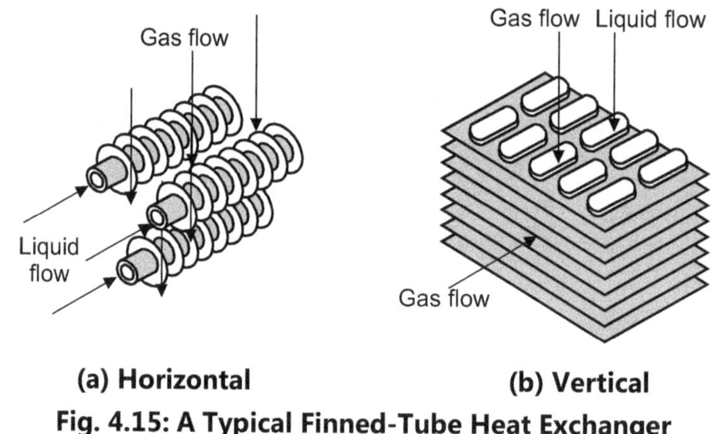

(a) Horizontal   **(b) Vertical**

Fig. 4.15: A Typical Finned-Tube Heat Exchanger

Finned tube heat exchangers are used for heat transfer between air, gas and liquids or steam. Heat exchangers with finned heating surfaces (finned tube) are significantly space-saving and is more efficient than exchangers with straight tubes. These heat exchangers are designed to transfer heat from clean air and gases with high efficiency on liquids or vapours, and vice versa.

Applications:

Finned tube heat exchangers are often used in power plants as an exhaust gas heat exchanger to increase the efficiency factor. Further applications in power plants are the preheating of combustion air as well as the condensation of exhaust steam from steam or turbines. In industrial dryers these heat exchangers are used for heating air by hot water, steam or thermal oil in large quantities. In many industrial production processes, such as for the air conditioning of buildings, these heat exchangers are used as an air cooler for cooling down or re-cooling of liquids.

Advantages:

(i)   Robust construction of finned tube heat exchanger can withstand contrarious operating conditions over a long period.

(ii) They have maximum transmission quality and high condensation rate.

(iii) The have wide application and temperature spectrum (range) thus value for money.

(iv) They are ideal for gas-liquid or gas-vapor heat transfer.

(v)   They show highest reliability of operation.

4.6.6 Plate Type Exchangers

The plate heat exchanger is a specialized design well suited for transferring heat between medium- and low-pressure fluids. Welded, semi-welded and brazed heat exchangers are used for heat exchange between high-pressure fluids or where a more compact product is required.

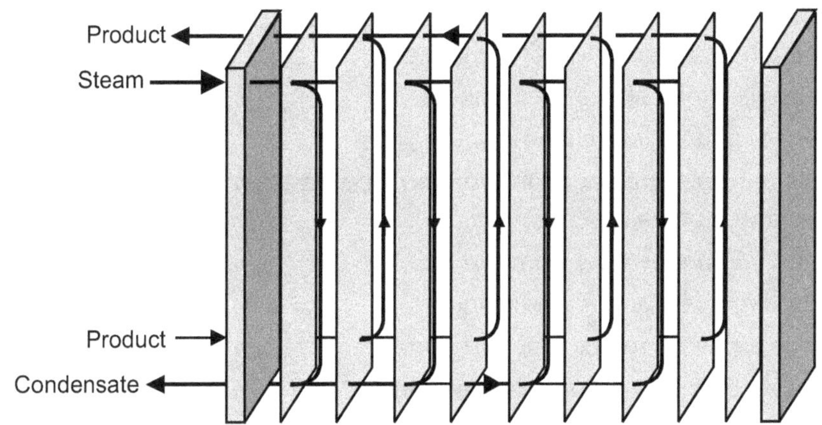

Fig. 4.16: Plate Type Exchangers

In this exchangers the media can be heated, cooled or condensed, in a closed space. Plate type heat exchangers can be used for different applications and in a variety of designs. Several forms of plate heat exchangers are available. These essentially consist of standard plates which serve as heat transfer surfaces, Fig. 4.16. Plates are provided with grooves for rubber gaskets. A number of such plates are supported on a frame and assembled in such a way that the plates can be separated individually for cleaning or replacing. A corrugated plate design is also used to impart rigidity to the plate. In place of a pipe passing through a chamber, there are instead two alternating chambers, usually thin in depth, separated at their largest surface by a corrugated metal plate. The plates used in a plate and frame heat exchanger are obtained by one piece pressing of metal plates. Stainless steel is a commonly used metal for the plates due to its ability to withstand high temperatures, its strength, and its corrosion resistance.

REVIEW QUESTIONS

1. What is heat transfer? What are its objectives?
2. Explain basic mechanisms of heat transfer.
3. What is the difference between diffusion and radiation heat transfer?
4. What is natural and forced convection?
5. How is natural convection different from forced convection?
6. State Fourier law. Write about its assumptions.
7. Explain Stefen-Boltzman law of thermal radiation.
8. Discuss pharmaceutical applications of heat transfer.
9. Write about thermal conductivity of metals.
10. Discuss convection type of heat transfer with heat transfer coefficients.
11. What do you mean by emissivity?
12. What are heat exchangers? Classify them.
13. What are heat interchangers? Enlist them.
14. Write applications of heat exchangers.
15. Write uses of heat interchangers.
16. Discuss principle, construction, working, applications, advantages and disadvantages of shell and tube heat exchangers.
17. What do you understand from the 1-1, 1-2 and 2-4 heat exchangers?
18. Discuss direct contact heat exchangers.
19. Describe indirect contact heat exchangers.
20. Short note on fluidized bed heat exchanger.
21. What are baffles? Write its function in heat exchangers.
22. Discuss construction, working and uses of double pipe heat interchangers.
23. Write short note on scraped surface exchangers.
24. What are finned tubes? Explain their importance in heat transfer.
25. What are advantages and applications of fin tube heat exchangers?
26. Discuss plate type heat exchangers.

✍ ✍ ✍

Chapter ...5

EVAPORATION

Evaporation is a surface phenomenon, wherein mass transfer takes place from the surface. It is the process of vaporization of a liquid. In this process, liquid state of a substance is changing to a gaseous state due to an increase in temperature and/or pressure. It is a fundamental part of the water cycle and is constantly occurring throughout nature. During evaporation water changes from a liquid to a gas or vapour. Water boils at 100 °C but in reality it begins to evaporate at 0 °C but extremely slowly. As the temperature increases, the rate of evaporation also increases. The amount of evaporation depends on the temperature, and it also depends on the amount of water to evaporate.

Pharmaceutical industries use evaporator for the vaporization of a solvent from a solution. The evaporation is so important operation that it is considered an individual operation. If we continue the evaporation process, the residual mater will be solid, which is known as drying. However, the aim of evaporation is not to dry but to concentrate the solution. In addition, it is not the crystallization, in which the evaporation leads to formation of crystal in the solution. It is expected that students should learn the difference between evaporation, drying and crystallization. The driving force in evaporation is temperature difference between steam chest temperature and product temperature that result in to removal of solvent from the feed that solution is concentrated.

To understand the evaporation process, few facts about the solution properties must be known. Knowledge of solution properties is important for the design of the equipment for evaporation. Some of the important properties of the solution are given below,

(i) Concentration: Initially, the solution may be quite dilute and the properties of the solution may be taken as the properties of solvent. As the concentration increases, the solution becomes viscous and heat transfer resistance increases. The crystal may grow on the heating coil or on the heating surface. The boiling points of the solution also rise considerably. Solid or solute contact increases and the boiling temperature of the concentrated solution became higher than that of the solvent at the same pressure (i.e. elevation in boiling point).

(ii) Foaming: Many of the materials like organic substance may foam during vaporization. If the foam is stable, it may come out along the vapor known as entrainment. Heat transfer coefficient changes abruptly during foaming for such systems.

(iii) Degradation: Some of the products in pharmaceutical industries are very temperature sensitive and may get degraded during evaporation. Thus, special case or technique is required for concentrating such solution.

(iv) Scaling: Many solutions have tendency to deposit the scale on the heating surface, which may increase the heat transfer resistance. These scales produce extra thermal resistance of significant value. Therefore, scaling in the equipment should not be ignored thus de-scaling becomes an important and routine matter.

(v) Equipment material: The material of the equipment must be chosen considering the solution properties so that the solution should neither be contaminated nor react with the equipment material.

Advantages:

(i)   Evaporation reduces transportation and storage cost.

(ii) It prepare material for the next unit operation, for example, drying, crystallization etc.

(iii) It reduces rates of deteriorative chemical reactions.

(iv) It gives better microbiological stability.

(v) It helps in recovery of solvent.

5.1 OBJECTIVES

The primary objective of evaporation is to concentrate a solution consisting of a non-volatile solute and a solvent. In the majority of evaporations the evaporating solvent is water. When the liquid phase is agitated, mass-transfer in the liquid phase is sufficiently rapid that the rate of evaporation of solvent can be determined by the rate of heat transfer from the heating medium, usually condensing steam, to the solution. Mineral-bearing water often is evaporated to give a solid-free product for boiler feed, for special process requirements, or for human consumption. This technique is often called water distillation, but technically it is evaporation.

Another objective of evaporation is to reduce the volume of the product by some significant amount without loss of other components. This reduction of volume permits more efficient transportation of the important product components and efficient storage of the solids. An equally important objective of evaporation is to remove large amounts of moisture effectively and efficiently before the product enters a dehydration process. The evaporation operation may be used for products which vary widely in characteristics, and in many cases these characteristics influence the evaporator design considerably. Evaporation involves vaporization of portion of the solvent to produce a concentrated solution of thick liquor. This thick liquor is the valuable product and the vapour is condensed and/or discarded.

In summarizing, objectives of the evaporation are to generate a sense of the never-ending equilibrium condition of water vapour and to know the speed at which humidify is transferred from one system to the other.

5.2 APPLICATIONS

(i) Evaporation is used in concentration and recovery of dissolved solutes like sodium chloride from aqueous solutions to produce salt.

(ii) It is used in ether recovery from fat extraction.

(iii) It is also used in concentration of solutions. For example, concentration of milk to produce condensed milk and to obtain concentrated juices.

(iv) It is used in concentrating pharmaceutical herbal extracts in herbal industry.

(v) It is used in pharmaceutical industries to eliminate excess moisture, providing an ease of handling products and improving product stability.

(vi) It is used in preservation of long-term activity or stabilization of enzymes in laboratories.

(vii) Evaporation process is used in the manufacture of bulk drugs.

(viii) Evaporation is used in the manufacture of biological products. For example, insulin, enzymes, hormones etc..

(ix) It is used in demineralization of water.

(x) It is also used in concentration of chromatographic fractions, glucose and fructose syrups.

(xi) It has applications in concentration of effluents.

5.3 FACTORS INFLUENCING EVAPORATION

The main factors that have an effect on evaporation are as follows:

(i) Surface area: If the surface area of evaporating solution is increased, then the amount of liquid that is exposed to air is larger. More molecules can escape with a wider surface area.

For example, if we spread out clothes to dry it speeds up the process of evaporation. The larger the exposed surface area, the more molecules can escape from the liquid. Thus larger the surface area faster is the evaporation.

(ii) Temperature: The water molecules move rapidly when the water is heated. This makes the molecules escape faster. Higher temperatures lead to increase in evaporation as more molecules get kinetic energy to convert into vapour.

For example, boiling water evaporates faster than normal water.

(iii) Humidity: Humidity means the amount of vapour present in the air. The air around can only holds a certain amount of vapour at a certain time and certain temperature. If the temperature increases and the air speed and humidity stay constant, then the rate of evaporation will increase since warmer air can hold more water vapour than colder air. Thus, the rate of evaporation decreases with increasing humidity and increases with vice versa.

(iv) Moving air: Particles of vapour move away when the speed of air increases. This leads to a decrease in the amount of water vapour in the atmosphere.

For example, we use hand dryers to dry our hands. Here the air is expelled from the hand dryer which dries our hand.

(v) Boiling point of liquid: Liquids with a lower boiling point evaporate faster. Mercury hardly evaporates at room temperature as it has a boiling point of 357 °C.

(vi) Density of liquid: As the density increases, the rate of evaporation decreases. Liquids with a higher density have a lower rate of evaporation.

For example, honey has a lower rate of evaporation as compared to water, which has a lower rate of evaporation as compared to alcohol. This is because honey is denser than water, and water is denser than alcohol.

5.4 DIFFERENCES BETWEEN EVAPORATION AND OTHER HEAT PROCESS

Table 5.1: Difference between Vaporization and Evaporation

Vaporization (Boiling)	Evaporation
(i) It is a process in which a substance changes its state from the liquid state to the gaseous state with boiling.	(i) It is process in which a substance changes its state from the liquid state to the gaseous state without boiling.
(ii) It is a fast process.	(ii) It is slow process.
(iii) Bubbles are formed while vaporization.	(iii) No bubbles formed during evaporation.
(iv) Occurs throughout the liquid.	(iv) Takes place only from the exposed surface of the liquid.
(v) Vaporization does not depend on surface area of liquid.	(v) Evaporation depends on the surface area of the liquid.
(vi) It occurs at a definite temperature i.e. at boiling point.	(vi) It occurs at all temperatures.
(vii) Heating source of energy is needed.	(vii) Energy is supplied by surroundings.

Table 5.2: Difference between Distillation and Evaporation

Distillation	Evaporation
(i) Distillation is a process of separating the component substances from a liquid mixture by selective evaporation and condensation.	(i) Evaporation is a type of vaporization of a liquid that occurs from the surface of a liquid into a gaseous phase.
(ii) In the distillation, vaporization takes place at the boiling point	(ii) In evaporation, vaporization takes place below the boiling point.
(iii) Distillation is taking place from the whole liquid mass.	(iii) Evaporation takes place only from the surface of the liquid.

... (Contd.)

Distillation	Evaporation
(iv) At the boiling point in distillation the liquid forms bubbles.	(iv) No bubble formation in evaporation.
(v) Distillation is a separation or purifying technique.	(v) Evaporation is not necessarily the separation or purifying technique.
(vi) In distillation, heat energy should be supplied to liquid molecules to go in to the vapour state.	(vi) In evaporation, molecules get energy when they collide with each other and is used to escape to the vapour state.
(vii) In distillation, the vaporization happens rapidly.	(vii) The evaporation is a slow process.
(viii) It involves boiling and condensation.	(viii) It involves only evaporation.
(ix) Process of purification and separating components with fractional distillation based on boiling point.	(ix) Process of purification and separating components without fractionation independent of boiling point.
(x) Example is water and alcohol mixture at boiling point of alcohol.	(x) Example is water below boiling point.

Table 5.3: Difference between Drying and Evaporation

Drying	Evaporation
(i) Drying is removal of water from a substance.	(i) Evaporation is the changing of phase of liquid water to gaseous water.
(ii) It is possible to dry a substance without evaporation. For example, using air, adsorbent, absorbent and freeze drying.	(ii) Evaporation is a physical phenomenon that may form part of the mechanisms that effect such a change, but there are others too.
(iii) Separation of moisture content from any type of biological, chemical and metallurgical materials due to temperature gradient.	(iii) In evaporation the surface molecules skip to the atmosphere by gaining extra energy, especially in the form of heat.
(iv) Drying follows evaporation.	(iv) Evaporation results in drying.
(v) Drying is a process of removing moisture from any object. Drying can occur due to evaporation as well as external factors such as wind.	(v) Evaporation is a process in which the surface molecules skip to the atmosphere by gaining extra energy, especially in the form of heat.
(vi) Drying is the evaporation or conversion of water molecules to the gaseous state for more stability.	(vi) Evaporation takes place in all liquids content, when left in open, tend to lose its water usually to atmospheric air.

... (Contd.)

Drying	**Evaporation**
(vii) Drying is removal of traces of water from material by just sending a hot dry air over it.	(vii) In evaporation mass of liquid at room temperature loses some of the water in it to adjoining environment.
(viii) Drying involves removal of volatile matter by evaporation. In short drying mass transfer takes place by means of evaporation process.	(viii) Evaporation is process to concentrate slurry of solid by removal of volatile matter. It is heat transfer operation.

Table 5.4: Difference between Sublimation and Evaporation

Sublimation	**Evaporation**
(i) Phase change is from solid to gas.	(i) Phase change is from liquid to gas.
(ii) No liquid state involves in this process.	(ii) In this liquid is involved.
(iii) It involves solid as starting material.	(iii) It involves liquid as starting material.
(iv) Requires external energy equal to achieve sublimation.	(iv) Requires external energy equal to achieve evaporation.
(v) Example: Camphor, iodine.	(v) Example: Water to vapor.

5.5 EQUIPMENTS USED FOR EVAPORATION

In evaporation, heat is added to a solution to vaporize the solvent, which is usually water. The heat is generally provided by steam on one side of a metal surface, with the evaporating liquid on the other side. The equipment used for evaporation is called as evaporator. The type of evaporator used depends primarily on the configuration of the heat-transfer surface and on the means employed to provide agitation or circulation of the liquid. Evaporator equipment may be classified, in general, as horizontal-tube, calandria type vertical, basket-type vertical, forced-circulation, and long-tube or film type vertical evaporators.

The general types of equipment are classified either based upon movement of heating medium or type of heating surfaces.

(i) Classification based on heating medium movement:
    (a)   Simple evaporators: Example: Evaporating pan (Steam jacketed kettle).
    (b)   Natural circulation evaporators. Example: Climbing film evaporator.
    (c)   Forced circulation evaporators. Example: Forced circulation evaporator.
    (d)   Film evaporators. Example: Horizontal tube evaporator.

(ii) Classification based on type of heating surfaces:
    (a)   Evaporators with heating medium in jacket. Example: Evaporating pan.
    (b)   Evaporators with horizontal tubes. Example: Horizontal tube evaporator.
    (c)   Evaporator with long tubes and natural circulation. Example: Climbing film evaporator.
    (d)   Evaporator with long tubes and forced circulation. Example: Forced circulation evaporator.
    (e)   Multiple effect evaporators.

5.5.1 Evaporating Pan

The evaporating pan is also called as steam jacketed kettle. In this type of evaporator the movement of the liquid to be evaporated is due to the convection currents set-up by the heating process. It is a type of natural circulation evaporator. It consists of a hemispherical pan surrounded by a steam jacket. The hemispherical shape provides a large surface area for the evaporation to takes place. The evaporation pan may be fixed and the contents are discharged from the outlet provided at the bottom of pan. In some cases the evaporators are mounted in such a way that they can be tilted on either side to remove the concentrated product. The evaporating pans are heated by the steam which enters the jacket through inlet and leaves it from outlet. The heat from the steam in jacket is utilized for evaporating liquid in pan.

Principle:

The mechanism involved in this evaporation process is conduction and convection so that the heat is transferred by this mechanism to the extract. Evaporating pan containing aqueous extract is provided with the steam which gives out heat to a jacketed kettle. The temperature raises and the escaping tendency of the solvent molecules in to the vapour increases and enhances the vaporization of the solvent molecules.

Construction:

Steam evaporating pan consists of hemispherical structure with an inner pan called kettle which is enveloped with an outer pan called jacket, Fig. 5.1. These two pans are joined to enclose a space through which steam is passed. Several metals have been used for the construction of the kettle. Copper is an excellent material for the kettle due to its superior conductivity. If acidic preparation evaporated in copper kettle, some of the copper gets dissolved in preparation. In order to avoid this, for acidic preparation is tinned copper kettle is used. Iron is also used for the construction of the jacket because it has low conductivity. Rusting of iron with use is major problem and to prevent this iron jacket is tinned or enameled on the inner surface. An inlet for the steam and non-condensed gases are provided near the top of the jacket. Condensate leaves the jacket through the outlet provided at the bottom. The kettle is provided with the outlet for the product discharge at its bottom.

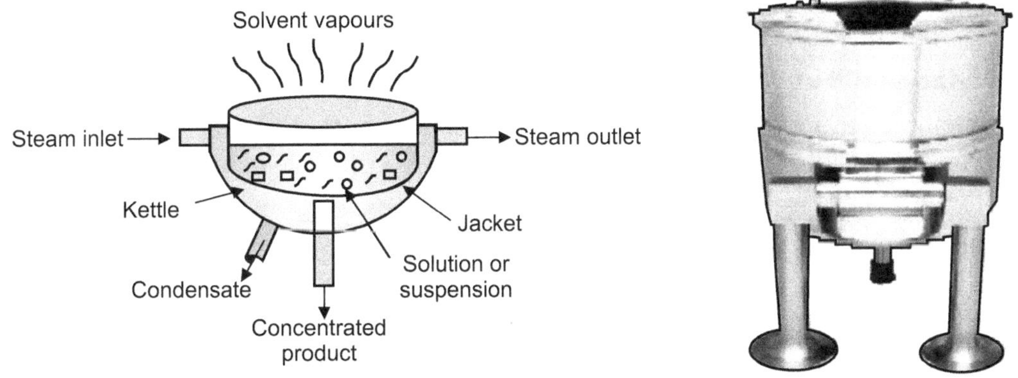

Fig. 5.1: Steam Jacketed Kettle

Working:

The solution to be evaporated is placed in the kettle and steam which gives out heat to the content is supplied through the inlet and condensate leaves through the outlet. For smaller volumes the contents must be stirred manually and mechanically for larger volumes. The rate of evaporation is fast in the initial stages. The room where evaporation is carried must have good ventilation to remove the vapour to avoid fog formation of condensed vapour. To prevent condensation in the room and also to accelerate the rate of evaporation fans are fitted. The kettle may be fixed or made to tilt. A kettle of capacity up to about 90 liters may be made to tilt. The bottom outlet is used to collect the concentrated products.

Applications:

(i)   Evaporating pan is suitable for concentrating aqueous liquids.

(ii)   It is suitable for concentrating thermostable liquors, for example, liquorices extracts.

Advantages:

(i)   Evaporating pan is constructed both for small scale and large scale batch operations.

(ii)   It is a simple in construction and easy to operate, clean and maintain.

(iii) Its cost of installation and maintenance is low.

(iv) Wide variety of materials such as copper, stainless steel and aluminium etc can be used for the construction of evaporating pan.

(v)   Stirring the contents in pan and removal of the products is easy.

Disadvantages:

(i)   Natural circulation of the product makes poor heat transfer.

(ii)   Deposition of solid may cause decomposition of the product.

(iii) Heating surface is limited and decreases proportionally to increase in size of the pan.

(iv) It is not suitable for the concentration of thermolabile materials.

(v)   It has no provision to operate under a reduced pressure.

(vi) No provision to recollect the costly organic solvents.

(vii) Being the evaporating pan open vapours directly pass in to the atmosphere. This may cause discomfort to the worker.

(viii) Saturation of surrounding environment with vapours may slow down the process.

5.5.2 Horizontal Tube Evaporator

Horizontal tube evaporator frequently found to be the most adaptable choice for simple evaporation wherein liquids are not viscous and do not deposit scale or salt on surface.

Principle:

The principle mechanism involved in this type of evaporator is that steam is passed through tubes arranged horizontally. Heating causes evaporation of the feed outside the tubes discharging concentrate at the bottom and vapours passed out from the outlet at top. The vapour is removed from the top of the chamber and the product circulation take place by natural circulation over the heating coil.

Construction:

Horizontal-tube evaporators are designed with either rectangular or circular cross-sections, with tubing of stainless steel, aluminium, nickel, carbon, spellerized iron pipe, lead-covered copper, or special bronze, Fig. 5.2 (a). The tubes are extended between two steam chests and arc is fastened to tube. Four-hole packing plate's force down conical gaskets around the tube ends into counter-sunk holes in the tube sheets. Secure sealing is obtained, with facility for quick and easy renewal. Horizontal tubes of 2 to 3 cm diameter are extended across the bottom of a cylindrical chamber with 1 to 3 meters diameter and 2.5 to 4.5 meter height. In case of vertical tube evaporators the tubes are arranged vertically in calendria, Fig. 5.2 (b). A calendria is a heating part in evaporator consisting of large number of smaller diameter tubes wherein liquid is concentrated while rising or falling.

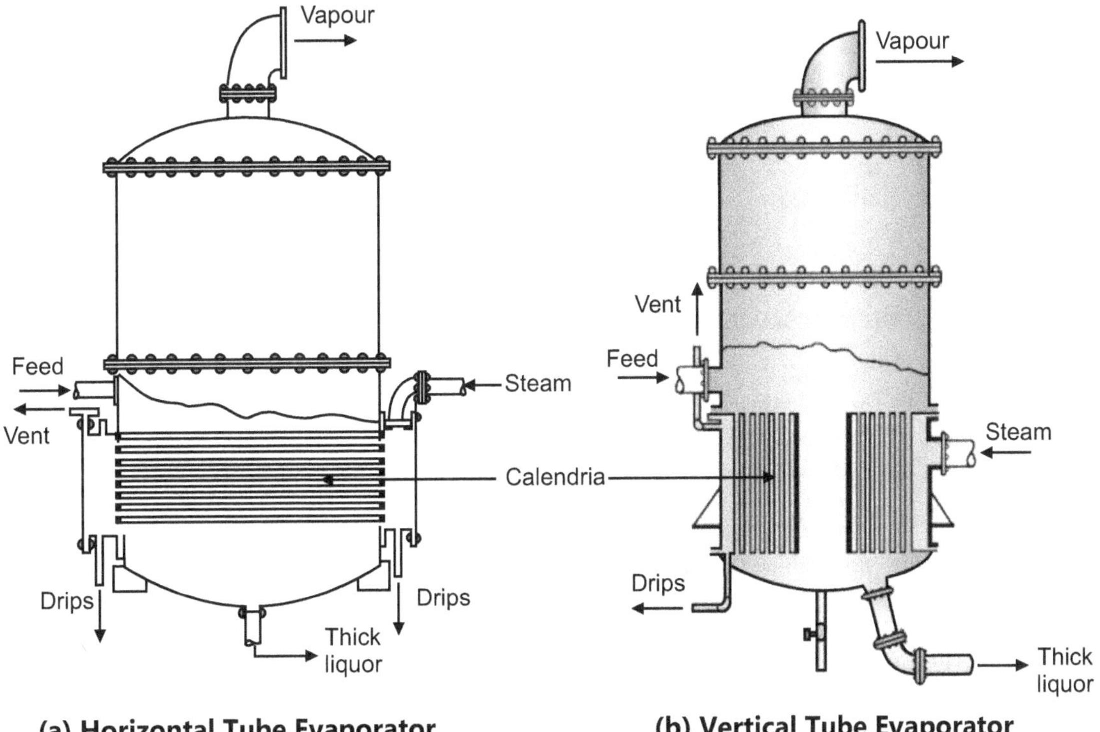

(a) Horizontal Tube Evaporator   **(b) Vertical Tube Evaporator**

Fig. 5.2: Short Tube Evaporators

Working:

In the horizontal-tube evaporator, steam is fed into steam chest and is directed through the horizontal tubes to heat the liquid surrounding the tube in the bottom of the evaporator body. The definite path followed by the steam assures that all non-condensed gases and condensate are swept to the opposite steam chest, where they are withdrawn. The velocity and paths of circulation of the liquid depend upon the distribution, size, anti shape of the heating surface in the liquid compartment.

Applications:

   (i)   It is used in the manufacture of the cascara extract.

  (ii)   It is used in the manufacture of caustic soda.

 (iii)   It is used in the manufacture of salts.

Advantages:

   (i)   A number of units can be joined to obtain more efficient effect.

  (ii)   It has low cost per unit of heating surfaces.

 (iii)   It has extreme simplicity.

 (iv)   Easy renewal of heating surfaces.

  (v)   Sectional construction with low maintenance cost.

 (vi)   Ease of operation.

 (vii)   Ability to carry large volume of liquor in the body.

(viii)   It requires low headspace.

 (ix)   Small cargo space required for shipment.

Disadvantages:

   (i)   Cleaning and maintenance is difficult when compared with steam jacketed kettle.

  (ii)   During operation the pressure inside the evaporator increases that reduces the effective temperature gradients and may affects heat sensitive materials.

 (iii)   It may be used only when rigorous boiling can be obtained with natural circulation.

 (iv)   It is not suitable for viscous liquids.

  (v)   Since the boiling liquid is outside of the tubular heating surface, it is not easily cleaned by mechanical means.

 (vi)   It is not suitable when scaling or salting liquids are involved.

5.5.3 Climbing Film Evaporator

A climbing film vertical long tube evaporator is a type of evaporator that is an essentially shell and tube heat exchanger. Thus, it is also known as rising film evaporator. This evaporator is superior to falling film evaporator as the upstream film movement causes some particles to remain in the feed stream. The absence of any kind of distributor makes it suitable for such variety of applications.

Applications:

   (i)   A climbing film is used for effluent treatment.

  (ii)   It can be used in production of polymers and for juice concentration and food processing.

 (iii)   It is used in thermal desalination of sea water.

 (iv)   It has many applications in pharmaceuticals especially for solvent recovery.

  (v)   It is used as reboilers for distillation columns.

 (vi)   It is used as pre-concentrators or flash evaporators or pre-heaters to remove volatile components prior to stripping.

Principle:

The theory of climbing film evaporator is that the ascending force of the steam produced during the boiling causes liquid and vapours to flow upwards in parallel flow. At the same time the production of vapour increases and the product is pressed as a thin film on the walls of the tubes, and the liquid rises upwards. This co-current upward movement against gravity has the beneficial effect of creating a high degree of turbulence in the liquid.

Construction:

A Rising Film Evaporator (RFE) is a vertical shell and tube heat exchanger with a vapour-liquid separator mounted at the top, Fig. 5.3. Tubes carrying the steam internally are placed vertically in the bottom of the cylindrical evaporator chamber. The length of the boiling tubes is typically not more than 23 ft (7m). This type of unit is known as the Roberts evaporator in Europe and is the calandria evaporator in the United States.

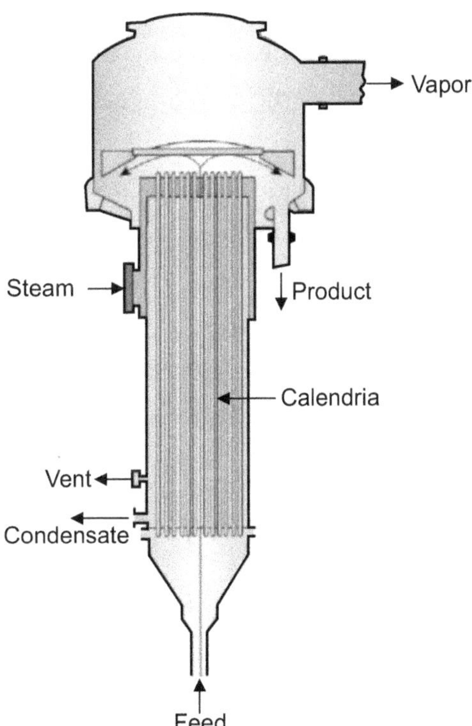

Fig. 5.3: Climbing Film Evaporator

Working:

The liquid to be concentrated is fed at the bottom of the heated tube bundle. The feed is heated with steam condensing on the outside of the tube from the shell side. This produces steam and vapour within the tube bringing the liquid inside to boil. The product circulation is by natural convection. The vapour so produced pushes the liquid against the walls of the tubes and causes the upward force that feed moves up. As more vapours are formed, the centre of the tube will have a higher velocity which forces the remaining liquid against the tube wall forming a thin film which moves to the top above the calandria. The velocities generated by the vapour lift are quite high, giving good thermal performance. This is useful while evaporating highly viscous products and products that have a tendency to foul the heating surface. Usually there must be a high temperature difference between the heating and boiling sides of evaporator and is required to convey the liquid and to produce the rising film. The vapour and balance liquid are separated in the vapour-liquid separator.

Advantages:

(i) The main advantage of the rising film evaporator is the low residence time of the liquid feed in the evaporator compared to other evaporators.

(ii) It has relatively high heat transfer coefficient that reduces the overall heat transfer area requirement which in turn will lower the initial capital cost of the evaporator.

(iii) It is easier to clean the tubes.

(iv) Thermosiphon action eliminates the need for circulation pump.

(v) Trace quantities of suspended particles in the feed are tolerated.

(vi) Can operate under reasonable vacuum.

(vii) Multiple effect arrangement provides steam economy.

(viii) It is relatively inexpensive evaporator.

Disadvantages:

(i) It requires large floor space and is heavy.

(ii) It has poor heat transfer at low temperature differences.

(iii) Not suitable for thermolabile materials.

(iv) It evaporates products of low viscosity and have minimal fouling tendencies.

Applications:

(i) The thermal desalination of sea water.

(ii) Concentration of dilute solutions such as plant extracts.

(iii) It is used as a reboiler to distillation column.

(iv) It is an economical alternative to falling film evaporator for moderate vacuum.

5.5.4 Forced Circulation Evaporator

Forced circulation evaporator uses force to drive the liquid through the evaporator tubes thus produces high tube velocities. A high efficiency circulating pump, designed for large volume and sufficient head, is used to supply the force. Proper design results in controlled temperature rise, controlled temperature difference and tube velocities that give optimum heat transfer. Forced circulation evaporator conducts evaporation under reduced pressure which is used to evaporate thermolabile substances.

Principle:

In forced circulation evaporator liquid is circulated through the tubes at high pressure by means of a pump. Hence boiling does not take places because boiling point is elevated. Forced circulation of the liquids also creates some form of agitation. When the liquid leaves the tubes and enters the vapor head, pressure falls suddenly. This leads to the flashing of super heated liquor leading to evaporation of feed.

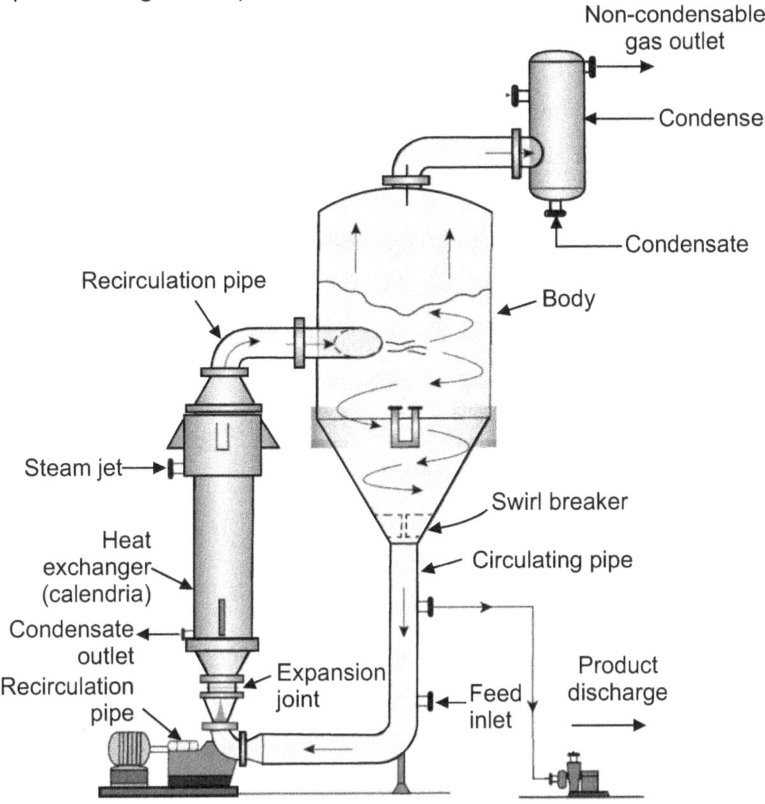

Fig. 5.4: Vertical Forced Circulation Evaporator

Construction:

In these types of evaporators pumps are fitted to circulate the contents heating in it. The forced circulation evaporator consists of steam jacketed tubes held between two tube sheets, Fig. 5.4. The tube measures 0.1 m inside diameter and 2.5 m long. The parts of the tubes projects in to the vapor head which consists of a deflector. The vapour head is connected to a return pipe which runs downwards and enters in to the inlet of a pump. The liquid is circulated by means of a pump. As it is under pressure in the tubes the boiling point is raised (but no boling take places) and it enters into the body of the evaporator.

Working:

Steam is introduced in to the calendria. Pump sends the liquid to the tube with a positive velocity. As the liquid move up through the tube it gets heated and begins to boil. As result the vapour and liquid mixture rushes out of the tubes at a high velocity. This mixture strikes the deflector in a manner that effective separation of liquid and vapour takes place. The vapour enters the cyclone separator and leaves the equipment. The concentrated liquid is circulated through the pump for further evaporation. Finally the concentrated product is collected at the bottom from discharge outlet.

Advantages:

(i)   There is a rapid movement of liquid due to high heat transfer coefficient.

(ii)   The liquid entering the circulation evaporator boils in the separator and not on a heating surface hence minimizes fouling.

(iii) Salting, scaling and fouling are not possible due to forced circulation.

(iv)   These evaporators are suitable for thermolabile substances because of rapid evaporation.

(v)   It is suitable for the viscous preparation because pumping mechanism is used.

(vi)   These evaporators are also used for liquids with high solids content.

(vii) Circulation evaporators are fairly compact and are easy to clean and operate.

Disadvantages

(i)   The hold up time of liquids is high.

(ii)   The equipments is expensive as well as power requirement is high.

(iii) It has high maintenance costs.

(iv)   The increased velocity can cause the equipment to corrode at a faster rate, which increases the overall maintenance cost.

Applications:

(i)   Forced circulation evaporator is used to concentrate thermolabile substance solutions.

(ii)   It is used for concentration of insulin and liver extracts.

(iii) It is well suited for crystallizing operation where crystals are to be suspended at all times.

(iv)   These evaporators are used in production of salt, corn steep water and calcium carbonate.

(v)   It is used for effluent treatment in pharmaceutical industries.

(vi)   Forced circulation chambers can be superimposed on each other to form a multi effect tower which can be utilized for increasing concentration of refined sugar and syrups.

5.5.5 Multiple Effect Evaporators

As we know, evaporator is a heat exchanger wherein liquid is boiled to produce vapour and simultaneously it generates a low pressure steam. This steam is further used as heating medium for another following evaporator. Thus the second evaporator is a low pressure boiler. Utilization of steam in first evaporator is called as first effect. The vapours generated in first evaporators are used for following second evaporator as heating source so it is called as second effect. All individual evaporators are single effect evaporators. To be used them as multiple they need to be connected within series.

For example, consider two evaporators are connected in such a way that vapors from first evaporator are supplied to the steam chest of the following evaporator as shown in Fig. 5.5, making-up a two effect evaporator.

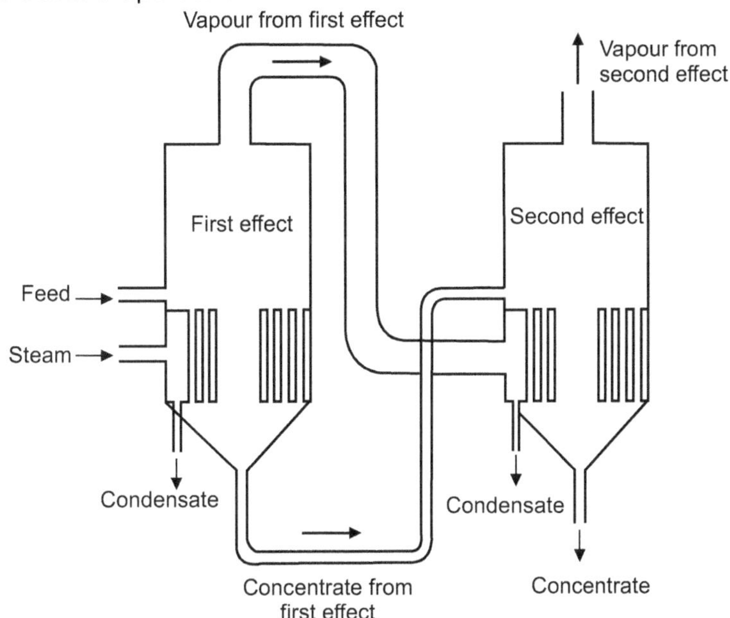

Fig. 5.5: Forward Feed Arrangement in Multi Effect Evaporator

If liquid is to be evaporated in each effect, and if the boiling point of this liquid is unaffected by the solute concentration, then a heat balance for the first evaporator is written as:

$$q_1 \;=\; U_1 A_1 (T_s - T_1) \qquad\qquad .... (5.1)$$

$$=\; U_1 A_1 \Delta T_1 \qquad\qquad .... (5.2)$$

Where,

q_1 = Rate of heat transfer

U_1 = Overall heat transfer coefficient in evaporator 1

A_1 = Heat-transfer area in evaporator 1

T_s = Temperature of condensing steam from the boiler

T_1 = The boiling temperature of the liquid in evaporator 1

ΔT_1 = $(T_s - T_1)$ = Temperature difference in evaporator 1.

Similarly, in the second evaporator the "steam" is a vapor from the first evaporator and this condensates at approximately the same temperature at which it boiled, since pressure changes are negligible. Thus, using subscript 2 for the conditions in the second evaporator the rate of heat transfer in second effect can be calculated using equation (5.4).

$$q_2 \;=\; U_2 A_2 (T_1 - T_2) \qquad\qquad .... (5.3)$$

$$=\; U_2 A_2 \Delta T \qquad\qquad .... (5.4)$$

If the evaporators are operating in balance that all of the vapors from the first effect are condensing and in their turn evaporates vapors in the second effect. In addition, if it is assumed that heat losses are least, no boiling-point elevation of concentrated solution and the feed input is at its boiling point, then at this condition the heat transfer relation can be expressed as:

$$q_1 = q_2 \qquad \qquad \text{... (5.5)}$$

If the evaporators are of same type and size (i.e. $A_1 = A_2$), above equations can be combined as:

$$\frac{U_2}{U_1} = \frac{T_1}{T_2} \qquad \qquad \text{... (5.6)}$$

Equation (5.6) states that the temperature differences are inversely proportional to the overall heat transfer coefficients in the two effects. This relation may be applicable to any number of effects operated in series, in the same way.

Steam feeding in multiple effect evaporators:

In case of two effect evaporators, the temperature in the steam chest of first evaporator is higher than in the second evaporator. The vapours generated in the first evaporator will the effect boiling of liquid in second evaporator; the boiling temperature in the second evaporator must be lower so that effect must be under lower pressure. The pressure in the second effect must be reduced below that in the first effect.

Forward feed multiple effect evaporators:

In some cases, the first effect may be at a pressure above atmospheric; or the first effect may be at atmospheric pressure and the second and subsequent effects have therefore to be under further lower pressures. Under lower pressures, the liquid feed progress is simplest if it passes from first effect to second effect, to third effect, and so on. In these situations the feed flows without pumping. This is called forward feed, Fig. 5.6. The most concentrated liquid products occur in the last effect of the process.

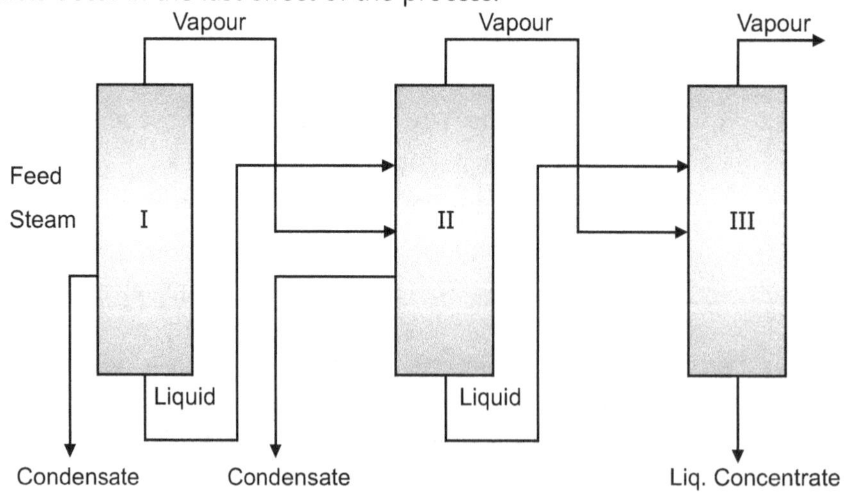

Fig. 5.6: Forward Feed Arrangement in Multi effect Evaporator

Backward feed multiple effect evaporators:

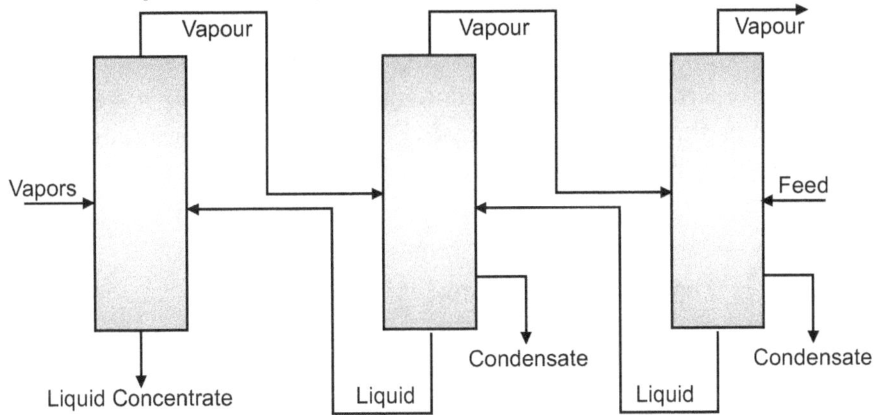

Fig. 5.7: Backward Feed Arrangement in Multi effect Evaporator

In backward feed evaporator the feed may pass the last effect and proceeds to the first. This is in reverse of forward feed multiple effect evaporators. In backward feed the liquid is pumped from one effect to the next against the pressure drops, Fig. 5.7. The concentrated viscous liquids are at the highest temperatures in the first effect and thus have larger evaporation capacity than forward feed systems.

Parallel feed:

In this method a hot saturated solution of the feed is directly fed to each of the three effects in parallel without transferring the materials from the one effect to the other. The parallel feed arrangement is commonly used in the concentration of the salts solution where the solute crystallizes on concentration without increasing the viscosity.

Construction:

A multiple effect evaporator system for concentrating a process liquid consists of more than one evaporator effects arranged in series, each effect includes a process liquid inlet and a process liquid outlet; a heating fluid inlet and heating fluid outlet and an evaporative condenser provided with liquid inlet. Two effect evaporators are connected together with the piping arrangement so that the vapors from the calandria of the first effect are used to heat the calandria of the second effect. The calandria of the second effect is used as a condenser for the first effect. The latent heat of vaporization is used to evaporate more quantity of the liquid. The vapour from the second effect then taken to a condenser and converted in to the liquids. In general not more than two or three effects are combined together to have economical and efficient evaporation of liquids. The construction of the multiple effect evaporators uses three evaporators so it is called as triple effect evaporators. The vapour from the first evaporator serves as heating medium for the second evaporator. Similarly, vapour from the second evaporator serves as a heating medium for the third evaporator. Last evaporator is connected to a vacuum pump.

Working:

Multiple effect evaporators (3 - stages) is a long tube forced circulation type evaporators where in the first effect high pressure steam is used to evaporate solvent from the feed. The evaporated solvent in the form of vapor is used for evaporating the feed in the second effect at atmospheric pressure. Evaporated solvent from the second stage is used for evaporating concentrating feed in the third effect under vacuum. Finally evaporated solvent from the third effect is condensed in the steam condenser using cooling water on other side. Condensate from all the three effects is collected in condensate receiving tanks, which is pure solvent and hence reused in the process.

Advantages:

(i)   It is suitable for large scale and continuous operation.

(ii)   It is highly economical when compared with single effect.

(iii) About five evaporators can be attached in series.

(iv)   Minimizes the energy input required to evaporate undesirable solvent.

Applications:

(i)   Used in the manufacture of the cascara extract.

(ii)   Used in the manufacture of salts and caustic soda.

(iii) Used in the manufacture of salts.

(iv)   Used in order to recover expensive solvents such as hexane which would otherwise be wasted.

(v)   Recovery of sodium hydroxide in Kraft pulping.

(vi)   Cutting down waste handling cost is another major application

(vii) To get a concentrated product and to improve the stability of the products.

(viii) Used in the concentration of the sodium salts that is obtained as a by-product from the production of p-cresol.

(ix)   In the food and drink industry, for example, coffee, need to go through an evaporation step during processing.

5.6 ECONOMY OF MULTIPLE EFFECT EVAPORATORS

The performance of a multiple effect evaporators is measured in terms of its capacity and economy. Capacity of evaporator is defined as the number of kilogram of water vaporized per hour. Its economy is the number of kilograms of water vaporized from all the effects per kilogram of steam used. For single effect evaporator, the steam economy is approximately about 0.8 (<1). The capacity is about n-times that of a single effect evaporator and the economy is about 0.8 n for an n-effect evaporators. However, pumps, interconnecting pipes and valves required for transfer of liquid from one effect to another effect increases both the equipment and the operating costs.

The economy of multiple effect evaporators is greater than single effect because vapors generated in first effect are used as a heating medium for second effect and so on. Thus, efficiency increases as steam consumption decreases and evaporative capacity increases.

At first sight, it may seem that the multiple effect evaporator has all the advantages, the heat is used over and over again and it appears to be getting the evaporation in the second and subsequent effects for nothing in terms of energy costs. However, fact is that there is a price to be paid for the heat economy. For example;

In the first effect, $q_1 = U_1 A_1 \Delta T_1$ .... (5.7)

In the second effect, $q_2 = U_2 A_2 \Delta T_2$ .... (5.8)

We shall now consider a single-effect evaporator, working under the same pressure as the first effect

$$q_s = U_s A_s \Delta T_s$$ .... (5.9)

Where, subscript 's' indicates the single-effect evaporator.

Since the overall conditions are the same,

$$\Delta T_s = \Delta T_1 + \Delta T_2$$ .... (5.10)

As the overall temperature drop is between the steam-condensing temperature in the first effect and the evaporating temperature in the second effect. Each successive steam chest in the multiple-effect evaporator condenses at the same temperature at which the previous effect is evaporating. Now, consider the case in which $U_1 = U_2 = U_s$, and $A_1 = A_2$. The A_s for the single-effect evaporator that will evaporate the same quantity as in the two effects is obtained as follows. From the given conditions and from equation (5.6),

$$\Delta T_1 = \Delta T_2$$ .... (5.11)

and $$\Delta T_s = \Delta T_1 + \Delta T_2$$ .... (5.12)

$$= 2\Delta T_1$$

$$\Delta T_1 = 0.5\Delta T_s$$ .... (5.13)

Now, $$q_1 + q_2 = U_1 A_1 \Delta T_1 + U_2 A_2 \Delta T_2$$

$$= U_1 (A_1 + A_2) \frac{\Delta T_s}{2}$$ .... (5.14)

But, $q_1 + q_2 = q_s$ and $q_s = U A_s \Delta T_s$

So that, $$\frac{A_1 + A_2}{2} = \frac{2A_1}{2} = A_s$$ .... (5.15)

That is $A_1 = A_2 = A_s$

The analysis shows that if the same total quantity is to be evaporated, then the heat transfer surface of each of the two effects must be the same as that for a single effect evaporator. In multiple effect evaporators, steam economy has to be paid for by increased capital costs of the evaporators. Since the heat transfer areas are generally equal in the various effects and since in a sense what you are buying in an evaporator is suitable heat transfer surface, the n effects will cost approximately n times as much as a single effect.

Table 5.5: Steam Consumption and Running Costs of Evaporators

Number of effects	Steam consumption (kg steam/kg water evaporated)	Total running cost (relative to a single-effect evaporator)
One	1.1	1
Two	0.57	0.52
Three	0.40	0.37

Comparative costs of the auxiliary equipment do not altogether follow the same pattern. Condenser requirements are less for multiple effect evaporators. The condensation duty is distributed between the steam chests of the effects, except for the first one, and so condenser and cooling water requirements will be less. The optimum design of evaporation plant is based on a balance between operating costs which are lower for multiple effects because of their reduced steam consumption, and capital charges which will be lower for fewer evaporators. The comparative operating costs are illustrated by the figures in Table 5.5. If the capital costs are known they would reduce the advantages of the multiple effects, but certainly not remove them.

REVIEW QUESTIONS

1. What is evaporation? Explain its mechanism.
2. Discuss properties of the solution that must be considered in selection of proper evaporator.
3. What are objectives of evaporation?
4. What are advantages of evaporation?
5. What are limitations of evaporation?
6. What are applications of evaporation?
7. What is rate of evaporation? Discuss factors affecting evaporation.
8. Differentiate between evaporation and drying.
9. Differentiate between evaporation and distillation.
10. Differentiate between evaporation and vaporization.
11. Differentiate between evaporation and sublimation.
12. Classify evaporators based on heating medium movement.
13. Classification evaporators based on type of heating surfaces.
14. Discuss principle, construction working, uses, advantages and disadvantages of
    (a) Evaporating pan   (b) Horizontal tube evaporator
    (c) Climbing film evaporator   (d) Forced circulation evaporator
15. Explain construction, working and advantages and applications of multiple effect evaporators.
16. What is multiple effect evaporator? What is its significance?
17. Comment on economy of multiple effect evaporators
18. What are forward feed and backward feed multiple effect evaporators? Explain wit diagrams.
19. How economy of multiple effect evaporator is determined?
20. Compare horizontal and vertical tube evaporators.
21. Compare falling film and rising (climbing) film evaporators.
22. What is mechanism and significance of forced circulation evaporator?
23. Discuss role of vacuum pump in evaporators.

☙ ☙ ☙

Chapter ...6

DISTILLATION

6.1 INTRODUCTION

Historically distillation was used since 1200 BC in perfumery operations. Early forms of distillation were batch processes using one vaporization and one condensation. Purity was improved by further distillation of the condensate. Greater volumes were processed by simply repeating the distillation. Chemists were reported to carry out as many as 500 to 600 distillations in order to obtain a pure compound. In the early 19th century the basics of modern techniques including pre-heating and reflux were developed. In 1877 U.S. Patent was granted for a tray column for distillation of ammonia and in the subsequent years for oil and spirits. With the emergence of chemical engineering as a discipline at the end of the 19th century, scientific rather than empirical methods were applied. More accurate designs were used during developments in petroleum industries. Today availability of powerful computers has allowed direct computer simulation of distillation columns.

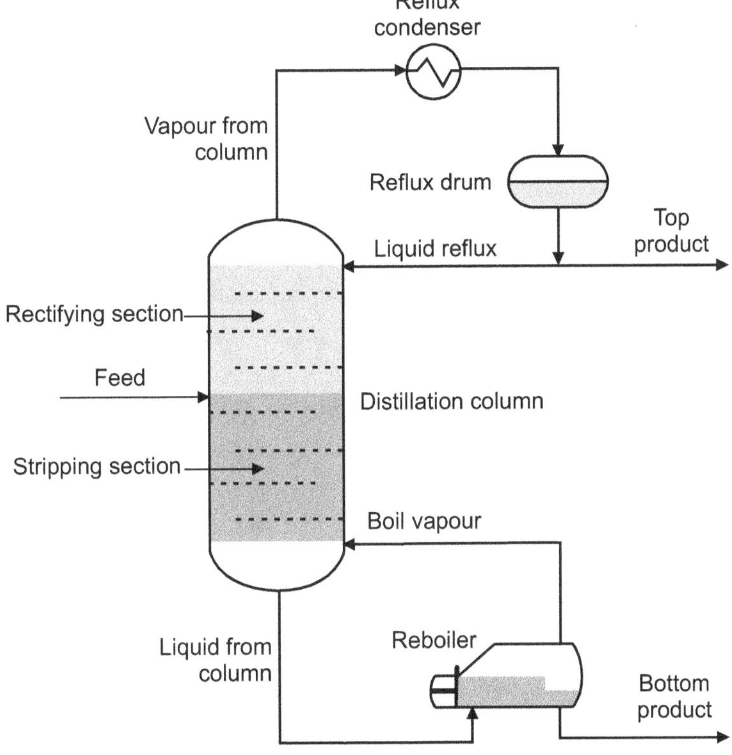

Fig. 6.1: Basic Distillation Unit Set-Up

Distillation is one of the most important processes for separating the components of a solution. The solution is heated to form a vapour of the more volatile components in the system, and the vapour is then cooled, condensed, and collected as drops of liquid, Fig. 6.1. By repeating vaporization and condensation, individual components in the solution can be recovered in a pure state. Essences and many pure products from the oil refinery industry are processed via distillation.

Objective of Distillation:

The basic objective of distillation is to separate liquid mixture into two or more components. In a basic distillation column a feed stream enters in the middle of the column and two streams leave, one at the top and one at the bottom. Components with lower boiling points are concentrated in the stream leaving the top while components with higher boiling points are concentrated in the stream leaving the bottom. Separation is achieved by controlling the column temperature and pressure to take advantage of differences in the relative volatility of the mixture components and therefore tendency to change phase. The lighter, lower boiling point components evaporate and travel up the column to form the top product and the heavier, higher boiling point components condense and travelling down the column to form the bottom product.

6.2 BASIC PRINCIPLES

Distillation is a process by which a liquid mixture is separated into fractions with higher concentrations of certain components by exploiting differences in relative volatility. Distillation has been used widely to separate volatile components from non-volatile compounds. In industrial settings such as oil refineries and natural gas processing plants this separation process is undertaken using a distillation column.

The mechanism involved in distillation is the differences in volatility between individual components. With sufficient heat applied, vapours are formed from the liquid solution. The liquid product is subsequently condensed from the vapour phase by removal of the heat. Therefore, heat is used as the separating agent during distillation. In general, distillation can be carried out either with or without reflux involved. For the case of single-stage differential distillation, the liquid mixture is heated to form a vapour that is in equilibrium with the residual liquid. The vapour is then condensed and removed from the system without any liquid allowed to return to the still pot. This vapor is richer in the more volatile component than the liquid removed as the bottom product at the end of the process. However, when products of much higher purity are desired, part of the condensate has to be brought into contact with the vapour on its way to the condenser and recycled to the still pot. This procedure can be repeated for many times to increase the degree of separation in the original mixture. Such a process is normally called "rectification."

Fractionation: It is another term for distillation also called fractional distillation.

Feed: The liquid and/or gas feed into the distillation column.

Feed tray: The tray below the inlet nozzle is called the feed tray.

Heavy Component: The component with the lower relative volatility, for example, simple hydrocarbon, this is a component with the higher molecular weight. It is found in higher concentration in the bottom product of the column.

Light Component: The component with the higher relative volatility, for example, simple hydrocarbon, this is a component with the lower molecular weight. It is found in higher concentration at the top of the column.

Stripping section: It is a section that consists of trays between the bottom of the column and the feed tray. In the stripping section the aim is to concentrate the heavier component in the liquid phase.

Rectifying section: It is a section that consists of trays between the feed tray and the top of the column. In the rectifying section the aim is to concentrate the lighter component in the vapour phase.

Top Product: It is a product which leaves from the top of the column, also called distillate. This product is usually passed through a heat exchanger and liquefied.

Bottom Product: It is the product which leaves through the bottom of the distillation column.

Reflux: A portion of vapour from the top of the column which has been condensed to a liquid and returned to the column as a liquid above the top tray.

Reboiler: A heat exchanger at the bottom of the column which boils some of the liquid leaving the column. The vapor generated returns to the column at the bottom of the stripping section.

Vapour-Liquid Equilibrium (VLE) Curve: A plot of the actual composition of the lighter component in the vapour phase for a given composition in the liquid phase. Usually it is derived from thermodynamic data.

Zeotropic mixture : It is a mixture of liquids with different boiling points. For example, nitrogen, methane, ethane, propane etc.

Azeotropic mixture : It is a mixture of two or more liquids that has a constant boiling point because vapour has same composition as liquid mixture.

Principle of Separation:

Distillation takes advantage of the difference in relative volatility of the feed mixture components. Generally for two or more compounds at a given pressure and temperature there will be a difference in the vapour and liquid compositions at equilibrium due to component partial pressure. Distillation exploits this by bringing liquid and gas phases into contact at temperatures and pressures that promote the desired separation. During this contact the components with the lower volatility (typically lower boiling point) preferentially moves into the liquid phase while more volatile components move into the vapour phase.

A distillation column may use either trays or a packed bed to bring the gas and liquid into contact. For a column using trays we can consider the changes to gas and liquid phase compositions as they both enter and exit a single tray. The liquid entering the tray will contact the gas exiting the tray, Fig. 6.2. The hotter vapour phase heats the incoming liquid phase as it bubbles through the tray, evaporating the light components which then leaves the tray with the vapour phase. Conversely the cooling of the vapor phase by the liquid phase will causes the heavier components of the vapour phase to condense and exit the tray with the liquid phase.

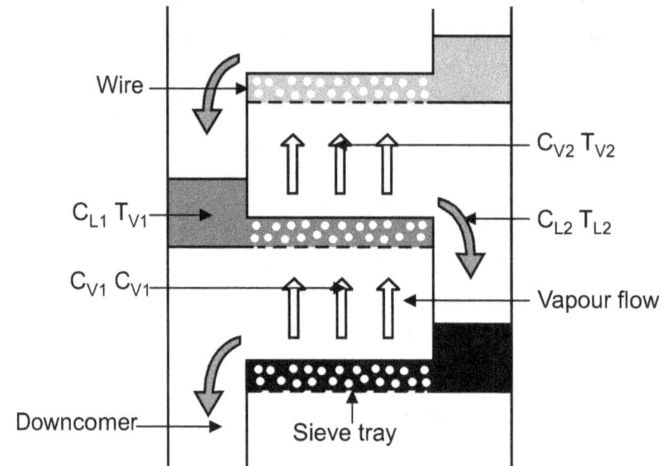

Fig. 6.2: Principle of Separation

For the liquid across the tray:

$$C_{L1,\ heavy} < C_{L2,\ heavy}$$
$$C_{L1,\ light} > C_{L2,\ light}$$
$$T_{L1} > T_{L2}$$

For the vapour through the tray:

$$C_{V1,\ heavy} > C_{V2,\ heavy}$$
$$C_{V1,\ light} < C_{V2,\ light}$$
$$T_{V1} > T_{V2}$$

Where, C is concentration and T is temperature.

When a packing is used rather than trays the principle remains the same, in fact packing is often referenced in terms of height equivalent to a theoretical plate (HETP) i.e. what height of packing is equivalent to one theoretical plate. The packing is just an alternative method to bring the liquid and vapour phases into contact with the liquid generally flowing over the surfaces of the packing material, while the vapour passes up through the space between packing elements.

Typical Operating Parameters:

The distillation process can be improved by understanding the following operating parameters.

(i) Temperature: The basic temperature profile of a distillation column is hotter at the bottom and cooler at the top. For a simple two component distillation the temperature at the bottom is just lower than the boiling point of the heavier component. The temperature at the top of the column is just above the boiling point of the lighter component. In order to have heavy component to remain as a liquid at the bottom of the column and the lighter component to stay as a gas we set the temperature at the bottom to match this requirement. This temperature is set by adding heat via a heat exchanger. Typically the heat added to the bottom of the column is easy to control, via steam or hot oil flow rates.

At the top of the column the situation is reverse. The light component remains as gas while the heavier component is condensed to a liquid and falls back down the column. The top temperature is set just above the boiling point of the lighter component. The temperature control situation is different at the bottom of the column, because the top product to be a liquid when we send it for storage. All of the gas coming out of the top of the column is condensed to liquid. This liquid stream is split with some returning to the column and some going to storage. The top temperature is often controlled by changing the reflux rate, i.e. the flow rate of liquid sent back to the top of the column. A higher reflux rate means cooler liquid falling down the column against the rising warmer gas, and the top temperature is lower. Overall heat is added at the bottom of the column and heat is extracted at the top of the column. Inside the column the temperature balance is created between the hot gas rising up the column and the cooler liquid falling down the column.

(ii) Pressure: There is typically a pressure gradient across the column with the pressure being higher at the bottom of the column than the top. This pressure gradient occurs as the liquid coming down the column hampers the flow of vapour up the column and imposes a pressure loss on the flow. In steady state distillations the pressure in the column is held constant, and the temperature is varied to control the composition of the product streams.

Applications:

   (i)   Distillation is used for many commercial processes, such as production of gasoline, distilled water, xylene, alcohol, paraffin, kerosene, and many other liquids.

   (ii)   Distillation is used for purifying solvents and liquid reaction products.

   (iii)   It is used in the manufacturing of distilled water, double distilled water used in Water for Injection and other pharmaceutical preparations.

   (iv)   Toxic and costly organic solvents are used in extraction, synthesis and analysis of drugs. These solvent can be recovered by distillation for economic as well as the environmental protection benefits.

   (v)   Distillation is used in the separation of volatile oils such as clove oil, anise oil, cardamom oil, eucalyptus oil etc. from the plant extracts.

   (vi)   It can be used in the separation of volatile components from a mixture of two or more volatile liquids.

   (vii)   It can be used as a quality control method for alcohol content in liquid formulations. The alcohol is separated from formulations by distillation and alcohol content is determined.

   (viii) It can be used to liquefy and separate gases from air. For example: nitrogen, oxygen, and argon are distilled from air.

   (ix)   Distillation is used in crude fermentation broths to separate alcoholic spirits.

   (x)   It can also be used in the fractionation of crude oil into gasoline and heating oil.

6.3 METHODOLOGY OF SIMPLE DISTILLATION

Simple distillation is a unit operation in which two liquids with different boiling points are separated.

Principle:

Simple distillation is a process of heating and cooling liquids in order to separate and purify them. As the liquid being distilled is heated, the vapours that form are richest in the component of the mixture that boils at the lowest temperature. Purified component boils, and thus turns into vapours, over a relatively small temperature range (2 or 3 °C). A careful observation of the temperature in the distillation flask helps to carry out a good separation. As distillation progresses, the concentration of the lowest boiling component steadily decreases. Eventually, the temperatures within the apparatus begin to change and a pure compound is no longer being distilled. As the temperature continues to increase the boiling point of the next-lowest-boiling compound is approached. When the temperature again stabilizes, another pure fraction of the distillate can be collected. This fraction of distillate is primarily the compound that boils at the second lowest temperature. This process can be repeated until all the fractions of the original mixture are separated. In order for simple distillation to perform, the two liquids' boiling points must have a difference of at least 25 °C (or about 77 °F).

Construction:

The set of simple distillation consists of distillation flask with side arm sloping downwards, Fig. 6.3. The mouth of the flask is fitted with cork closure with inserted thermometer. The condenser is attached to sloping arm for cold water circulation with inlet at lower side and outlet at upper side. The cold water pipe is attached to inlet while outlet discharges water to waste. The condenser outlet delivers liquid product that is collected in a collector or receiver.

Working:

1.   Calibration of thermometer: Calibration can be done by placing the thermometer in an ice bath of distilled water. Allow thermometer to reach thermal equilibrium. Now remove from ice water and place it in a beaker of boiling distilled water and again allow it to reach thermal equilibrium. If the temperatures measured does deviate from the expected values by more than two degrees then use it for recording temperature in distillation process.

2.   Filling the distillation flask: The flask is filled with not more than two third of its volumes to have sufficient space above the liquid surface so that when boiling begins the liquid will not be propelled into the condenser. This is important in view point of purity of the distillate. Porcelain chips should be placed in the distillation flask to prevent superheating of the liquid and to cause a more controlled boiling, eliminating the possibility of liquid to bump into the condenser.

3.   Heating the distillation flask: The distillation flask is heated slowly until the liquid begins to boil. The vapours rise up through the neck of the distillation flask and pass through the condenser and condense and drip into the collection receiver, Fig. 6.3. Generally rate of distillation is approximately 20 drops per minute. Distillation must occur slowly enough that all the vapours condense to liquid in the condenser. Many organic compounds are flammable and if vapours pass through the condenser without condensing, they may ignite as they come in contact with the heat source.

4.   Condensation of vapours: As the distillate begins to drop from the condenser, the temperature changes steadily. When it is stable, new receiver is used to collect all the drops that form over a two to three degree range of temperature. As the temperature begins to rise further, a third receiver is used to collect the distillate. This process is repeated; using a new receiver every time the temperature stabilizes or begins changing, until all of the distillate has been collected in discrete fractions. All fractions of the distillate should be saved until it is shown that the desired compound has been effectively separated by distillation.

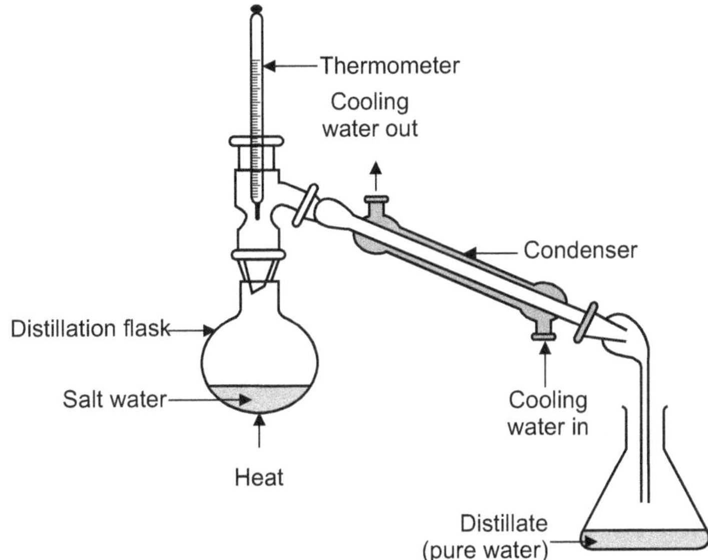

Fig. 6.3: Simple Distillation

Handling Precautions:

(i)   If direct heating is used stop the heat source from the distillation flask before all of the liquid is vaporized.

(ii)   When all of the liquid is evaporated, the temperature of the glass of the distillation flask rises very rapidly, possibly ignites whatever vapours still is present in the distillation flask.

(iii) Never distill to dryness. The residue left in the distillation flask may contain peroxides, which could ignite or explode after all the liquid has distilled away.

(iv)   Make sure that all joints are secured very tightly. If any vapour escapes at the connection points, it may come into direct contact with the heat source and ignite.

(v)   Never heat a closed system, the increasing pressure will cause the glass to explode.

(vi) If the distillation flask has a tapered neck, the thermometer may be placed in such a way as to block the flow of vapours up the neck of the flask; in effect creating a closed system; make sure that if using a tapered neck flask, the thermometer is not resting in the lowest portion of the neck.

(vii) If the liquids comprising the mixture that is being distilled have boiling points closer than 25 °C to one another, the distillate collected will be richer in the more volatile compound but not to the degree necessary for complete separation of the individual compounds.

Advantages:

(i)   It is simple, cheap, easy and economic method.

(ii)   It requires less energy.

(iii) This process requires single run and thus is comparatively faster.

Disadvantages:

(i)   The final product may contain impurities.

(ii)   Azeotropic mixtures cannot be separated by simple distillation.

(iii) Not suitable for mixtures containing thermolabile components.

(iv)   The volume of mixture should be not more than $2/3^{rd}$ of the container.

Applications:

(i)   Simple distillation is primarily used for production of distilled water.

(ii)   Many volatile oils are separated by simple distillation.

(iii) It is also used in the separation of organic solvents from mixtures.

(iv)   It is used to separate non-volatile components from volatile ones.

(v)   It is used in preparing pharmaceutical spirits.

6.4 FLASH DISTILLATION

Flash distillation, also called "equilibrium distillation", is a single stage separation technique. Simple flash separations are very common in industry, particularly petroleum refining. Even when some other method of separation is to be used, it is not uncommon to use a "pre-flash" to reduce the load on the separation itself.

Principle:

The separation using flash distillation is based upon the flash vaporization. In flash vaporization hot liquid mixture when passes from high pressure zone to low pressure zone suddenly get vaporized. Reduced pressure reduces the boiling point which leads to the vaporization of the liquid. The energy for vaporization is taken-up from the liquid itself, which causes decrease in temperature. The molecules in vapour phase with low boiling point get condensed while high boiling point molecules remain as vapour. The vapour and condensed liquid fraction remain in contact till saturation. The liquid falls at the bottom and is collected where as vapours are further allowed to condense.

Construction:

Flash distillation unit consists of pump attached to feed tank from where it pumps feed at high pressure, Fig. 6.4. This unit has a heating chamber through which the liquid mixture carrying pipe passes. The chamber is insulated to avoid heat loss during operation and maintain desired temperature. There is a pressure control valve fitted between heating chamber and the flash drum. The other end of the pipe directly opens into the flash drum. In single stage flash distillation unit liquid outlet is provided at the bottom. In case of multi-stage distillation the liquid and vapours are taken to next unit for further distillation. When designing a flash system it is important to provide enough disengaging space in the flash drum. Flash drum can also be designed as cyclone separators.

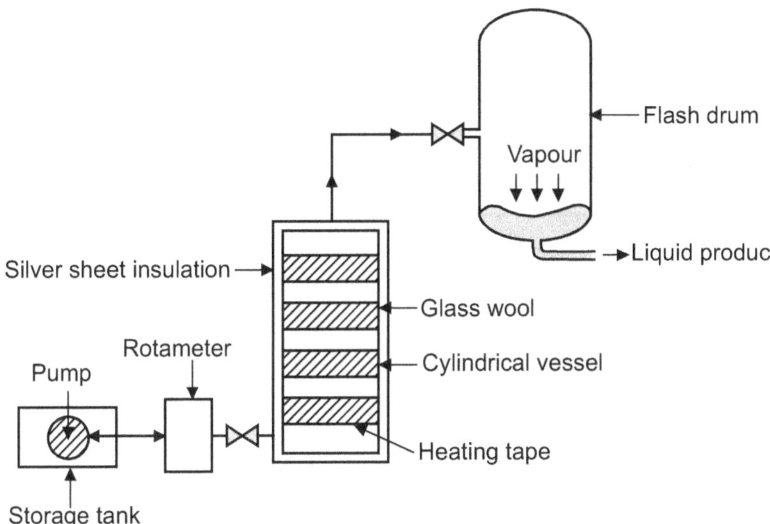

Fig. 6.4: Flash Distillation

Working:

A liquid mixture feed is pumped through a heater to raise the temperature and enthalpy of the mixture. It then flows through a valve and the pressure is reduced, causing the liquid to partially vaporize. Once the mixture enters in a big enough volume, the "flash drum", liquid and vapoors get separated. Because the vapoor and liquid are in such a close contact the "flash" occurs and the product liquid and vapoor phases approach equilibrium. Flash distillation can be operated in continuous mode as well as at multi-level. The operational setting are synchronized in such a way that input equals the output of the process and thus the vapour and liquid proportions at any instance remain constant in the flash drum.

Application:

(i)   Flash distillation is used in petroleum industry for refining crude oil.

(ii)   It is used in the desalination of ocean water by multi-stage flash distillation.

(iii)   It can also be used for separation of heptane from octane.

Advantages:

    (i)   Flash distillation is a continuous process.

    (ii)   The equipment is smaller than the multi-stage flash distillation.

    (iii) The operating costs are low compared to multi-stage flash distillation.

Disadvantages:

    (i)   Flash distillation is not effective in separating components of comparable volatility.

    (ii)   It is not suitable for two component systems.

    (iii) It is not an efficient distillation when nearly pure components are required, because the condensed vapour and residual liquid contain both components to some extent.

6.5 FRACTIONAL DISTILLATION

The basic idea behind fractional distillation is the same as simple distillation. The difference between simple and fractional distillation is the number of times that the liquid is vaporized and condensed. Simple distillation condenses the liquid once, so the boiling points of the two liquids must be far apart to make it efficient. Simple distillation is performed on a mixture of liquids with similar volatilities and the resulting distillate is in more concentrated form in the more volatile compound than the original mixture and it may contain a significant amount of the higher boiling compound. If the distillate of simple distillation is distilled again, the resulting distillate is again of further more concentrated form of the lower boiling compound, but still a portion of the distillate contain the higher boiling compound. The number of simple distillations in a fractional distillation depends on the length and efficiency of the fractionating column.

Fractional distillation is a process in which vaporization of liquid mixture gives rise to a mixture of constituents from which the desired one is separated in pure form. This method is also known as rectification, because a part of the vapour is condensed and returned as a liquid. This method is used to separate miscible volatile liquids, whose boiling points are close, by means of a fractionating column. Fractional distillation is different from simple distillation. In simple distillation, vapour is directly passed through the condenser. In fractional distillation the vapour must pass through a fractionating column in which partial condensation of vapour is allowed to occur. In simple distillation, condensate is collected directly into the receiver, while in fractional distillation condensation takes place in the fractionating column, so that a part of the condensing vapour returns to the still.

Principle:

When a liquid mixture is distilled, the partial condensation of the vapour is allowed to occur in a fractionating column. In the column, ascending vapours from the still are allowed to come in contact with the condensing vapour returning to the still. This result is enrichment of the vapours with the more volatile component. By condensing the vapour and reheating the liquid repeatedly, equilibrium between liquid and vapour is set-up at each stage, which ultimately results in the separation of a more volatile component.

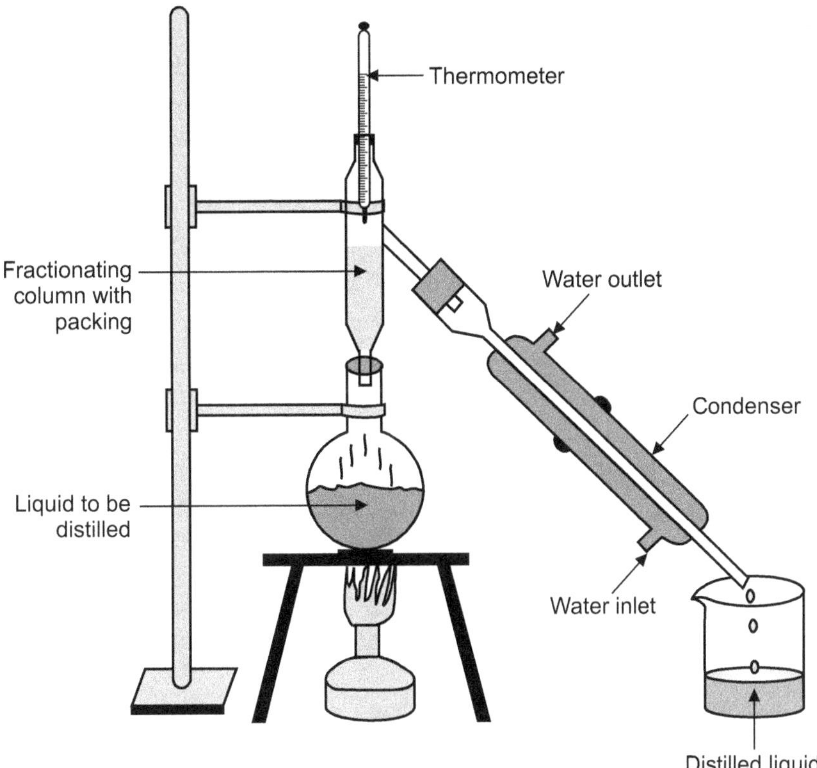

Fig. 6.5: Laboratory Set of Fractional Distillation

Construction:

The equipment used for fractional distillation consists of special type of still-heads known as fractionating columns. In still-heads condensation and revaporisation are affected continuously. Fractionating column is an essentially a long vertical tube in which the vapour moves upward and partially gets condensed. The condensate flows down the column and is returned to the flask. The columns are constructed to provide a large cooling surface for the vapour to condense and obstruct the ascending vapour to allow easy condensation. The obstruction also retards the downward flow of liquid, which is a high boiling component. Fractionating columns used are packed columns and plate columns.

Packed columns: In this column some form of packing is used to affect the necessary liquid/vapour contact. The packing consist of single turn helices (spirals) of wire or glass, glass rings, cylindrical glass beads, stainless steel rings etc. The column consists of a tower containing a packing that becomes wetted with a film of liquid, which is brought into contact with the vapour in the intervening spaces. The same type of fractionating columns can be obtained in various lengths. A long fractionating column is necessary when the boiling points of the constituents are lying fairly close together. A short fractionating column is necessary when the boiling point of the constituents differ considerably. Packing must be uniform so as to obtain proper channels. If packing is irregular, mass transfer becomes less effective. Example is Widmer column.

Plate columns: Many forms of plates are used in the distillation columns. These can be divided into Bubble cap plates and Turbo grid plates. The bubble cap column is used in large distillation plants. The column consists of a number of plates mounted one above the other. Caps are present on each plate, which allow the vapour to escape by bubbling through the liquid. Ascending vapour from the still passes through the bubble-caps on plate A and the rising vapour will be richer in the more volatile component. This vapour passes through the liquid on plate B and partially condensed. The heat of condensation partially vaporizes the liquid. The process of condensation and vaporization is repeated at plate C and so on all the way up the column. Each bubble-cap plate has the same effect as a separate still. The bubble cap plate is effective over a wide range of vapour-liquid proportions. There is an excellent contact as the vapour bubbles through the liquid. The major limitation is a layer of liquid on each plate that results in considerable hold-up of liquid over the entire column. There is a need to force the vapour out of the caps, through the liquid that leads to a large pressure drop through the column. In addition, column does not drain when it is not in use. The structure of bubble plate is so complicated that makes construction and maintenance expensive.

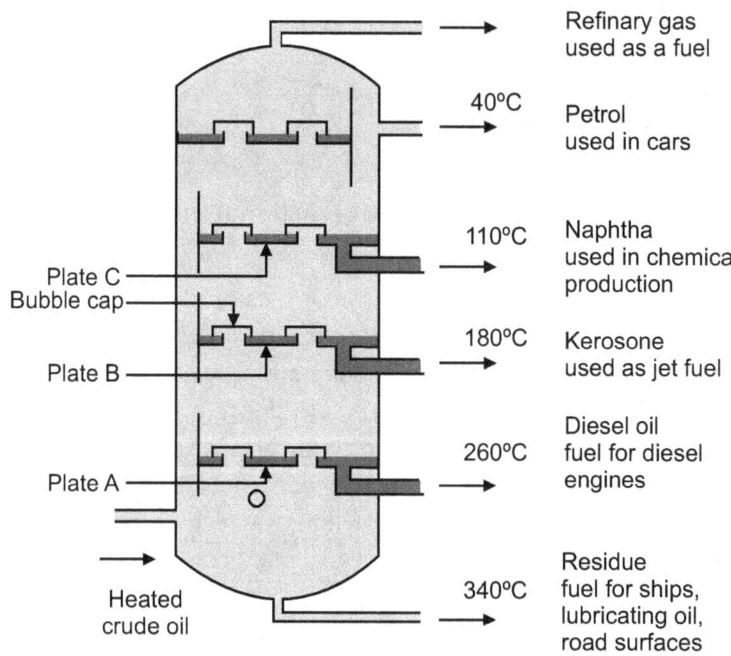

Fig. 6.6: Fractional Distillation Schematic for Crude Oil Separation

Working:

In fractional distillation, the vapors formed from the boiling mixture rise into the fractionating column where they condense on the column's packing. This condensation is similar to a single run of simple distillation; the condensate is more concentrated in the lower boiling compound than the mixture in the distillation flask. As vapors continue to rise through the column, the condensed liquid revaporizes. Each time this occurs the resulting vapours are more and more concentrated in the more volatile substances. The length of the fractionating column and the material it is packed with impact the number of times the vapors will recondense before passing into the condenser. The number of times the column will support this is referred to as the number of theoretical plates of the column. The procedures of simple distillation are so similar to those involved in fractional distillation; the apparatus that are used in the procedures are also very similar. In fractional distillation, a packed fractionating column is attached to the top of the distillation flask and beneath the condenser. This provides the surface area on which rising vapors condense, and subsequently revaporize.

The fractionating column is used to supply a temperature gradient over which the distillation can occur. In an ideal situation, the temperature in the distillation flask would be equal to the boiling point of the mixture of liquids and the temperature at the top of the fractionating column would be equal to the boiling point of the lower boiling compound; all of the lower boiling compound would be distilled away before any of the higher boiling compound. In reality, fractions of the distillate must be collected because as the distillation proceeds, the concentration of the higher boiling compound in the distillate being collected steadily increases. Fractions of the distillate, which are collected over a small temperature range, will be essentially purified; several fractions should be collected as the temperature changes and these portions of the distillate should be distilled again to amplify the purification that has already occurred.

Efficiency of Fractional distillation: The efficiency of separation by fractional distillation of a mixture may depend upon various factors that include fractionating column, reflux ratio, heat input and column temperature etc. Reflux ratio is the quotient of the amount of liquid returning through the column to the amount collected into the receiver during the same interval of time. A column that operates under total reflux will not yield distillate and thus it should be high. It is controlled by selecting proper still. Other experimental conditions necessary for good separation are comparatively large amount of liquid continuously returning through the column, thorough mixing of liquid and vapour and a large active surface of contact between liquid and vapour. The number of vaporization-condensation cycles that can occur within a fractionation column determines the purity which can be attained. The efficiency of a column depends upon column length and composition. Generally column is packed with copper sponge. This increases the surface area that the ascending vapour encounters and results in more vaporization-condensation cycles compared to an empty column.

Theoretical Plates: A measure of efficiency of a column is known as the number of theoretical plates of that column. One theoretical plate is equivalent to one vaporization-condensation cycle which is equivalent to the one simple distillation. Thus a fractionation column that can attain the equivalent of three simple distillations would be said to have three theoretical plates.

Applications:

(i)   Fractional distillation is used for the separation of miscible liquids such as acetone and water, chloroform and benzene.

(ii) Fractional distillation is suitable for a system when the boiling point of the mixture is always intermediate between those of pure components.

(iii) There is neither a maximum nor a minimum in the composition curves (zeotropic mixtures). Examples include benzene and toluene, carbon tetrachloride and cyclohexane, and water and methanol.

Advantages:

(i)   Frictional distillation gives good solvent recovery

(ii) Fractional distillation is easy to use and operate.

(iii) Fractional distillation is also highly efficient, especially for systems that use stacked distillation columns, which produce more output at lower costs.

(iv) It helps to produce much-needed fuel.

Disadvantage:

(i)   Fractional distillation cannot be used to separate miscible liquids, which form pure azeotropic mixtures.

(ii) It is expensive because it requires large structures, heavy-duty materials, and specialized machinery.

(iii) It also requires staff to be fully trained in the operation of systems to ensure they know how to use the distillation equipment and won't make mistakes.

(iv) It presents a wide range of risks for the people who are involved in it. For example, explosion.

(v)   It can contribute to environmental pollution. Fractional distillation in itself is not harmful but the types of mixtures that are distilled disturbs ecology. For example, refining crude oil.

6.6 DISTILLATION UNDER REDUCED PRESSURE

The boiling point of water increases when the external pressure is increased whereas decreased external pressure decreases the boiling point. This principle is used in the process of freeze drying. Many compounds cannot be distilled at atmospheric pressure because their boiling points are so high. At their normal boiling points, the compounds decompose. Thus, some of these materials can be distilled under reduced pressure because the required temperature to boil the liquid can be lowered significantly. If the boiling point is lowered by 10 °C each time the external pressure is halved. To vaporize a liquid, its temperature can be raised or its pressure can be decreased. Distillation under reduced pressure can also be called as vacuum distillation. During vacuum distillation, the pressure inside the distillation column is maintained at a vacuum to lower the temperature needed to vaporize the liquid. This method of distillation is used for heat sensitive products, liquids with low viscosities, and liquids that tend to foul or foam. In vacuum distillation, vacuum pumps are added to the distillation system to decrease the column pressure below atmospheric pressure, Fig. 6.7. Careful pressure control is important because the separation is dependent on the differences in relative volatility at a given temperature and pressure. Changes in relative volatilities could adversely affect the separation.

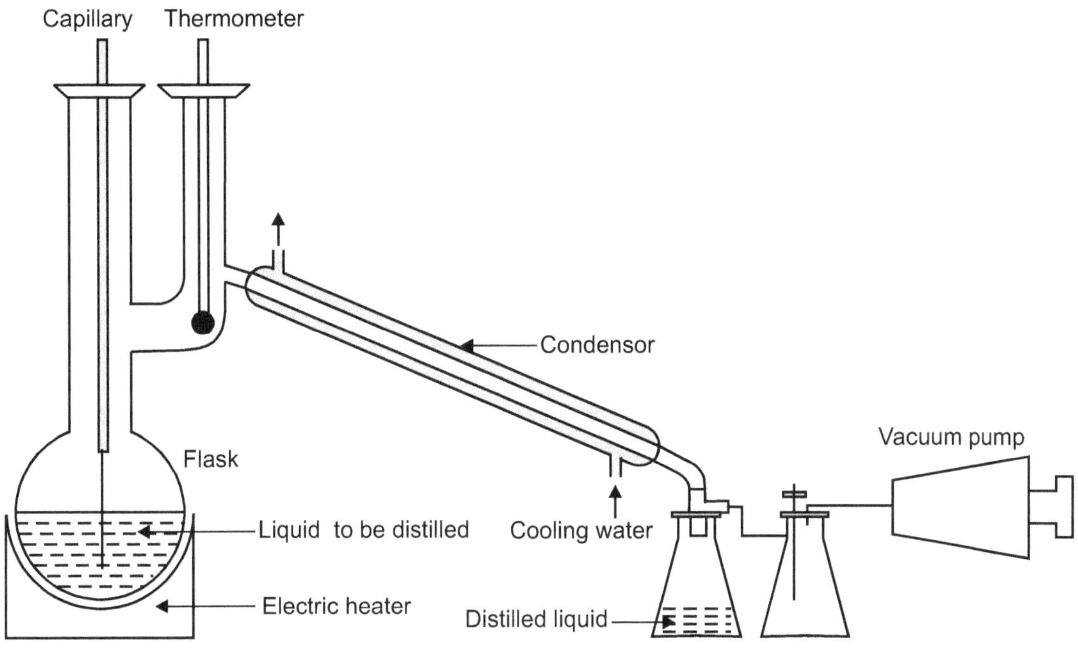

Fig. 6.7 : Distillation under reduced pressure

Principle:

This distillation method works on the principle that boiling occurs when the vapour pressure of a liquid exceeds the ambient pressure. Vacuum distillation is used with or without heating the mixture.

Construction:

The vacuum distillation unit consists of a distillation column, condensing distillate, and reboiler. Vacuum pumps and vacuum regulators are added to distillation columns to maintain the column at a vacuum. Many mixtures can be distilled at much more economical temperatures with the use of these vacuum distillation columns.

Working:

A vacuum distillation is also called as low temperature distillation. The target product in this distillation could either be the remaining product, the distilled product or a purified product. The vacuum pressure associated with a distillation depends on the product to be distilled. For example, volatile substances like those used in oil refineries are likely to undergo vacuum distillations at above 1 Torr, perhaps 20-50 mmHg.

Applications:

(i)   The products of normal distillation are further distilled using vacuum distillation. The high boiling point hydrocarbons, such as lubricants and waxes, are separated at economical temperatures.

(ii)   Vacuum distillation is also used in the separation of sensitive organic chemicals and recovery of organic solvents.

Advantages:

(i)   Vacuum distillation reduces the number of stages needed in distillation.

(ii)   The product output per day is very high.

(iii)   It increases the relative volatility of the key components in many applications. Lower pressures increases relative volatilities in most systems.

(iv)   It requires lower temperatures at lower pressures.

(v)   Vacuum distillation can improve a separation by prevention of product degradation because of reduced pressure leading to lower tower bottoms temperatures.

(vi)   It has very high capacity to handle liquid mixtures giving high yield and highest purity.

(vii)   It requires low capital cost, at the expense of slightly more operating cost. Using vacuum distillation one can reduce the height and diameter, and thus the capital cost of a distillation column.

(viii)   Columns can be operated at lower temperatures.

Disadvantages:

(i)   High energy costs of vacuum pumps.

(ii)   Pressure and energy losses due to any leaks or cracks.

(iii)   Large column diameters needed for the process to be efficient.

6.7 STEAM DISTILLATION

The steam distillation is a process in which concentration and isolation of an essential oil from reliable and often cheaper natural sources is carried out. This is an important technique and has significant commercial applications. Many compounds, both solids and liquids, are separated from complex mixtures by taking advantage of their volatility in steam. A compound must satisfy three conditions to be successfully separated by steam distillation. It must be stable and relatively insoluble in boiling water, and must have a vapor pressure in boiling water that is of the order of 1 kPa (0.01) atmosphere. If two or more compounds satisfy these three conditions, they will generally not separate from each other but will be separated from everything else.

Principle:

The principle behind steam distillation is a way of separating miscible liquid based on their volatilities. The boiling point of the products is so minimized that it permits the constituents to get vaporized. The vapour pressure exerted by the liquids differs in strength which is a function of temperature. The boiling of the liquids takes place and at a certain instance of time the boiling point of the natural products in the liquid form surpass the atmospheric pressure. The result is that the vapor pressure of the whole system increases.

Construction:

A large scale stainless steel steam distillation unit usually has capacity from 0.5 to 15 thousand liters. Its usual diameter varies from 1.5 to 5 meter. The still contains jacket through which steam can be passed for heating the content, Fig. 6.8. Steam vessel is hydrostatically tested at 125 psi to serve as the distillation tank. Low pressure or high pressure steam is supplied by a boiler. The steam vessel can hold extract approximately 3 to 5 liters of essential oil per distillation. The size of the tub is designed to provide oil in sufficient quantity for industrial evacuation or for analysis. The vapors of water and volatile oil are condensed in condenser attached. The distillate is collected as two layers which is separated by Florentine receiver. Following the distillation, the vessel can be disconnected from the cold-water condenser and rotated on swivels to a horizontal position, permitting easy removal and re-filling of plant material. The entire extraction unit (vessel, condenser, boiler and oil collector) is suitable for mounting and transportation. It is built to extract volatile essential oils from aromatic plants.

Working:

Steam distillation is a process employed to extract essential oils from organic plant matter by passing steam generated through the plant material. Usually a chamber is filled with holes (perforations) in the bottom for steam to come through with either fresh or dried herbs.

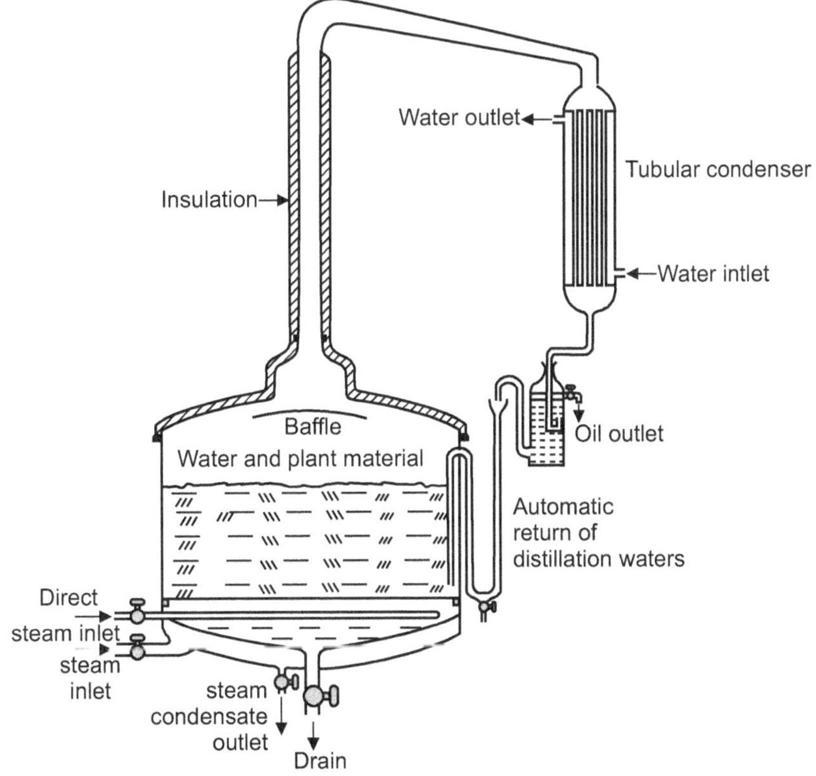

Fig. 6.8: Steam Distillation Unit

Temperature sensitive compounds which would normally decompose through simple distillation vaporize at lower temperatures when subjected to steam in the distillation column. This allows for the separation of essential oils, which tend to be less soluble in boiling water, from chemically complex materials. When the steam is passed through the organic material, tiny pockets holding the essential oils open to release the essential oil molecules without doing any damage to these delicate components. A lid keeps the oil from diffusing into the air when the steam is applied to it. The distillate obtained contain a mixture of water vapour and essential oils which returns to their liquid form in the condensing apparatus. The condensed water and oil droplets are collected and channeled them through a filter, which separates the water from the oil. They are separated using a Florentine separator. In case of essential oils, using steam allows the distillate to retain the more delicate flavours and aromas which would otherwise breakdown if high temperatures are applied.

Advantages:
  (i)   Steam distillation is useful for extracting most fats, oils and waxes. This process works well for types of substances that do not mix with water.
  (ii) It can be a cost-effective method to invest in to extract a diverse array of immiscible substances.
  (iii) Since steam temperature can remain at the boiling point of water; this process also has a cost benefit of requiring less fuel for the steam boiler.
  (iv) The amount of steam and the quality of the steam can be controlled.
  (v)   Lower risk of thermal degradation as temperature generally do not rise above 100 °C.
  (vi) Most widely used process for the extraction of essential oils on a large scale.
  (vii) It is the standard method of extracting flavour and fragrance.

Disadvantages:
  (i)   Need trained operator in order to operate the equipment.
  (ii) The process has a hidden cost of maintaining and repairing equipment.
  (iii) There is a much higher capital requirement and with low-priced oils the payback period can be over 10 years.
  (iv) Requires higher level of technical skill and fabrication and repairs and maintenance require a higher level of skill.

Applications:
  (i)   Steam distillation is used to extract essential oils from aromatic plants to flavour liqueurs.
  (ii) It is used at wide scale for the manufacturing of essential oils like perfumes.
  (iii) It is used in synthesis of complex organic compounds.
  (iv) Orange oil and eucalyptus oil are obtained at industrial scale using this method.
  (v)   It is also used in petroleum industries and in the production of consumer food products.
  (vi) It is used for extraction of peppermint and spearmint oils.

6.8 MOLECULAR DISTILLATION

Molecular distillation is a type of short-path vacuum distillation, characterized by an extremely low vacuum pressure ($\approx$ 0.01 torr). It is a process of separation, purification and concentration of natural products, complex and thermally sensitive molecules. This process is characterized by short term exposure of the distillate liquid to high temperatures in high vacuum in the distillation column and a small distance between the evaporator and the condenser around 2 cm. In molecular distillation, fluids are in the free molecular flow regime. The mean free path of molecules is comparable to the size of the equipment. The gaseous phase no longer exerts significant pressure on the substance to be evaporated, and consequently, rate of evaporation no longer depends on pressure. The motion of molecules is in the line of sight, because they do not form a continuous gas anymore. Thus, a short path between the hot surface and the cold surface is necessary.

Principle:

Molecular distillation is considered as the safest mode of separation and to purify the thermally unstable molecules and related compounds with low volatility and elevated boiling points. The process distinguishes the short residence time in the zone of the molecular evaporator exposed to heat and low operating temperature due to vacuum in the space of distillation. The separation principle of molecular distillation is based on the difference of molecular mean free path. The passage of free path for molecules should be collision free.

Langmuir and Knudsen derived an equation which describes the yield of distillate for molecular distillation.

$$Q = k \times P \times F \left(\frac{M}{T}\right)^{\frac{1}{2}} \qquad \ldots (6.1)$$

Where,

Q is the evaporated quantity kg/h,

P = pressure (mbar),

F = evaporator surface (m^2), k = 1577,

M = molecular weight g/mole and

T is absolute temperature (K).

Theoretically molecular distillation could be used for separating mixtures which have close boiling point or forming azeotrope.

According to the principle of thermodynamics under certain temperature and pressure conditions the molecular mean free path (L) is expressed as;

$$L = \frac{0.707\, K \times T}{\pi\, d^2 P} \qquad \ldots (6.2)$$

Where,

D is effective molecular diameter;

P is molecular space in which the pressure;

T is the molecular environment temperature;

K is the Boltzmann constant.

Construction:

A simple molecular distillation has a unit which is placed on a hot surface. The distillate moves a very short distance before it gets condensed, Fig. 6.9. If the substance is not too viscous, it will drip from the point on the glass condensing surface and run down to the receiving point. The sophisticated apparatus with a different design will have the liquid distilled down on a heated surface close to the condenser. The movement of a film prevents a build-up of non-volatile materials on the surface of the material to be distilled as this might cause the distillation to stop.

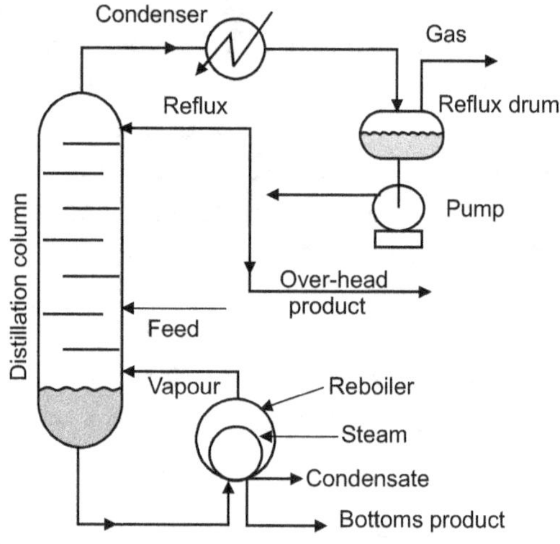

Fig. 6.9: Typical Molecular Distillation Unit

Centrifugal Molecular Distillation:

This is a technique of purification applied under molecular distillation utilized worldwide for food processing, pharmaceutical applications, petroleum industries, and chemical industries. The main principle behind the unit is low pressure and very short residence time. Degassing of feed material leads to the next stage where the material is flown into a spinning disc which is pre-heated. The entire process of distillation gets over in less than fraction of a second because the material that is feed into expands on the spinning pre-heated disc. The distillate finally condenses on the outer extremes of the shell and then slowly flow into the collecting vessel due to gravity. The residual matter is collected in the gutter around the spinning disc and finally into the collecting vessel below Fig. 6.10. The molecular distillation process occurs at a very low temperature and hence can avoid thermal decomposition. The high vacuum applied helps in eliminating the oxidation due to exposure to atmospheric air. The free path distillation is carried out at a very low pressure of 10^{-2} Torr while in molecular distillation the pressure is kept at 10^{-3} Torr.

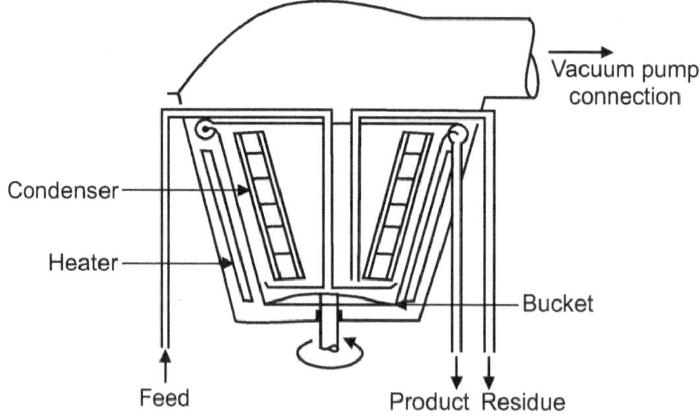

Fig. 6.10: Centrifugal Molecular Distillation Unit

Working:

The molecular distillation process is carried out at a very low pressure so that the distance between hot and condensing surface is less than the mean free path of the molecules. Each of the unit is a single stage but has several units in series. Molecular distillation is applied to thermally sensitive high molecular weight materials. The contact times in commercial units may be low as 0.001 seconds. The film thickness is of the order of 0.05 – 0.1 mm. In vacuum operations, the air ingress is very much possible, whereas in pressure operations the vapour emissions are likely to occur. The distillation process is inherently hazardous with flammables and the presence of huge volume of flammables in reboilers, in column internals and adjacent piping pose huge explosion hazards in these distillation units. Concentration gradient between top and bottom of the column has a bearing on safety. Concentration of impurities in the column can lead to hazards.

Advantages:

(i) **Toxicity:** Avoids the problem of toxicity of solvents used as the separating agent.

(ii) **Thermal stability:** Minimizes losses due to thermal decomposition.

(iii) **Continuous process:** It can be used in a continuous feed process to harvest distillate without having to break vacuum.

(iv) **Stability:** The vacuum allows oils to be processed at minimal temperatures, reducing the risk of oxidative damage.

(v) **Purity:** Separating the oil's components by weight allows contaminants to be reduced far below industry standards.

(vi) **Concentration:** Weight grouping allows the processor to concentrate fatty acids.

(vii) **Short residence time:** This process has short residence time of the feed liquid.

(viii) It works at a significantly lowered temperature due to high vacuum capability

(ix) It has optimal efficiency in mass and heat transfer.

(x) It is suitable for processing high value products.

Disadvantages:

(i) **Cost:** The cost for this complicated technology is relatively high.

(ii) **Natural form:** The starting natural triglyceride form is lost in the distillation process.

Applications:

(i) It is used for separation of vitamins and polyunsaturated fatty acids.

(ii) Molecular distillation is used industrially for purification of oils.

(iii) It is also used to enrich borage oil in γ-linolenic acid (GLA) and recover tocopherols from deodorizer distillate of soybean oil.

(iv) It can be used for the production of synthetic and natural vitamin E,

(v) Capsicum red pigment containing 1% to 2% of the solvent can be separated after two stage molecular distillation.

(vi) It is used for separation of strong spices like volatile substances.

(vii) It is used for highly heat sensitive materials.

(viii) It is a common process in deodorization, decolonization and purification.

(ix) It is used for deoxidation, level off odour or purification and for bleaching or purification.

(x) It is used in fractionation of dimers of fatty acids, separation of radioactive nuclides from melts of irradiated media, lanolin purification, preparation of high concentrated monoglycerides, recovery of carotenoids from palm oil,

(xi) It is used in synthesis of pure diglicyde ether of bisphenol-A.

REVIEW QUESTIONS

1. What is distillation? What are its objectives and applications?
2. Discuss mechanism of distillation.
3. Discuss principle of separation using distillation.
4. Describe significance of temperature and pressure in distillation.
5. What is simple distillation? Give its principle, construction, working, advantages, disadvantages and applications.
6. What is flash distillation? Write about its principle, construction, working, advantages, disadvantages and applications.
7. What is fractional distillation? Discuss its principle.
8. Write about working of fractional distillation unit with reference to its efficiency.
9. What are advantages, disadvantages and applications of fractional distillation?
10. Discuss distillation under reduced pressure. OR
11. What is vacuum distillation? Discuss its principle, construction, working, advantages, disadvantages and applications.
12. What is steam distillation? Give its principle. Comment on construction, working, advantages, disadvantages and applications of steam distillation.
13. What is molecular distillation? Give its principle. Comment on construction, working, advantages, disadvantages and applications of steam distillation.
14. Write short note on centrifugal molecular distillation.

☛ ☛ ☛

Chapter ... **7**

DRYING

7.0 INTRODUCTION

Drying is a mass transfer process in which water or another solvent is removed by evaporation from a solid, semi-solid or liquid. Drying is often a final step in production or packaging of pharmaceutical products. To material to be considered as "dried", the final product must be solid, in the form of a continuous sheet, long pieces, particles or powder. The drying process involves a source of heat and a facility to remove the produced vapours. In majority of pharmaceutical intermediates or finished products the solvent removed is water. Desiccation may be synonymous with drying or considered an extreme form of drying. In pharmaceutical industry final product quality is never be compromised. The deterioration of the product may be due to microbial infection, oxidation, and thermal decomposition, contamination by metallic particles or by presence of organic solvent. These solvents need to be removed at any cost.

The materials used in construction of dryers should be non-contaminating and should be like polished stainless steel or enameled iron. Closed dryers are often useful when moisture removed is organic solvent or their mixture. The oxidative decomposition is prevented by performing drying in an inert gas. Thermal decomposition can be reduced by drying by vacuum and freeze drying methods. All these requirements make dryers for pharmaceuticals use the most expensive.

A variety of drugs are produced in pharmaceutical companies worldwide in many different forms and for that dryers need to operate at batch and continuous mode. The manufacturing of drug in solid forms such as tablets, capsules etc. is carried out in three subsequent stages namely synthesis of intermediate products, final synthesis of the drug and manufacture of dosage form. After each stage the products are dried. Selection of a proper dryer for these products depends on the properties of materials. Adjustment and control of moisture levels in solid materials through drying is a critical process in the manufacture of products. Drying of solid materials is one of the most common and important unit operation in the pharmaceutical industries, where powders and granules handled and manufactured.

The effectiveness of drying processes has a large impact on product quality and process efficiency. For example, in the batch processing of pharmaceuticals drying is a key manufacturing step. The drying process can impact subsequent manufacturing steps such as tableting or encapsulation and can affect critical quality attributes of the finished products. Apart from drying of solids for a subsequent operation, it may be carried out to improve handling characteristics such as bulk powder filling and powder flow.

7.1 OBJECTIVES

The drying unit operation is used extensively in the pharmaceutical industry, but often a lack of understanding of the impact of the presence of moisture, environmental conditions and drying process parameters on active pharmaceutical ingredients critical quality attributes can create challenges during product development, manufacturing, storage and use. Thus, following are the objectives of drying :

(i)   To overcome common challenges in pharmaceutical drying development, including material constraints for scale-up studies and transferring to different equipment types and sizes.

(ii)   To understand drying development related to chemical and physical stability, drying kinetics, and powder properties and highlights common development gaps for improving drying development workflows within the industry.

(iii) To encourage further fundamental research and technological advancements for improving the drying process.

(iv)   Other objectives are to carry out size reduction, to avoid deterioration on storage, to dry the tablet granules to reduce the moisture, to reduce the bulk and weight to lower transportation charges and for certain preparations such as spray dried lactose.

(v)   To design and produce a dryer that conserves energy consumption for optimal utilization in terms of acquisition and operating cost and with optimal local content and versatility.

(vi)   To understand the impact of factors and establish the product specifications, as well as the nature and limits of residual solvents, in agreement with current regulations.

7.2 APPLICATIONS

In manufacturing of pharmaceuticals the last stage of processing is drying which is carried out for one or more of the following applications:

(i)   Drying is used to remove excess moisture or other volatiles from coatings and various substrates.

(ii)   It is used to reduce and control moisture levels in solid materials in the manufacture of many materials.

(iii) It is most important in the processing of highly thermolabile products which are not stable in liquid form. The lyophilization enables longer shelf life of thermolabile materials and make them suitable for storage and transport of the product. For example, drying of biological products such as blood plasma, vaccines, enzymes, microbiological cultures, hormones and antibiotics.

(iv) Drying is used to make the material easy or more suitable for handling and processing. In the manufacturing of bulk drugs or for large scale production of synthetic drugs, drying is essential to get free flowing materials. For example, dried aluminium hydroxide, spray dried lactose etc.

(v) It has applications in avoiding or eliminating moisture that initiates corrosion and decreases the product or drug stability.

For example, to avoid deterioration or contamination of crude drugs of animal and vegetable origin, synthetic and semi synthetic drugs.

(vi) It is used to maintain and improve good properties such as flowability, compressibility etc. of a materials.

For example, drying of fresh plants such as belladonna leaves, nux vomica before subjecting them to size reduction.

(vii) It is used in the production of tablets and granules to improve tablet properties especially, compression of viscous and sticky material.

(viii) Drying is used to improve solubility of materials by modifying their physical form.

For example, milk and coffee extract is dried to convert them into instant soluble power form.

(ix) Drying is necessary to make material light in weight that help to reduce the cost of transportation of large volume materials (liquids).

(x) Drying is used as the final step in evaporation, filtration, and crystallization and to preserve materials from environmental factors.

(xi) Drying is used to maintain and improve shelf life of thermolabile and hydrolytic substances for longer period of time. It is necessary to avoid deterioration of blood products, skin and tissue that undergo microbial decomposition.

(xii) Drying significantly decreases rate of chemical reactions as well as chances of microbial attack or enzymatic actions and thus improves stability.

7.3 MECHANISM OF DRYING PROCESS

The process of drying does not mean only removal of the moisture but the physical structure and the appearance of material has to be preserved. Drying is governed by the principles of heat and mass transfer. When a moist solid is heated to an appropriate temperature, moisture vaporizes at or near the solid surface. The heat required for evaporating moisture from the drying product is supplied by hot air or a gas. Drying involves diffusion in which the transfer of moisture to the surrounding medium takes place by the evaporation from the surface. As some of the moisture from the surface vaporizes more moisture is transported from bulk of the solid to its surface. This movement by diffusion of moisture in a solid takes place by a various mechanisms depending upon the nature and type of the solid and its state of aggregation. Wide variety of solids are handled for drying such as crystalline, granular, beads, powders, sheets, slabs, filter-cakes etc. The mechanism involved in moisture transport in those solids is classified as:

(i)   Transport by liquid or vapors diffusion.

(ii)   Capillary action, and

(iii) Pressure induced transport.

A specific mechanism that involves in drying a specific solid depends on its nature, pore structure and the rate of drying. More than one mechanism may come into play and dominate at different stages of drying of the same material.

There are various common terms used in designing of drying systems. Moisture content of a substance which exerts as equilibrium vapors pressure less than of the pure liquid at the same temperature is referred to as bound moisture. Moisture content of the solid which exerts an equilibrium vapour pressure equal to that of pure liquid at the given temperature is the unbound moisture.

7.4 EQUILIBRIUM MOISTURE CONTENT

The moisture contained in a material comprises all those substances which vaporize on heating and lead to weight loss of the sample. The weight is determined by a balance and interpreted as the moisture content. As per this definition, moisture content includes not only water but also other mass losses such as evaporating organic solvents, alcohols, greases, oils, aromatic components, as well as decomposition and combustion products. The moisture content is also called as moisture assays which is one of the most important analyses performed on most of the pharmaceutical products. Water activity measurements parallel to the moisture content is also an important parameter for quality and stability of pharmaceuticals.

The moisture in products can be present in different forms based upon type of bonding with solids, Fig. 7.1. It is called 'Free water' when water is on the surface of the test substance and it retains its physical form, 'Absorbed water' when water is present in large pores, cavities or capillaries of the test substance and 'Water of hydration' occluded in lattice ions or water of crystallization coordinately bonded to ions.

The loss on drying (LOD) is the amount of water and volatile matters present in a sample when the sample is dried under specified conditions. Moisture content (MC) is the quantity of water contained in a material, such raw materials, API and blend.

$$\% \text{ Loss of drying } = \frac{\text{Mass of water in sample (kg)}}{\text{Total mass of wet sample (kg)}} \times 100 \qquad \dots (7.1)$$

$$\% \text{ Moisture content } = \frac{\text{Mass of water in sample (kg)}}{\text{Mass of dry sample (kg)}} \times 100 \qquad \dots (7.2)$$

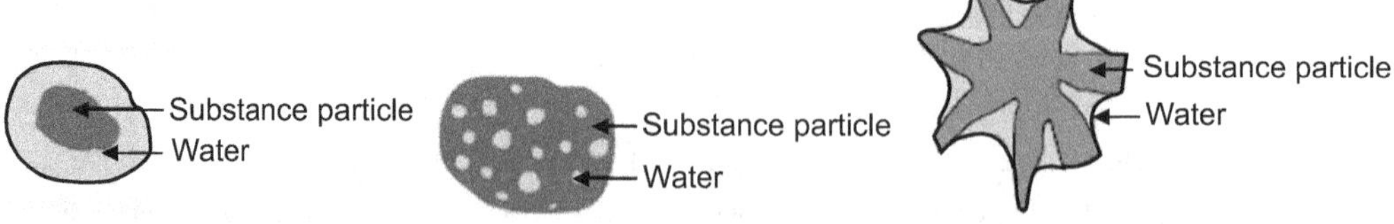

Fig. 7.1: Types of Bonding of Moisture in Pharmaceutical Products

The moisture content of solid in excess of the equilibrium moisture content is referred as free moisture (water). It must be noted that during drying only free moisture is evaporated. The free moisture content (FMC) of a solid depends upon the vapour concentration in the air above solid surface. The moisture contents of solid when it is in equilibrium with given partial pressure of vapour in gas phase is called as equilibrium moisture content (EMC). Similarly, the moisture content at which the constant rate drying period ends and the falling rate drying period starts is called critical moisture content (CMC). During the constant rate drying period, the moisture evaporated per unit time per unit area of drying surface remains constant and in falling rate drying period the amount of moisture evaporated per unit time per unit area of drying surface continuously decreases.

When the water vapour pressure of the air approaches the saturation water vapour pressure at the temperature of the gas, the EMC of materials rapidly increases. At these stages, the process undergone by the material is not only adsorption. Water vapour begins to condense within the pore structures of the materials. Theoretically, if the material is in contact with air that is 100 % saturated for a very long period, all pores of the material should be filled with the condensed moisture. The EMC that corresponds to that hypothetical state is called the saturation moisture content (SMC) of the material. But in practice the rate of this process becomes infinitesimally small at an EMC that is known as the capillary saturation moisture content (CSMC) and is often substantially less than the saturation moisture content referred to above.

7.4.1 Measurements

The moisture content is determined by several direct and indirect methods.

(i) Direct Methods:

The direct methods include mainly thermo gravimetric methods. The moisture content can be determined by an oven method directly. The solid is weighed and dried, then weighed again according to standardized procedures. In the Thermogravimetric method, moisture is always separated. Thus, there is no distinction made between water and other readily volatile product components. A representative sample must be obtained to provide a useful moisture content evaluation. Also, the moisture content of the product must be maintained from the time the sample is obtained until the determination is made by storing in a sealed container. Thermogravimetric techniques can be used to continuously measure the mass of a sample as it is heated at a controlled rate. The temperature at which water evaporates depends on its molecular environment. The free water normally evaporates at a lower temperature than bound water. Thus by measuring the change in the mass of a sample as it loses water during heating it is often possible to obtain an indication of the amounts of water present in different molecular environments. For many solids this method is mandatory particularly for granules. For granules the moisture content is measured by heating them in hot air oven at suitable temperature until weight becomes constant. For heat sensitive materials vacuum is applied in the oven to decrease the boiling point of liquid.

(ii) Indirect Methods:

Indirect methods are developed to determine the moisture content rapidly. For example, use of modern heating measurement methods like infrared, microwaves, ultra sound, and spectroscopy. These methods are developed due to requirements of rapid, non-destructive and precise moisture content determination. The indirect methods are generally faster than the direct methods for moisture determination. When done properly, the indirect methods can be accurate and precise. However, the accuracy and precision of the indirect methods depend on careful preparation and analysis of known standards to establish reliable calibration curves. Indirect methods require a large capital investment in equipment. Nevertheless, preparation of the standards and accurate calibration curves must be verified by a specific direct method to establish a reliable indirect method of instrumentation that can achieve accurate and precise predicted values.

The methods for moisture determination given in USP24 NF19 are the best, classical, and addresses only the determination of moisture content. The U.S.P. offers two methods for the determination of moisture content in solids:

(a) Titrimetry (Karl Fisher titration).

(b) Gravimetric (Thermal gravimetric analysis).

Moisture content is used in a wide range of scientific and technical areas, and is expressed as a ratio, which can range from 0 (completely dry) to the value of the materials' porosity at saturation. It can be given on a volumetric or mass (gravimetric) basis. Moisture content is expressed as a percentage of moisture based on total weight (wet basis) or dry matter (dry basis). Wet basis moisture content is generally used. The moisture content is expressed by following formulae.

$$M_w \text{ (wet basis)} = \frac{W_{water}}{W_{water} + W_{dry}} \times 100 \qquad \ldots (7.3)$$

$$M_d \text{ (dry basis)} = \frac{W_{water}}{W_{dry}} \times 100 \qquad \ldots (7.4)$$

where,

$$M = \text{Moisture content on a percent basis,}$$
$$W_{water} = \text{Total weight as wet weight}$$
$$d = \text{Total as dry weight}$$

Based on the different forms of moisture present in the material the method used for measurement of moisture may estimate more or less moisture content. Therefore, for different pharmaceutical products Official Methods of moisture measurement have been given by agencies.

Example: Accurately 10 g of granules are transferred into a 4 g container and after drying the container with granules weighs 6.3 g. What is percent moisture content in the granules on wet basis.

$$\textbf{Solution:} \qquad M_w = \frac{W_{water}}{W_{water} + W_{dry}} = \frac{10 - 2.3}{(10 - 2.3) + (6.3 - 4)}$$

$$= \frac{7.7}{7.7 + 2.3}$$

$$= 77\%$$

7.4.2 Applications of Moisture Content Determination

Accurate per cent moisture content is essential for maintaining stability of drug products. If a product is too moist or too dry, it may not be suitable to be administered and will not exert desired therapeutic effect. Most of the pharmaceutical products contain moisture. The per cent moisture content is seldom of interest. Rather, it shows whether a product intended for trade and production has standard characteristics such as storage ability, agglomeration, microbiological stability, flow properties, viscosity etc. The dry substance content, concentration or purity, compliance with quality agreements, therapeutic value of the product and legal conformity are other important issues. In addition, determination of moisture content has following applications:

(i) **Freshness:** Fresh products has specified characteristic features. Moisture induces changes in the state of solid. As they age and begin to degrade, some dry out and some pick-up excess moisture and begin to mold.

(ii) **Labeling:** Pharmaceutical industries require a minimum or maximum percentage of moisture in certain products in order for them to be packaged and labelled. If they don't fit to these standards, the products cannot pass the quality standards and unfit for commercial release. For example, freeze dried products, hard gelatine capsules etc.

(iii) **Cost:** In processed pharmaceutical products, the percentage of water can determine its final price. Generally, a product with more water will cost less.

(iv) **Processing:** The moisture has effect on the performance of excipients thus manufacturers and physicians need to know the moisture content of product to ensure that it is processed and packaged in a safe, stable way.

(v) **Quality:** Moisture content determines the way most product appropriate to administer, taste, feel and look. It is one of the important ways to measure product quality.

(vi) **Shelf life:** The physicochemical stability of bioactive agents alone and in combination with excipients is affected by moisture. Thus, shelf life of product depends on its moisture content at the time of packaging and rate of moisture gain during storage. Stability of products depends upon the per cent moisture in finished products.

7.5 RATE OF DRYING

When a wet non-porous granular solid material is placed in a tray and dried with a carrier gas like air under constant drying conditions of velocity, temperature, humidity and pressure of air at the inlet, the experimental data can be plotted as drying rate vs. free moisture content or time, Fig. 7.2. The obtained typical drying rate curve is divided into a constant rate period (AB), a first falling rate period (BC) and a second falling rate period (CD). The free moisture content at the end of the constant rate period (B) is known as CMC. During drying process, the moisture content is plotted based on the entire material. In general, at the start of drying process there is an unsteady state of warming-up period during which wet solid keep changing till the beginning of the constant rate period.

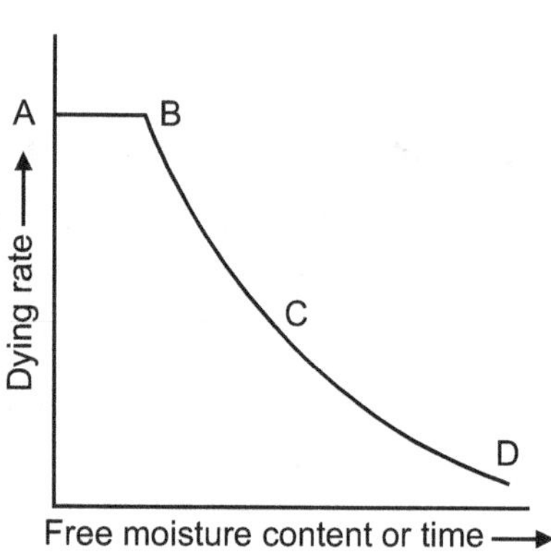

Fig. 7.2: Rate of drying

The drying rate curves are not smooth and continuous which indicates that the drying process involves a single mechanism throughout. In drying calculations, the water content in the wet solid is usually expressed on a dry weight basis, i.e. Kg of water/Kg of dry solid.

7.6 DRYING CURVE

For each and every product, there is a representative curve that describes the drying characteristics for that product at specific temperature, velocity and pressure conditions. This curve is referred to as the drying curve for a specific product. Variations in the curve will occur principally in rate relative to carrier velocity and temperature. The curve is extremely valuable in understanding unusual behaviour associated with the drying of each unique product. Drying process can be divided in to three periods:

   (a)   Constant drying rate period.

   (b)   First falling drying rate period.

   (c)   Second falling rate period.

(a) Constant Drying Rate Period:

In a constant drying rate period, a material or mass of material contain much of water that liquid surface exists which dries in a similar fashion to an open faced body of water. Diffusion of moisture from within the droplet maintains saturated surface conditions and as long as this lasts, evaporation takes place at constant rate. When a solid is dried under constant drying conditions, the moisture content (MC) typically falls. The graph is linear at first, then curves and eventually levels off. Constant rate drying period (B-C) will proceed until free moisture appears from the surface, the moisture removal rate will then become progressively less. At CMC the drying rate ceases and remains constant. During the constant rate period, the moisture from interior migrates to the surface by various means and is vaporized.

As the moisture content is lowered, the rate of migration to the surface is also lowered. If drying occurs at too high temperatures, the surface forms closely packed shrunken cells which are sealed together. This acts as a barrier to moisture migration and tends to keep the moisture sealed within. This condition is known as 'case hardening'. The constant rate period is characterized by a drying independent of moisture content. During this period, the solid is so wet that a continuous film of water remain over the entire drying surface, and this water acts to lower the drying rate. The temperature of the wetted surface attains the wet bulb temperature.

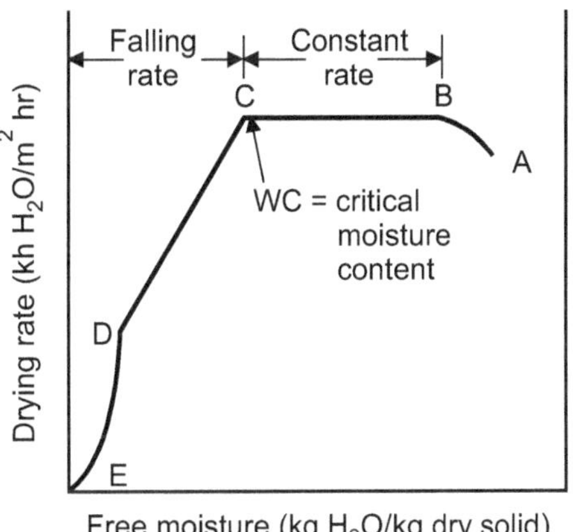

Fig. 7.3: A Typical Drying Curve for a Solid (Drying Rate Vs. Free Moisture)

Web Bulb Temperature (WBT): *WBT is the steady state temperature shown by the thermometer whose bulb is covered with a wet wick and from which water is evaporating into a high velocity air stream. The quantity of water evaporated is not high enough to alter the temperature and humidity of the air stream. The air is blown at high velocity (minimum 300 m/min) to cause evaporation of water from the wick. Evaporation requires latent heat. This heat comes from surface of glass bulb of thermometer. So the temperature of the glass bulb decreases. The heat comes from the temperature difference between T_w and T_a (large). It is the case of simultaneous heat and mass transfer. This heat is latent heat for phase change of water to water vapour.*

(b) Falling Rate Periods :

The constant rate period ends when the migration rate of water from the interior of the surface becomes less than the rate of evaporation from the surface. The period subsequent to the critical point is called 'the falling rate period'. Following this point, the surface temperature rises, and the drying rate falls-off rapidly. The falling rate period takes a far longer time than the constant rate period, even though the moisture removal may be much less. The drying rate approaches zero at some equilibrium moisture content.

Drying in falling rate period involves two processes:

(a)   Movement of moisture within the material to the surface.

(b)   Removal of the moisture from the surface.

The method used to estimate drying rates and drying times in the falling rate period depends on whether the solid is porous or non-porous. In a non porous material, once there is no superficial moisture, further drying can occur only at a rate governed by diffusion of bulk moisture to the surface. In a porous material other mechanism appears, and drying takes place in the bulk of solid instead of at the surface.

(i) First falling drying rate period

The moisture content at the end of the constant rate period (point c), is the 'critical moisture content'. At this point the surface of the solid is no longer saturated, and the rate of drying decreases with the decrease in moisture content. At point C, the surface moisture film evaporates fully, and with the further decrease in moisture content, the drying rate is controlled by the rate of moisture movement through the solid.

(ii) Second falling drying rate period:

Period C to D represents conditions when the drying rate is largely independent of conditions outside the solid. The moisture transfer may be due to any combination of liquid diffusion, capillary movement, and vapour diffusion.

Effect of Shrinkage:

A factor that often greatly affects drying rate is the shrinkage of the solid as moisture is removed. Rigid solids do not shrink appreciably, but colloidal and fibrous materials do undergo shrinkage. The most serious effect is development of a hard layer on the surface which is impervious to the flow of liquid or vapour moisture and slows down drying rate. In many materials, if drying occurs at too high temperature, a layer of closely packed, shrunken cells, which are sealed together, forms at the surface that presents a barrier to moisture migration. Another effect of shrinkage is to cause the materials to warp and change its structure. Sometimes, to decrease these effects of shrinkage, it is desirable to dry with moist air. This decreases the rate of drying so that the effects of shrinkage on warping or hardening at the surface are greatly reduced.

7.7 DRYING EQUIPMENTS

Drying equipments are classified in different ways, according to design and operating features or based on mode of operation such as batch or continuous. In case of batch dryer the material is loaded in the drying equipment and drying proceeds for a given period of time, whereas, in case of continuous mode the material is continuously fed to the dryer and dried material is continuously discharged. In some cases vacuum may be used to reduce the drying temperature. Some dryers can handle almost any kind of material, whereas others are severely limited in the size and style of feed they can accept.

Drying equipments also can be categorized according to the physical state of the feed such as wet solid, liquid, and slurry and the type of heating system i.e. conduction, convection, radiation. Heat may be supplied by direct contact with hot air at atmospheric pressure, and the water vaporized is removed by the air flowing. Heat may also be supplied indirectly through the wall of the dryer from a hot gas flowing outside the wall or by radiation.

Dryers can also be classified on the basis of exposure of material to be dried. Dryers exposing the solids to a hot surface with which the solid is in contact are called adiabatic or direct dryers, while when heat is transferred from an external medium it is known as non-adiabatic or indirect dryers. Dryers heated by electric, radiant or microwave energy are also non adiabatic. Some units combine adiabatic and non- adiabatic drying; they are known as direct-indirect dryers. They can also be categorized on the basis of energy efficiency. To reduce heat losses most of the commercial dryers are insulated and hot air is recirculated to save energy. Modern designs have energy-saving devices, which recover heat from the exhaust air or automatically control the air humidity. Computer control of dryers in sophisticated driers also results in important savings in energy.

Classification of Dryers:

There are numerous criterion used to classify dryers. Table 7.1 lists the criteria and typical dryer types.

Table 7.1: Classification of dryers

Criterion	Types of dryer	Examples
Mode of operation	• Batch • Continuous	• Tray dryer • Rotary drum dryer
Heat input-type	• Convection, conduction, radiation, electromagnetic fields, combination of heat transfer modes • Intermittent or continuous • Adiabatic or non-adiabatic	• Hot air oven, Tray dryer • Rotary drum dryer • Tray dryer
State of material in dryer •	• Stationary • Moving, agitated, dispersed	• Hot air oven • Rotary dryer
Operating pressure	• Vacuum • Atmospheric	• Vacuum dryer • Rotary dryer
Drying medium (convection)	• Air • Superheated steam • Flue gases	• Hot air oven • Steam dryer • Flue gas dryer
Drying temperature	• Below boiling temperature • Above boiling temperature • Below freezing point	• Freeze dryer, spray dryer • Vacuum dryer • Freeze dryer
Relative motion between drying medium and drying solids	• Co-current • Counter-current • Mixed flow	• Rotary dryer • Counter current flow dryer • Mixed flow dryer
Number of stages	• Single • Multi-stage	• Spray dryer • Spray dryer
Residence time	• Short (< 1 min) • Medium (1 – 60 min) • Long (> 60 min)	• Spray dryer • Hot air oven • Freeze dryer

7.7.1 Tray Dryer

Tray drying is a batch process used to dry materials that are liquid or wet cake. Tray drying works well for material that requires more gentle processing or cannot be atomized in an air stream due to viscosity. This dryer is well utilized for drying of the wet products like crude drugs, chemicals, powders or the granules, etc. It is the most conventional dryer used very widely and still being used where the moisture content is more and where the product has to be dried at low temperature for long hours.

Principle:

A laboratory oven is the elementary form of tray dryer which contains a cabinet with a heater at the bottom. The values of these ovens are very less because of its uncontrollable heat transfer or humidity. When we fit a fan in the oven, the circulation of the forced hot air gets started. This process is beneficial for reducing the local flour concentrations and also for increasing the heat transfer. In the direct circulation form the air is heated and then focused on the object in a controlled flow. The material to be dried is dispersed on the tiers of the trays. For the circulation of the air across the drying materials, the screen in trays are perforated and lined with paper. A limited amount of heat is provided to every shelf at that time when the air passes over it to provide the latent heat of vaporization. This kind of dryers provides proper control of humidity and temperature.

Construction:

Tray dryer can be electrically or steam heated. It consists of any number of trays that varies with customer requirement. It is fabricated out of rigid angle iron frame with double walled panels insulated with best quality compressed fiber glass and with a rigid door fitted with strong hinges and best chosen locking system. There may be facility to circulate hot air such as fans. A control panel is fixed in the front of the oven to facilitate easy operation. It has a large functional space and is made of mild steel and in good finishing outside with synthetic enamel colour and inside painted with heat resistant paint to resist temperature up to 300 °C.

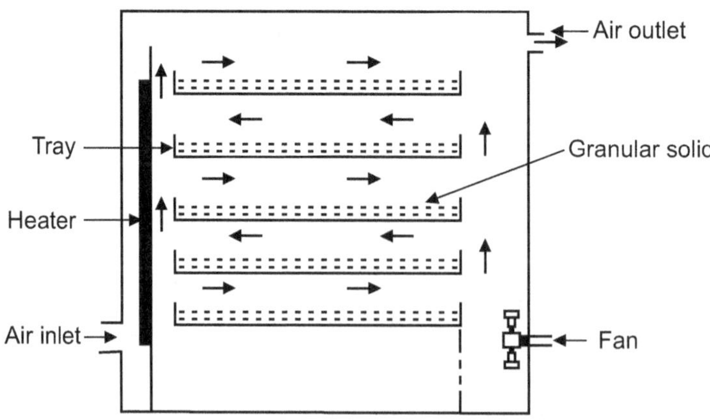

Fig. 7.4: A Typical Spray Dryer

Working:

Tray dryer is widely used in pharmaceutical industries. The material to be dried is placed on the trays. The heat in the dryer is produced by the heater along a side or at base. Other than the hot air generated by the oven, the other method is to employ radiator coils that use steam for heat circulation. During the heating process the material to be dried is spread out on the trays. The heated air is directed to flow in a circulation form. It flows over the material in the trays in a controlled flow. Trays can have a solid, perforated or wire mesh base. A paper lining could be used to reduce chances of contamination through contact with the tray. The efficiency of the dryer depends on recirculation of the hot air. Apart from a regular supply and presence of heated air, it also depends on supply of fresh air. The fresh air is combined with the heated air in fixed proportion for an efficient performance. Such regulated drying is important to ensure uniform drying in the dryer at the bottom as well as at the top. Apart from the double-walled construction insulation is achieved by heating coils.

Advantages:

(i)   It is operated on batch mode so each batch can be handled as a separate entity.

(ii)   It is energy efficient dryer as it consumes less energy.

(iii) It's simple to use and clean.

(iv)   Tray dryer is available in different sizes thus capital cost can be controlled.

(v)   Chamber walls are heated externally thus prevents condensation.

(vi)   It is available in unique single chamber and multi chamber design with lowest leakage.

(vii) It has excellent surface contact between tray and shelf.

(viii) It is best option in small scale production and drying valuable pharmaceutical materials such as drying wet lumpy solids and wet cakes.

(ix)   It has heavy duty hollow shelf design with all connection outside the chamber.

(x)   Operating parameter can be controlled more easily.

(xi)   Using vacuum systems tray dryers can be best suited for drying of heat sensitive materials.

Disadvantages:

(i)   As it is operated at low to intermediate temperatures the process is time-consuming.

(ii)   Only a fraction of the solid particles are directly exposed. Heat transfer and mass transfer are comparatively inefficient.

(iii) It provides tendency to over-dry contents in the lower trays.

(iv)   The operation is long during cycle (5 to 45 h per batch) and expensive to operate due to high labour requirement for loading and unloading.

(v)   Plastic substances can also be dried using this dryer.

(vi)   It is not suitable for large scale production.

(vii) Thermolabile drugs, liquids, slurries, cannot be dried.

Applications:

(i)   Tray dryer has industrial applications such as in chemical and pharmaceuticals.

(ii) Sticky materials, granular mass or crystalline materials, precipitates and paste can be dried in a tray dryer.

(iii) It has been used in agricultural drying because of its simple design and capability to dry products at high volume.

7.7.2 Drum Dryer

The drum dryer has been used since long time for drying sheets of paper or cloth and, more recently, for drying liquids and pastes. Drum dryers in general and the various types of drum dryers (atmospheric single drum, vacuum single-drum, and the double-drum dryers) in particular are selected or rejected for any given drying requirement on the basis of their individual operating characteristics and costs.

Principle:

Drum dryers operate by applying a thin layer of the product to be dried to the outside of a rotating drum. The drum is internally heated by steam which quickly evaporates any liquid from the product. After almost one full revolution the remaining dried material is removed from the drum by a knife as a film or powder.

Construction:

Drum dryer is a moving bed dryer. The unit is constructed from cast iron and stainless steel, providing cleanliness and resistance to chemical attack. The drums are engineered with hard chrome plating or chrome plated over nickel to ensure maximum heat transfer and to accommodate high steam temperatures and pressures, precision machined to provide maximum and reproducible heat transfer throughout its life. The drums are hollow horizontally mounted 0.6 to 3.0 meter in diameter and 0.6 to 4.0 meter in length, whose external surface is smoothly polished. Steam or heating coils can be used inside the drum for heat generation. Heat is transferred by conduction to the material that can be controlled with a thermostat. Drum is rotated with a motor device at 1-10 r.p.m.

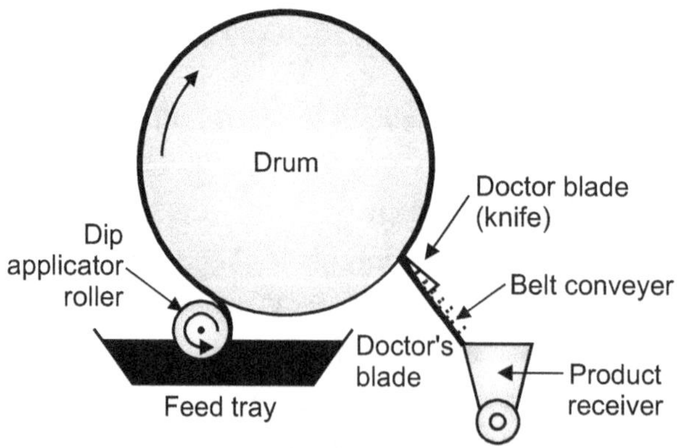

Fig. 7.5: Single Drum Dryer with Dip Roller Feed

Double drum dryer: The extra capacity can be provided by using double drum dryer. A double drum dryer is also called as dual drum and is often used for products with low to medium viscosity. In this system, the product is fed into a pool between the two drums which always turn in opposite directions. The small space between the drums can be set accurately so that a desired film layer can be obtained. Other combinations are possible depending on the product and the desired end-result.

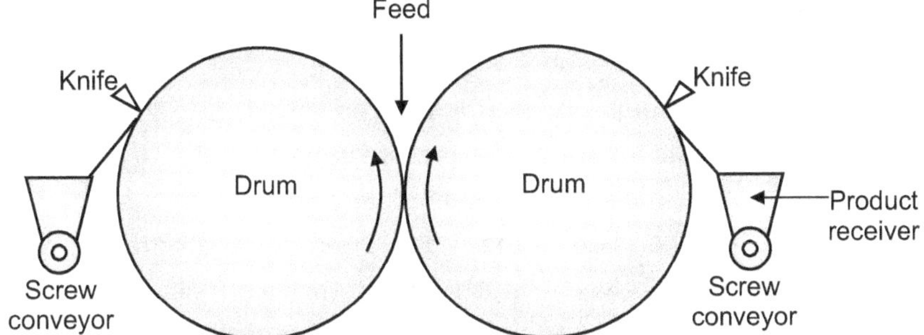

Fig. 7.6: Double Drum Dryer with Nip Feed.

Vacuum drum dryer: A drum dryer that operates under vacuum allows the product to be dried at lower temperatures. These drum dryers provide a higher capacity and less product loss under vacuum. Two steam-heated drums turn in an air-tight casing under high vacuum. The liquid is fed between the drums from the top, dried and scraped-off before the drums have fully rotated. There is no accumulation of product residues and no recirculation of the material. The drum dryer is easily accessed for inspection and maintenance. There is a wide range of applications, including damage prevention to heat-sensitive product components or evaporation of solvents at low temperatures. The vapours collected are condensed elsewhere. Absence of atmospheric pollution and climatic conditions gives reproducible product quality. Feed materials can benefit from such careful treatment. Evaporation takes place within a few seconds without risk of oxidation. Thermolabile materials such as, enzymes and proteins are preserved and blockage of proteins is prevented. The end product can be dissolved easily into a liquid. Chemical products, too, can be processed in the dryer from using vacuum process and undergo the drying treatment. It can use a gas such as nitrogen to keep the environment inert.

Accessories: Dryers for pharmaceutical applications are generally provided with vapour canopy and extract system to remove the vapours from the operating area. Dryers for hazardous materials may be provided with complete dust and fume tight enclosures.

Working:

Single drum dryer: The robust construction of drum dryers made them to be used efficiently over last 60 years and still are in use today. The drum body of the drum dryer is heated on the inside by steam. Steam heating gives a uniform temperature distribution over the drum surface to provide consistent product quality. The steam condenses on the inside of the drying drum. The condensate is continuously removed from the drum, so that the largest possible surface area remains available on the inside of the drum for condensation of the steam. The steam system is a closed system, which means that the product cannot come into contact with the steam or condensate. Depending on the design of the drum dryer, the product is applied continuously as a thin film on the underside or top of the main drum. As the drum turns it is heated on the inside and the product dries on the outside of the drum dryer. The short exposure to a high temperature reduces the risk of damage to the product. The water or solvent evaporates and leaves from the surface of drum. If necessary, the vapour can also be suctioned-off locally around the drum. The dried product layer finally reaches the knife and is scraped-off.

Double drum dryer: The liquid to be dried is fed into the valley created by the two drums, where it is applied to the drums as they rotate together. The dry product is removed by a knife on each drum. Wet materials are completely dried during slightly less than one rotation from one side to another side of the drum. Dried materials are scrapped by a knife, which then falls into a product receiver. Contact time of the material with hot metal is 6 to 15 seconds only. Therefore, processing conditions such as film thickness and drum temperature are closely monitored and controlled. The shaft-mounted main drive speed is adjusted by electronic inverter in the control panel. The liquid or paste material present in the feed pan adheres as a thin layer to the external surface of the drum during its rotation.

Product Removal: Product is removed from the drum dryer surface by means of an alloy steel doctor blade or knife rigidly clamped in a cast iron knife bar assembly. The knife is applied to the surface of the drum by pneumatic cylinders located at each end of the dryer. For improved knife life and reduced drum maintenance an oscillating knife system is fitted with either conventional or disposable knives. After removal from the drum the product is collected by a transverse screw conveyor specially designed to break up the product film or flakes into easy-to-handle particles. For products that may require cooling after removal from the drum air.

Advantages:

(i)   Drum dryer gives a rapid (few seconds) drying and its mass transfer rate is higher.

(ii)   The entire material is continuously exposed to uniform heat. This process is characterized by short drying time and minimum product heating.

(iii)   The equipment is compact 100% closed system and tailored models are available.

(iv)   Their simple operation makes them run with the minimum of training and require no specialist maintenance.

(v)   Drum dryers are economical with cheap installation and 24 hour a day continuous production.

(vi)   It can have vacuum facilities to prevent dust emission thereby giving a guarantee of optimal hygiene during the complete production process.

(vii)   This dryer work with minimum energy consumption and does not require large dust recovery systems such as filters.

(viii) The heat is transferred by steam to the (metal) wall, which in turn transfers it to the product on the other side of the wall. All the heat transferred by the wall is used to dry the product and does not leave the machine or chimney unused making this dryer a much more efficient process.

(ix) Using these dryers product supply can be controlled. Furthermore, drums create a kneading effect that prevents the formation of lumps in sticky products.

(x) A perfect distribution over the entire length of the drum makes the system ideal for processing doughy or pasty products.

(xi) The temperature of the drum can be controlled independently for the required drying task by setting the steam pressure and thus are best suited for processing certain heat-sensitive products,

Disadvantages:

(i) The operating conditions are critical and need to be monitored.

(ii) Skilled operators are needed to control feed rate, film thickness, speed of rotation and temperature.

(iii) It is not suitable for low concentration solutions or suspensions of low viscosity.

Applications:

(i) Drum dryer is used in drying of liquids and pastes of sticky and highly viscous products.

(ii) It is used under vacuum for drying temperature sensitive products such as vitamins, proteins, yeasts, pigments, malt extracts, hormones and antibiotics.

(iii) It has closed process area that protects the product and/or the environment.

(iv) Drum dryer is used for drying solutions, slurries, suspensions etc.

(v) Used to dry products such as starch products, ferrous salts, suspensions of zinc oxide, suspension of kaolin, calcium, insecticides, barium carbonates etc.

(vi) Vacuum drum drying is used for instant beverages, chocolate products, chemicals and recovery of solvents, foods and beauty soaps etc.

7.7.3 Spray Dryer

Spray drying is a method of producing a dry powder from a liquid or slurry by rapidly drying with a hot gas. This is the preferred method of drying of many heat-sensitive pharmaceuticals. A consistent particle size distribution can be achieved using spray drying of some industrial products such as catalysts.

Principle:

Spray drying is the continuous transformation of feed from a fluid state into dried particulate form by spraying the feed into a hot drying medium. The feed is either solution, slurry, emulsion, gel or paste which is provided through pump in atomized form.

Construction:

Many different types of spray dryers exist, each with different features for meeting various spray drying needs. A spray dryer consists of a feed pump, atomizer, air heater, air dispenser, drying chamber and systems for exhaust air cleaning and powder recovery/separator and process control systems. It consists of a large cylindrical drying chamber with a short conical bottom, made-up of glass (lab scale) or stainless steel (large scale). The diameter of the chamber is 2.5- 9 meters and height 25 meters or more. An inlet for hot air is placed in the roof of the chamber and another inlet carrying spray disk atomizer is set in the roof. The spray disk atomizer is about 300 mm in diameter and rotates at a speed of 3000 to 50,000 r.p.m. Bottom of the dryer is connected to a cyclone separator.

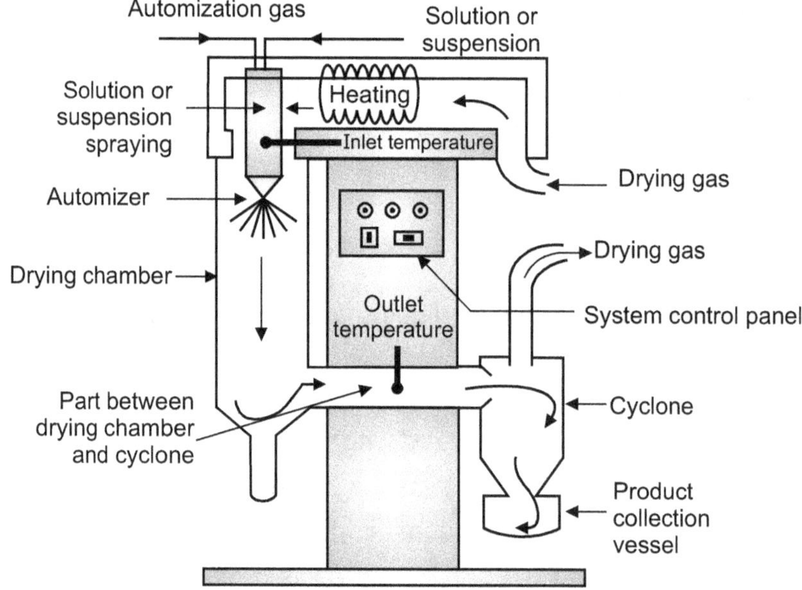

Fig. 7.7: Spray Dryer and Its Stepwise Working Sequence

Working:

Spray drying is a one-step continuous unit operation that employs liquid atomization to produce droplets that are dried to individual particles when moved in a hot gaseous drying medium. The three stages that occur in a spray dryer before drying is accomplished include atomization, spray-air mixing and moisture evaporation and dry product separation from the exit air. The spray drying process begins with atomization. During atomization, a nozzle or rotary atomizer turns the liquid feed stock into small liquid droplets. This is followed by separation of the solute or suspension as a solid and the solvent into a vapour. It is during this stage that many of the desired product qualities such as particle size and viscosity are developed. When droplets exit the nozzles or atomizer, they are dried to form a powder which is easily packed and transported. Solids form as moisture quickly leaves the droplets. The solid is usually collected in a drum or cyclone. The nature of the final product depends on the design and operation of the spray dryer and the physicochemical properties of the feed. Drying of the powder is commonly completed using hot air. Final moisture content in the powder is controlled by adjusting the hot air temperature. The recovery process is last step that takes a few seconds to recover the powder from the exhaust gas within the cyclone.

Advantages:

The main advantage of spray drying is its versatility of the technology. Spray drying offers multiple opportunities that no other single drying technology provides. The flexibility and reproducibility of spray dryer makes spray drying the process of choice for many industrial drying operations. It has following other advantages :

(i)   This technique has ability to operate in aseptic pharmaceutical processing.

(ii) Feed rates in spray drying can range from a few pounds per hour to over 100 tons per hour and thus can be designed to any capacity required.

(iii) The spray drying process is very rapid, with the major portion of evaporation taking place in less than a few seconds.

(iv) It is adaptable to fully automated control system that allows continuous monitoring and recording of very large number of process variables simultaneously.

(v)   Wide ranges of equipment designs are available to meet various product specifications.

(vi) It has few moving parts and careful selection of various components can result in a system having no corrosion and wear and tear problems.

(vii) It can be used with both heat-resistant and heat sensitive products.

(viii) It can handle feed for drying in solution, slurry, paste, gel, suspension or melt form.

(ix) It can have control over properties such as particle size, bulk density, and degree of crystallinity, impurities and residual solvents.

(x)   It has ability to produce nearly spherical particles with uniform size and thus reduces the bulk density of the product. Powder quality remains constant during the entire run of the dryer.

Disadvantages:

(i)   The equipment is very bulky and the ancillary equipment components are expensive to install.

(ii) The overall thermal efficiency is low, thus large volumes of heated air is wasted as pass through the chamber without contacting a particle.

(iii) It is difficult maintain and clean after use.

(iv) It needs material in liquid form and thus solid materials cannot be dried using spray dryers.

(v)   Product degradation or fire hazard may result from product deposit in the drying chamber.

Applications:

Spray drying technology is widely applied in pharmaceutical fields as well as non-pharmaceutical fields.

(i)   Many pharmaceutical and biochemical products are spray dried, including antibiotics, enzymes, vitamins, yeasts, vaccines, and plasma.

(ii) It can be used for drying algae, antibiotics and moulds, bacitracin, penicillin, streptomycin, sulphathiazole, tetracycline, dextran, enzymes, hormones, lysine (amino acids), pharmaceutical gums, sera, spores, tableting constituents, vaccines, vitamins, yeast products, tannin products etc.

(iii) Spray drying stands out as unique method in making granules and tablets. The composite particles with good compactibility and excellent micrometric properties as filler for direct tableting of controlled release matrix tablets. It has been used for granulating, for slow-release granulations of magnesium carbonate, theophylline and acetaminophen. The spherical composite particles consisting of amorphous lactose and sodium alginate are prepared by spray drying.

(iv) It can be used in preparing dry powder aerosol formulations.

For example, salbutamol sulphate particles prepared by spray drying, using a mini spray dryer and liposomal ciprofloxacin powder for inhaled aerosol drug delivery.

(v)   It can be used in preparing micro particles for the preparation of dried liposomes, amorphous drugs, and mucoadhesive microspheres, microcapsules, gastro-resistant microspheres, and controlled-release systems.

(vi) Spray drying has proved extremely useful in the coating and encapsulation of both solids and liquids. Spray-dried micro particles of theophylline were prepared with a coating polymer in an aqueous system.

(vii) Dry emulsions can be prepared by spray drying of various liquid. For example, o/w emulsions containing fractionated coconut oil dispersed in aqueous solutions of HPMC (solid carrier).

(viii) It can also be used to prepare dry elixirs. For example, Flurbiprofen Dry Elixir.

(ix) Non-pharmaceutical applications of spray drying includes drying of various materials in food, chemical and ceramic industry.

For example, detergents, soaps and surface-active agents, pesticides, herbicides, fungicides and insecticides, dyestuffs, pigments, fertilizers, mineral floatation concentrates, inorganic chemicals, organic chemicals, spray concentration (purification), milk products, egg products, food and plant products, fruits, vegetables, carbohydrates and similar products, slaughterhouse products, fish products and many others.

7.8 FLUIDIZED BED DRYER

Fluidized bed dryer (FBD) is well known and widely used equipment in the pharmaceutical manufacturing. It is used in granulation process for drying the material to get desired moisture content in the granules or powders required for perfect compression of tablet formulation. Conventional fluidized bed dryers include batch fluidized bed dryer, semi-continuous fluidized bed dryer, well-mixed continuous fluidized dryer and plug flow fluidized bed dryer.

Principle:

The equipment works on a principle of fluidization of the feed materials. In fluidization process, hot air is introduced at high pressure through a perforated bed of moist solid particulate. If air is allowed to flow through a bed of solid powdered material in the upward direction with the velocity greater than the settling rate of the particles, the solid particles are blown-up and remain suspended in the air stream. At this stage, the solid bed looks like the boiling liquid; therefore this stage is called as fluidized. Heat transfer is accomplished by direct contact between the wet solid and hot gases. Use of hot air for fluidizing the bed increases the drying rate of the material. The vaporized liquid is carried away by the drying gases. Sometimes to save energy, the exit gas is partially recycled.

Construction:

A fluidized bed dryer contains a stainless steel chamber having a removable perforated bottom known as the bowl. A typical FBD consists of the air handling unit, product container, exhaust filter, exhaust blower, control panel, air distribution plate, spray nozzle, and solution deliver. The appropriate choice of distributor used during drying process ensures uniform and stable fluidization. The pressure drops across the distributor must be high enough to ensure good and uniform fluidization.

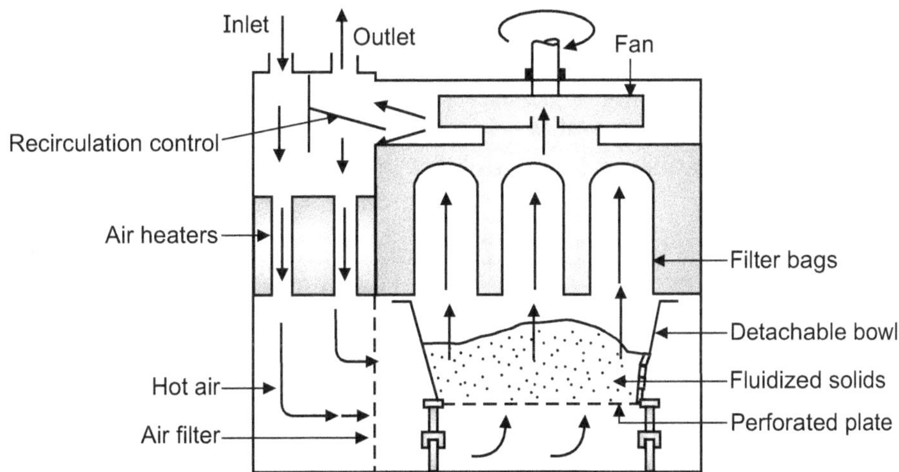

Fig. 7.8: A Typical Vertical Fluidized Bed Dryer

Working:

Material to be dried is placed in the bowl type vessel. Air is introduced from the top and heated at required temperature by the heaters. The air is filtered through the filter and then passes through the bed of the material at the bottom. The airflow is generated by the fans fitted at the top of the equipment. The air flow rate and the operating temperature are adjusted by the control panel. As the flow of air increases, the bed expands and particles of powder start to rise up in a turbulent motion. The regular contact with air causes the material to dry. The air leaving the FBD passes through the filter to collect the fine particles of the material. Fluidized bed dryer has a high drying rate and the material is dried in a very short time. Material remains free-flowing and uniform. FBD bags have finger-like shape to increase the volume of the drying bed that helps to increase the drying rate and decrease the drying time.

Advantages:

(i)   FBD has high rates of moisture removal due to excellent air-particle contact which results in high heat and mass transfer rates thus has fast and homogeneous drying.

(ii)   High thermal efficiency is usually achieved if part of the thermal energy for drying is supplied by the internal heat exchanger.

(iii)   It has low capital and maintenance cost.

(iv)   Minimum contact time for drying is best suited for heat sensitive products.

(v)   FBD is highly efficient in material drying to desired level.

(vi)   Handling FBD is easy due to simple system control panel and thus requires less labour.

(vii)   FBD designs come in a wide range of capacities and sizes.

(viii)   It shows no hot spots on the final products.

(ix)   It is suitable for both continuous and batch material processing.

Disadvantages:

(i)   The high pressure drop requires more energy to suspend particles.

(ii)   Requires increased air handling due to extensive recirculation of exhausts air for high thermal efficiency operation.

(iii)   It has poor fluidization and low flexibility in operation, especially if the feed is too wet.

(iv)   Not the best choice of equipment when organic solvents are to be removed during drying.

(v)   Non-uniform product quality for certain types of materials.

(vi)   There may be entertainment of fine particles.

(vii)   It has high potential for attrition; and in some cases agglomeration of fine particles.

(viii)   The conventional hot air FBD is not a good choice of dryer when handling toxic or flammable solids since there is danger of fire or explosion of flammability limits are exceeded.

(xi) It has a possibility of product loss.

(x) There are high chances of electrostatic force build-up.

(xi) Using FBD drying of sticky material is quite difficult.

Applications:

(i) Fluidized bed dryers are used in chemical, pharmaceutical, food, dairy, metallurgical, dyes and other process industries for drying of powders, mixing of powders and agglomeration of various materials such as powders, tablets, granules, coals, fertilizers, plastic materials etc.

(ii) This process being fast is used in granulation of pharmaceutical powders.

(iii) Fluidized bed coaters are used widely used for coating of powders, granules, tablets, pellets, beads that are held in suspension by column of air.

(iv) FBD is used for several purposes, such as fluidized bed reactors (types of chemical reactors), solids separation, fluid catalytic cracking, fluidized bed combustion, heat or mass transfer or interface modification, such as applying a coating onto solid items.

(v) The three types (Top spray, Bottom spray, Tangential spray) of FBD are mainly used for aqueous or organic solvent-based polymer film coatings.

(vi) Top-spray fluidized bed coating is used for taste masking, enteric release and barrier films on particles/tablets. Bottom spray coating is used for sustained release and enteric release and Tangential spray coating is used for SR and enteric coating products.

(vii) FBD is efficiently employed for applications in chemical, pharmaceutical, dyestuff, foodstuff, dairy and various other process industries with the spray dryers and granulation systems for effective drying, mixing, granulation, finishing and cooling of powdered substances.

(viii) It has been preferred over rotary dryers for drying and cooling a wide range of polymer materials which require precise control of residence time and temperature for effective processing.

(ix) It is used for drying moist dibasic calcium phosphate anhydrous (DCPA).

(x) It is suitable for the formulation, development and production of clinical materials.

(xi) The modified versions of FBD are used as precision granulators, top spray granulators, spray drying granulator and granulator coater.

(xii) Various types of modified fluidized bed dryers have been developed and are applied in many industrial processes to overcome some of the problems encountered while using conventional fluidized bed dryer and for a drying process.

(A) Batch Type FBD:

(i) **Reverse turning bed type:** In this FBD, by turning the air dispersion plate (the reverse turning bed) in 90° direction with the control motor, all the dried material can be discharged at once.

(ii) Rotating discharge type: Dried material is discharged by opening the discharge gate equipped at the side of the dryer. Since the perforated plate is used as the air dispersion plate, the air inside the equipment whirls and pushes the dried material out from the discharge gate.

Example: Vertical FBD with granulating option

Characteristics of batch FBD:

(i)   The residence period of the dried material can be controlled which results in uniform drying.

(ii) It is most suitable in case where an accurate control of the residence period is required at the decreasing rate drying zone.

(iii) Small destruction of particle occurs therefore suitable for granular or crystallized material.

(iv) Easy operation can be achieved by an automatic control of material feeding, drying discharging etc.

(v)   When multiple stage system is adopted, the exhaust air heat can be used efficiently.

(B) Continuous Type FBD:

Residence time in any drying zone is dependent on length of the zone, the frequency and the amplitude of the vibration and use of dams. Heat transfer units such as tube or plate are built inside the equipment. These units supply 60-80 % heat necessary for drying.

Example: Horizontal vibrating conveyor fluid bed dryer

Characteristics of continuous FBD:

(i)   The materials with relative high moisture content can be dried.

(ii)   At and after a second drying chamber piston flowability can be achieved by arranging numbers of the partition plates as per the required residence period.

(iii) The perforated plate at the fixed direction ensures easy discharging.

(iv)   It causes small destruction of particles and thus are suitable for drying granules or crystalline materials.

(v)   In multiple zone, fluid bed dryers heating and cooling occurs in same unit.

(vi)   Each zone has independent control for temperature, dew point and velocity of air.

(vii) By adjusting the weir height for each zone, residence time can vary up to four fold in the unit.

7.8.1 Vacuum Dryer

Vacuum drying is a viable technology used successfully for many years in the pharmaceutical, food, plastics and textile industries. It is an indirect-heat dryer and best used for drying heat sensitive materials at comparatively low temperature. These materials are dried by applying vacuum to evaporate the water or solvent. The use of vacuum lowers down the environmental pressure and hence lowers the boiling point of solvents and hence this process is known as vacuum drying. The combination of heat and vacuum together is very effective source of the drying at relatively lower temperature. The moisture content in the material dried via vacuum dryers is comparatively lower to those of normal dryers without vacuum.

Principle:

Vacuum drying is the mass transfer operation in which the moisture present in wet solid is removed by means of creating a vacuum. The principle involved is creating a vacuum to decrease the pressure below the vapour pressure of the water. With the help of vacuum pumps, the pressure is reduced around the substance to be dried. This decreases the boiling point of water inside that product and thereby increases the rate of evaporation significantly. The result is a significantly increased drying rate of the product. The pressure maintained in vacuum drying is generally 0.0296 –0.059 atmospheres and the boiling point of water is 25 - 30 °C. The vacuum drying process is a batch operation performed at reduced pressures and lower relative humidity compared to ambient pressure, enabling faster drying.

Construction:

In the pharmaceutical industry vacuum dryer is also known as vacuum oven. Vacuum dryers are made-up of stainless steel or cast iron so that they can bear the high vacuum pressure without any kind of deformation. The oven is divided into hollow trays which increases the surface area for heat conduction. The oven door is locked air tight and is connected to vacuum pump to reduce the pressure. Heat is usually supplied by passing steam or hot water through hollow shelves.

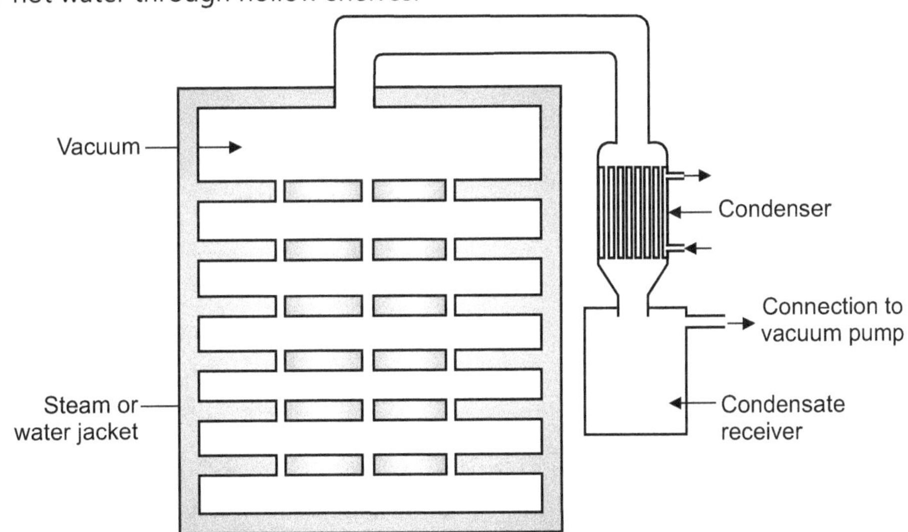

Fig. 7.9: Vacuum Dryer

Working:

The materials to be dried are kept on the trays inside the vacuum dryer and pressure is reduced by means of vacuum pump. The dryer door is tightly shut and steam is passed through the space between trays and jacket so that the heat transfer occurs by conduction. Water vapours from the feed are sent into the condenser. After drying vacuum pump is disconnected and the dried product is collected from the trays. The reduced pressure lowers the heat needed for rapid drying. Drying temperatures can be carefully controlled and, for the major part of the drying cycle, the material remains at the boiling point of the wetting agent. Drying times are long, usually about 12 to 48 h. The heat is transferred to the material as it contacts the dryer's heated surface, drying the material by conduction.

Advantages:

(i) Vacuum dryers offer low temperature drying of thermolabile materials and are suitable for solvent recovery from solid products containing solvents.

(ii) Materials can be dried in final containers or enclosures with removing large amount of moisture compared to normal dryers.

(iii) Average drying temperature is much lower than normal standard dryers and the quality of dried material is much better than that of the normal dryers.

(iv) Drying action becomes faster as heat is easily transferred throughout the body of the dryers, due to its large surface area.

(v) A major advantage is its energy conservation. It requires less energy for drying, cutting down on the economic and environmental costs associated with drying a product for storage, sale or other purposes.

(vi) Vacuum-drying processes also tend to work faster than other drying methods, cutting down on processing times.

(vii) Another advantage of drying materials using this dryer is that it is a less damaging drying process. Vacuum drying tends to retain the integrity of the original item without damaging it with heat.

(viii) It is predominately a batch unit operation however it can be integrated as continuous process.

(ix) This equipment reduces risks to workers from vented fumes and particles that can usually make people sick or that force people to wear protective garments while operating other dryers.

Disadvantages:

(i) In general vacuum drying process is batch type drying process with low efficiency.

(ii) Vacuum dryers are expensive in terms of its cost and there is requirement of skilled labour to operate it.

(iii) Cost of maintenance is comparatively high.

(iv) Its upper temperature limit (typically about 600 °F) is lower than that of a direct-heat dryer. Thus the rate at which material temperature can be raised in a vacuum dryer is also limited. The vacuum pump is primarily responsible for the vacuum level inside the dryer.

Applications:

The following examples describes areas in which vacuum-drying is employed.

  (i) Type of industries: Vacuum drying equipment has many applications across most industrial sectors such as chemical, pharmaceutical, food and plastics.

 (ii) Type of operation: It is typically used for batch operation as it removes water or removes and recovers solvents from a moist material.

(iii) Changing physical state: It can be used to change a material's molecular and physical chemistry (called a phase change) in specialized operations such as chemical reactions and polymer solid stating.

 (iv) Separation: It is typically used for separating volatile liquid by vaporization from a powder, cake, slurry, or other moist material.

  (v) Indirect-heat drying: The heat is transferred to the material as it contacts the dryer's heated surface, drying the material by conduction.

 (vi) Safety: With a vacuum dryer, ventilation does not require and personnel working near the dryer are safer. It is also possible to recover the precipitated moisture collected during the drying for further use.

(vii) Drying pharmaceuticals: It is used in the preparation of mouth-dissolving tablets and granules of nimesulide, camphor, crospovidone and lactose by a wet granulation. Camphor sublimes from the granules by exposure to vacuum. The porous granules are compressed to get superior tablets.

(viii) Drying proteins: Vacuum-drying overcome long processing times (typically 3–5 d), and the inherent steps in freeze drying that lead to instabilities in the protein structure. Due to the complex structural properties, proteins have a tendency to denature and undergo irreversible aggregation during various processing steps of freeze drying. Vacuum drying is used in the formulation of proteins as dry powders using mannitol as the bulking agent.

 (ix) Drying bacteria: Normally, probiotic bacterial strains and starter cultures are dry-frozen to preserve them until use. It consumes a very high amount of energy and some bacterial strains do not survive temperatures below 0 °C. Thus low-temperature vacuum drying can be used to dry probiotic at moderate temperatures above 0°C without causing too much damage to the cell structure.

  (x) Vaccines and other injectable: Freeze drying involves use of vacuum to produce pharmaceutical products. Freeze-drying is used to increase the shelf life of products, such as vaccines and other injectable. By removing water from the material and sealing the material in a vial under vacuum, the material can be easily stored, shipped, and later reconstituted to its original form for injection.

7.8.2 Freeze Dryer

Freeze drying, also called lyophilization, is a process in which water is frozen, followed by its removal from the sample, initially by sublimation followed by desorption. The equipment used to dry solutions or suspensions at or below freezing points of liquids is called as freeze dryer or lyophilizer. This drying process utilized in the manufacture of pharmaceuticals and biologicals that are thermolabile or otherwise unstable in aqueous solutions for prolonged storage periods, but that are stable in the dry state.

Principle:

The main principle involved in freeze drying is a phenomenon called sublimation, where water passes directly from solid state (ice) to the vapour state without passing through the liquid state. Sublimation of water can take place at pressures and temperature below triple point of water (4.579 mm of Hg and 0.0099 °C). The material to be dried is first frozen and then subjected under a high vacuum to heat (by conduction or radiation or by both) so that frozen liquid sublimes leaving only non-volatile solid, dried components of the original liquid. The concentration gradient of water vapour between the drying front and condenser is the driving force for removal of water during freeze drying.

Construction:

Generally, there are three types of freeze dryers. There are manifold freeze-dryer, the rotary freeze dryer and the tray style freeze-dryer. The components common to all of them are a vacuum pump to reduce the ambient gas pressure in a vessel containing the substance to be dried and a condenser to remove the moisture by condensation on a surface cooled to − 20 to − 80°C. The manifold, rotary and tray type freeze-dryers differ in the method by which the dried substance is interfaced with a condenser.

(a) In manifold freeze-dryers a short usually circular tube is used to connect multiple containers with the dried product to a condenser.

(b) The rotary freeze-dryers have a single large reservoir for the dried substance. Rotary freeze-dryers are usually used for drying pellets, cubes and other pourable substances. The rotary dryers have a cylindrical reservoir that is rotated during drying to achieve a more uniform drying throughout the substance.

(c) The tray freeze-dryers also have a single large reservoir for the dried substance. They usually have rectangular reservoir with shelves on which products, such as pharmaceutical solutions and tissue extracts, can be placed in trays, vials and other containers.

A freeze dryer consists of a vacuum chamber wherein product to be dried are kept on shelves and capable of cooling and heating containers and their contents. A vacuum pump, a refrigeration unit, and associated controls are connected to the vacuum chamber.

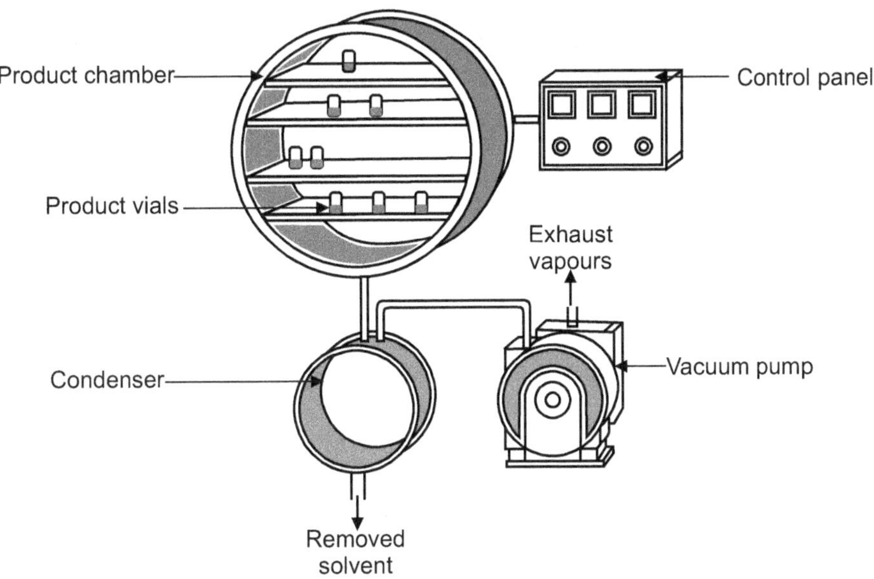

Fig. 7.10: A Typical Freeze Dryer

Working:

Traditional freeze drying is a complex process that requires a careful balancing of product, equipment, and processing techniques. In this process water is removed from a product after it is frozen and placed under a vacuum, allowing the ice to change directly from solid to vapour without passing through a liquid phase. It is performed at temperature and pressure conditions below the triple point of liquid, to enable sublimation of frozen material. The entire process is performed at low temperature and pressure. Steps involved in lyophilization start from sample preparation followed by freezing, primary drying and secondary drying, to obtain the final dried product. The concentration gradient of water vapour between the drying front and condenser is the driving force for removal of water during lyophilization. The vapour pressure of water increases with an increase in temperature during the primary drying. Therefore, primary drying temperature should be kept as high as possible, but below the critical process temperature, to avoid a loss of cake structure.

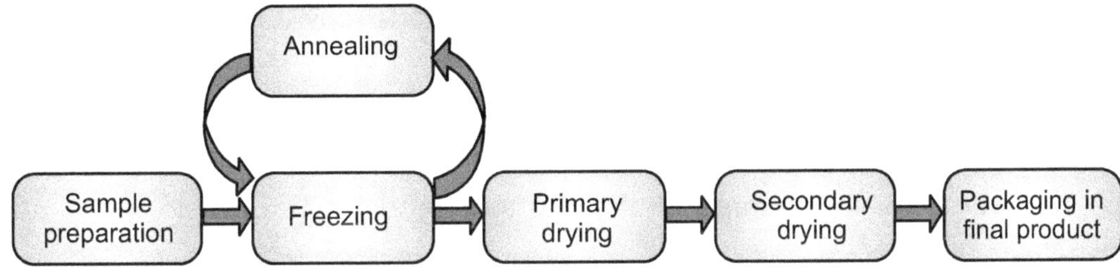

Fig. 7.11: Freeze Drying Cycle- Sequence of Operational Steps

There are four important stages in the complete freeze drying process namely pretreatment, freezing, primary drying and secondary drying.

(i) Pretreatment: In this stage product is treated for freeze concentration, solution phase concentration, preserve product appearance, stabilize reactive products, increase surface area, and decrease high vapour pressure solvents concentration prior to freezing. In many instances the decision to pre-treat a product is based on theoretical knowledge of freeze-drying and its requirements, or is demanded by cycle time or product quality considerations.

(ii) Freezing: During freezing stage the liquid sample is cooled down to -40 to $-60\,°C$ until pure crystalline ice forms from part of the liquid and the remainder of the sample is freeze-concentrated into a glassy state where the viscosity is too high to allow further crystallization.

(iii) Primary drying: In primary drying the ice formed during the freezing is removed by sublimation under vacuum at low temperatures, leaving a highly porous structure in the remaining amorphous solute that is typically 10% water. This step is carried out at pressures of 10^{-4} to 10^{-5} atmospheres, and a product temperature of -45 to $-20\,°C$. The sublimation during primary drying is the result of coupled heat- and mass-transfer processes.

(iv) Secondary drying: This is last step wherein most of the remaining water is desorbed from the glass as the temperature of the sample is gradually increased upto 10 - 15 °C while maintaining low pressures. Ideally, the final product is a dry, easily reconstituted cake with a high surface area and low moisture content (below 5% w/w).

Advantages:

(i)   Oxidizable substances are well protected under vacuum conditions.

(ii)   Long drying period owing to 95%-99.5% water removal.

(iii) Loaded quantities are accurate and has content uniformity.

(iv)   Little contamination owing to aseptic process.

(v)   Minimal loss in volatile chemicals and heat-sensitive nutrient and fragrant components.

(vi)   Minimal changes in the properties because microbe growth and enzyme effect can not be exerted under low temperature.

(vii) Transportation and storage of thermostable products is possible under normal temperature.

(viii) Rapid reconstitution time, usually less than 10 sec.

(ix)   Constituents of the dried material remain homogenously dispersed.

(x)   Sterility of product can be achieved and maintained.

Disadvantages:

(i) Removing volatile compounds may require high vacuum.

(ii) Most expensive unit operation.

(iii) Stability problems such as low temperature stress are associated with individual drugs.

(iv) There are some issues associated with sterilization and sterility assurance of the dryer chamber and aseptic loading of vials into the chamber.

Applications:

(i) Pharmaceutical companies often use freeze-drying to increase the shelf life of products, such as vaccines and other injectable.

(ii) By removing the water from the material and sealing the material in a vial under vacuum, the material can be easily stored, shipped, and later reconstituted to its original form for injection.

(iii) Freeze-drying is used to preserve biologicals and make it very light weight.

(iv) It is used to preserve blood products in freeze-dried form.

(v) It is used in chemical synthesis where products are often freeze dried to make them more stable, or easier to dissolve in water for subsequent use.

(vi) As freeze-drying can effectively remove solvents that can be used in bio-separations as a late-stage of purification procedure.

(vii) In addition, it is capable of concentrating substances with low molecular weights that are too small to be removed by a filtration membrane.

REVIEW QUESTIONS

1. What is drying? What are its objectives?

2. Give pharmaceutical and other applications of drying.

3. Discuss in detail mechanism of drying process.

4. What are various types of moistures? Define them.

5. What is equilibrium moisture content? How it is determined? What are its applications in drying?

6. Write note on rate of drying.

7. Discuss in detail drying curve and its parts. What is importance of knowing CMC?

8. Classify drying equipments used in pharmaceutical industries.

9. Discuss in details principle, construction, working, advantages, disadvantages and applications of either of following dryers.

    (a) Tray dryer

    (b) Drum dryer

    (c) Spray dryer

    (d) Fluidized bed dryer

    (e) Vacuum dryer

    (f) Freeze dryer.

10. What are stages of freeze drying? Explain them in detail.

11. Explain what makes vacuum dryer superior to conventional dryers.

12. Compare principle working and applications of single drum and double drum dryer.

13. Discuss "FBD is most commonly used dryer in pharmaceutical manufacturing".

☙ ☙ ☙

Chapter ...8

MIXING

8.0 INTRODUCTION

In pharmaceutical processing mixing involves certain heterogeneous components to be manipulated with the intent to make them more homogeneous. The term mixing is defined as a process that results in randomization of dissimilar particles within a system. Mixing is defined as an operation in which two or more components in a separate roughly mixed condition are treated so that each particle lies as nearly as possible in contact with a particle of each of the other ingredient. Mixing may be performed between any two phases ranging from mobile liquids to viscous liquids, semi-solids and solids. It is performed to allow heat and/or mass transfer to occur between one or more streams, components or phases. Even modern industrial processing involves chemical reactors as mixers. Mixing can be between one component with different particle size.

The operation opposite to the mixing is 'segregation'. The terms 'mixing' and 'blending' are often used synonymously, but technically they are a bit different. Blending is a process of combining materials, but is a relatively gentle process compared to mixing. In terms of the phase of material, blending is the process of solid-solid mixing or mixing of bulk solids with small quantity of liquid whereas mixing is more closely associated with liquid-liquid, gas-liquid, and viscous materials.

Mixing and blending are the most demanding unit operations in the pharmaceutical, chemical and food process industries. For example, chemical process industries involves mixing and blending of specialty chemicals, explosives, fertilizers, dry powdered detergents, glass or ceramics, and rubber compounds. Pharmaceutical industry employs blending of active ingredients of a drug with excipients like starch, cellulose, or lactose whereas in food industry preparation of cake mix, spices, and flavours. In practice mixing is a critical process because the quality of the final product and its attributes are derived by the quality of the mix. Improper mixing results in a non-homogenous product that lacks consistency with respect to desired attributes like chemical composition, colour, texture, flavour, reactivity, and particle size.

With the proper equipment selection it is possible to mix a solid, liquid or gas into another solid, liquid or gas. For example, a biofuel fermenter requires mixing of microbes, gases and liquid medium for optimal yield; organic nitration requires concentrated (liquid) nitric and sulfuric acids to be mixed with a hydrophobic organic phase whereas production of pharmaceutical tablets requires blending of solid powders. The wide variety and ever increasing complexity of mixing processes encountered in industrial applications requires careful selection of design, and scale-up to ensure effective and efficient mixing. Improved mixing efficiency leads to shorter batch cycle times and operational costs. In order to increase productivity and survive in today's competition there is a need of selecting robust equipment capable of fast blend times, lower power consumption, equipment flexibility, ease of cleaning and other customized features. In addition to blending components, many modern mixers are designed to combine different process steps such as coating, granulation, heat transfer and drying, in single equipment etc.

Agitation is the process of keeping a mixture that has been mixed in the proper mixed state required for the 'end' product. Mixing refers to the actual stirring of different liquids and/or materials to blend them together into an end product or mixture. Once this mixture is 'mixed' it may require agitation to keep the mixture in the proper 'mixed' state.

Generally mixing can lead to three types of mixtures that are fundamentally different in their behaviours:

(i) **Positive mixtures:** Positive mixtures formed when two or more components are irreversibly mixed together by diffusion process. In this case no energy input is required and the time allowed for the components to mix is sufficient. In addition, these types of materials do not create any problem during their mixing process.

(ii) **Negative mixtures:** Negative mixtures are formed when components are mixed to form a heterogeneous system, for example, emulsion or suspension. The components of these mixtures have high tendency to separate out as they are not continuously being stirred. Thus, such mixtures are more difficult to prepare as they need high degree of mixing with external force.

(iii) **Neutral mixtures:** Neutral mixtures are stable in behavior. The components of these mixtures do not have tendency to mix spontaneously but once mixed, they do not separate out easily. Pharmaceutical products such as pastes, ointments and mixed powders are the examples of neutral mixture.

8.1 OBJECTIVES

The aim of mixing is to ensure that there is uniformity of composition between the mixed ingredients that represent overall composition of the mixture. The primary objective of mixing is to make homogeneous product using the minimum amount of energy and time. The other objectives are as follows:

(i) **To produce single physical mixture:** This may be simply the production of a blend of two or more miscible liquids or two or more uniformly divided solids. In pharmaceutical practice the degree of mixing must commonly be of high order as many of such mixtures are dilutions of active substances and must be in accurate amount for dose uniformity in dosage forms.

(ii) **To produce physical change:** Mixing can be performed to produce physical as well as chemical change, for example, solution of a soluble substance. In such cases a lower efficiency of mixing is often acceptable because mixing merely accelerates a dissolution and diffusion process that could occur by simply agitation.

(iii) **To produce dispersion:** Mixing is also aimed to include dispersion of two immiscible liquids to form an emulsion or dispersion of a solid in liquid to give a suspension or paste. Usually good mixing is required to ensure stability and effectiveness.

(iv) **To promote chemical reaction:** Mixing encourage and at the same time control a chemical reaction. Mixing ensures uniform product such as reactions where accurate adjustment to pH is required and the degree of mixing will decide the possibility of reaction.

Mixing fulfills many objectives beyond simple combination of raw ingredients. These include preparing fine emulsions, reducing particle size, carrying out chemical reactions, manipulating rheology, dissolving components, facilitating heat transfer etc. So even within a single pharmaceutical product line, it is a common practice to employ a number of different style mixers to process raw ingredients, handle intermediates and prepare the finished product.

8.2 APPLICATIONS

(i) **Dry mixing:** Mixing help various powders to be mixed in varying proportions prior to granulation or tableting. Dry mixing of the materials makes them suitable for direct compression in to tablets.

(ii) **Product features:** The mixing help to deliver accurate dosage that has an acceptable appearance and texture, or to maintain formulation stable for the appropriate length of time. The importance of proper mixer selection and its optimal operation can hardly be over-estimated.

(iii) **Dry blending:** Mixing is used for dry blending in the manufacture of many vitamins, dietary supplements and drugs in powders (insufflations, face powders, and tooth powders), capsules and tablets. Dry blending operation combines the active ingredient with other solid excipients in most appropriate way. Sometimes relatively small amounts of liquid may be added to the solids in order to coat or absorb colouring and flavouring agents, oils or other solutions.

(iv) **Emulsions:** Throughout the pharmaceutical industry, high shear mixing is widely used in the preparation of emulsions such as creams and medicated lotions.

(v) **Heterogeneous mixtures:** Mixing is used when different powders behave differently when added into liquid, and some require more coaxing in order to dissolve, hydrate or disperse completely than others. The 'easier' ones need only gentle agitation but more challenging powders needs higher speed devices that generate a powerful vortex into which the powders are added for faster wet-out.

(vi) Tough agglomerates: It is used to deal solids that tend to form tough agglomerates which do not easily break apart. A high shear mixer is often used to resolve such issues and many solutions and dispersions are made. For example, tablet coatings, vaccines and disinfectants.

(vii) Fluid blending: Mixing is used for continuous blending of fluid streams, emulsification, and dispersion of gases into liquid, pH control, dilution and heat exchange. A static mixer is unique with no moving part that relies on external pumps to move the fluids through it. For example, dissolution of soluble solids in viscous liquids for dispensing in soft capsules and in the preparation of syrups.

(viii) Viscous fluids: Mixing is used for batch mixing of viscous formulations. Mixers are used in the pharmaceutical industry for batch manufacturing of moderate to relatively high viscosity applications such as syrups, suspensions, pastes, creams, ointments and gels.

(ix) Uniformity in size distribution: Mixing helps in particle size distribution and other related parameters which depends on cycle time and mixer design. Thus selection of proper mixer along with product chemistry, operating temperature, pressure/vacuum conditions, quality of raw materials, presence of additives etc. help to obtain appropriate product features.

8.3 FACTORS AFFECTING MIXING

There are factors that can influence the efficiency of mixing leading to non-uniform distribution of materials which can result in inaccurate dosage production. These factors are as follows:

(i) Material density: If the mixture components are of different density, the denser material will sink through the lighter one, the effect of which will depend on the relative positions of the material in the mixer. To maximize mixing, the denser material is placed at lower layer in the mixer during the mixing process so as to enhance degree of mixing to equilibrium state.

(ii) Particle size: Different particle sizes in materials to be mixed can cause segregation that lead to non-uniform distribution. The smaller particles fall within the voids between the lager particles. During mixing process the particles in bed might dilate and the greater porosity of open packing allows a large particle to slip into void that eventually results in non-uniform distribution. As the particle size increases, flow properties also increases due to the influence of gravitational force on the size. It is easier to mix two powders having approximately the same particle size.

(iii) Particle shapes: The particles with spherical shape are easier to mix uniformly whereas other shape particles face increase in difficulty in mixing process. The ideal particle is spherical in shape, and further the particles depart from this theoretical form, there is greater difficulty of mixing. If the particles are of irregular shapes, then they can become interlocked leading to a decrease in the risk of segregation once mixing has been achieved.

(iv) Particle attraction: Some particles exert attractive forces due to adsorbed liquid films or electrostatic charges on their surfaces and tends to aggregate. Since these are surface properties, the aggregation increases as particle size decreases. The interaction forces between drug and carrier surface are predominately van der Waals' forces, but electrostatic and capillary forces may also play a role. These forces vary with the size, shape, crystallinity, hardness of the adhering particle, surface roughness and contamination of the carrier particles, the intensity and duration of shear forces during mixing and the relative humidity.

(v) Proportion of materials: The proportion of substances in a given mixture is one of the crucial factors that result in the efficacy of mixing. The proportions of materials to be mixed play a very important role in powder mixing. It is easy to mix the powders if they are available in equal quantities but it is difficult to mix small quantities of powders with large quantities of other ingredients or diluents. However, to ensure uniform mixing, the substance should be mixed in geometric and ascending order of their weights.

(vi) Mixer volume: In mixing process, the mixer must reserve sufficient space for dilation of bed during mixing process. If this condition is maintained the powder samples are getting enough space for the free mixing to achieve uniform mix with increased efficacy. Overfilling reduces the efficiency and may prevent mixing entirely.

(vii) Mixing mechanisms: The suitable and sufficient shear force and a convective movement is prime requirement for the mixer to ensure efficient mixing of bulk material. The mixer selected based on its mechanism must apply suitable shear forces to bring about local mixing as well as convective movement to ensure that the bulk of the material passes through this area.

(viii) Mixing time: Mixing must be carried out for an appropriate time so that the degree of mixing will approach its limiting equilibrium value. Since, there is an optimum time for mixing of any particular mixture it must be noted that the equilibrium condition may not represent the best mixing if there is segregation. While handling uniformly mixed powders after completion of operation enough care need to be taken to avoid segregation. The vibration caused by subsequent handling, transport or during use is likely to cause segregation.

(ix) Method of handling: When mixing is completed, the product is required to be handled according to standard operating procedures to minimize the risk of segregation. A common factor that causes segregation is vibration throughout the handling, transport, or packaging. This results into fact that all bulk powder should undergo remixing before taking them into use.

(x) Nature of the product: Rough surface of the powder components may result in to ineffective mixing. The active substances which are generally very fine in size may enter into the pores and cavities on the surfaces of the other larger ingredients.

If such substances get adsorbed on the surface of other powders there is decrease in aggregation as well as segregation. For example, addition of colloidal silica to strongly aggregating zinc oxide help to maintain fine dusting powder that can be easily mixed.

(xi) Mixing Conditions: The theory of powder mixing shows four conditions that should be observed in the mixing operation. Those conditions affects mixing.

8.4 DIFFERENCE BETWEEN SOLID AND LIQUID MIXING

Industrial applications involve mixing of solids to solids such as free flowing solids to pasty materials, solids to liquids, and solids to gas, liquids to liquids, and liquids to gas.

Liquid mixing	Solid mixing
(i) Fluid mixing is generally associated with liquid – liquid mixing and liquid-gas mixing.	(i) Mixing of solids to some extent resembles the mixing of low-viscosity liquids.
(ii) Liquid mixing depends on the creation of flow currents, which transport unmixed material to the mixing zone adjacent to the impeller.	(ii) In heavy masses of particulate solids there are no such currents possible and mixing is accomplished by some other means.
(iii) Power required for mixing and blending of liquids is less.	(iii) Power required for mixing of dry solids is comparatively higher.
(iv) In liquid mixing, a well-mixed product is usually a truly homogenous liquid phase.	(iv) In solid mixing the product often consists of two or more easily identifiable phases, each of which may contain individual particles of considerable size.
(v) A "well-mixed" liquid product samples are homogenous in nature.	(v) A "well-mixed" solid product samples differ markedly in composition.
(vi) Design, construction and operation of fluid mixing equipment are specific and are termed as liquid agitators.	(vi) Design, construction and operation of solid mixing equipment are different than liquids and are commonly referred to as mixers and blenders.
(vii) The liquid mixing technology has been extensively studied and understood.	(vii) The understanding of solid mixing, and the design of solid mixers is an art rather than a science.
(viii) The liquid mixing technology is simple.	(viii) Solid mixing is more complex.

8.5 MECHANISMS OF MIXING

In general mixing involves one or more of the following mechanisms:

Convective Mixing: Convective mixing is a process of transferring groups of particles in bulk from one part of powder bed to another. It is also known as micro-mixing and is regarded as analogous to bulk transport. Depending on the type of mixer employed, convective mixing may occur by an inversion of the powder bed or by means of blades and paddles or by means of a revolving screw, or by any other method of moving a relatively large mass of material from one part of the powder bed to another.

Shear Mixing: During this process, shear forces are created within the mass of material by using agitator arm or a blast of air. As a result of forces within the particulate mass slip and planes are set-up. Depending on the flow characteristics of the powder, these can occur singly or in such a way as to give rise to laminar flow. When shear occurs between regions of different composition and parallel to their interface, it reduces the scale of segregation by thinning the dissimilar layers. Shear that occurs in a direction normal to the interface of such layers is effective as it also reduces the scale of segregation.

Diffusive mixing: Diffusive mixing is also known as micro mixing. In diffusive mixing, the materials are tilted to ensure that the upper layer slips and diffusion of individual particle take place at the new developed surfaces. This occurs when random motion of particles within a powder bed causes them to change position relative to one another. Such an exchange of positions by single particles results in a reduction of the intensity of segregation. Diffusive mixing occurs at the interfaces of dissimilar regions that undergo shearing and therefore it results from shear mixing. It may also be produced by any form of agitation that results in interparticulate motion.

8.5.1 Solid Mixing

In solid mixing two different dimensions in the mixing process are convective mixing and intensive mixing. In convective mixing material in the mixer is transported from one location to another. This leads to less ordered state inside the mixer. The mixing components are distributed over the other components. With time the mixture becomes more random and after certain time the ultimate random state is reached. This type of mixing is observed for free-flowing and coarse solid materials. Physical properties of material that affects solid mixing are density, particle size and its distribution, wettability, stickiness and particle shape or roughness. Usually these factors contribute for the demixing of macromixed solids. If solids are in fine form with cohesive nature or if it is wet convective mixing is not enough to obtain random state. The relative strong inter-particle forces form lumps. The decrease in size of lump requires more intensive energy which is provided either as impact force or shear force.

8.5.2 Liquid Mixing

The liquid mixing occurs in two stages; first, localized mixing which applies sufficient shear to the particles of the fluid and second, a general movement sufficient to take all parts of the material through the shearing zone and to ensure a uniform final product.

There are four essential mechanisms involved in liquid mixing as follows:

1. **Bulk Transport:** Movement of a relatively large portion of material being mixed from one location in the system to another.

2. **Turbulent flow:** It is characterized by the fluid having different instantaneous velocities at the same instant of time. The temporal and spatial velocity differences resulting from turbulence produce randomization of fluid particles.

3. **Laminar Flow:** In this mechanism a streamline flow is encountered in highly viscous liquids.

4. **Molecular diffusion:** It is a primary mechanism responsible for mixing at the molecular level which results from the thermal motion of molecules. It is governed by Fick's fist law of diffusion that describes concentration gradient across the system as:

$$\frac{dm}{dt} = - DA \frac{dc}{dx} \qquad \qquad ... (7.1)$$

Where, $\dfrac{dm}{dt}$ = Rate of transport of mass across a surface area

D = Diffusion co-efficient

A = Area across which diffusion is occurring

$\dfrac{dc}{dx}$ = Concentration gradient

There is decrease in concentration gradient with time which approaches zero at completion.

Liquid mixing as a process that can either be carried out batch to batch or can be a continuous one. Impellers, air-jets, fluid-jets and baffle mixers are the major types of mixing equipments used for batch mixing. Impellers operate using a combination of radial, axial and tangential flow. These might be classified into two further types, propellers and turbines, the former being used for low viscosity liquids while the latter for high viscosity liquids.

8.5.3 Semisolids Mixing

The mechanisms involved in mixing semi-solids depend on the properties of the material which generally may show considerable variations. Many semi-solids form neutral mixtures having no tendency to segregate although sedimentation may occur. Three most commonly used semi solid mixers are:

(i) **Sigma blade mixer:** This mixer has two blades which operate in a mixing vessel which has a double trough shape. These blades moving at different speeds towards each other. It can be used for products like granulation of wet masses and ointments.

(ii) **Triple-roller mill:** The triple roller has differential speed and narrow clearance between the rollers which develops a high shear over small volumes of semi-solid material. This type of mills are generally used to grind semisolids to achieve complete homogeneity in the material for example, ointments.

(iii) Planetary mixers: This mixer has a mixing arm rotating about its own axis and also about a common axis usually at the centre of the mixing wheel. The blades attached to the arm provide the kneading action, while the narrow passage between the blades and the wall of the container provides shear.

8.6 EQUIPMENTS USED IN PHARMACEUTICAL MIXING

The operation of the mixing equipment may be batch or continuous depending upon the required production capacity, product quality, pre and post mixing equipment condition, type of mixer, etc. The most common classification of mixers is based on the type of dosage form to be handled. Physical properties of materials to be mixed such as density, viscosity and miscibility and economic considerations such as operating efficiency, cost and maintenance are some important factors to be taken into consideration while selecting mixing equipment. Other factors include whether it is intended to be a batch or a continuous process, load to be handled, size for the optimal working volume, fill level and residence time. The optimal working volume generally lies between 50 to 70 % of the total volume of the mixer. Similarly, type of agitator is other important factor which is based on nature of material to be mixed and degree of mixing desired. Following are various agitator types and their respective uses.

    (i)   Ribbon mixer - Powders, granules, some slurries, mainly free flowing.

    (ii)   Paddle mixer - Powders, granules, some slurries, free flowing, light pastes.

    (iii) Sigma mixer - Sticky materials, thick pastes and slurries.

Classification of Mixers:

Mixing equipments are most commonly classified on the basis of type of materials being mixed. The three main classes of mixing equipment are described below:

(i) Blenders: These are mixers used for solid-solid blending. Considering the multitudes of industrial operations that require blending of bulk solids, there are wide ranges of blenders available. Based on the principle mechanism of mixing, mixer blenders are classified as follows:

    (a) Tumbler Blenders: Double cone blender, V-cone blenders, Octagonal blender.

    (b) Convective Blender: Ribbon blender, Paddle blender, Vertical screw blender.

    (c) Fluidization Blenders / Mixers: Plow mixer, Double paddle mixer (Forberg mixer).

(ii) Agitators: These mixers are employed for liquid-liquid and liquid-gas mixing. A variety of processing like blending of miscible liquids, contacting or dispersing of immiscible liquids, dispersing of a gas in a liquid, heat transfer in agitated liquid, dispersion of solids in liquids etc. are carried out in agitated vessels by rotating impellers. The impellers based on the angle that the impeller/agitator blade makes with the plane of impeller rotation are classified as:

    (a) Axial flow impellers: This impeller blade makes an angle of less than 90° with the plane of impeller rotation. As a result the locus of flow occurs along the axis of the impeller (parallel to the impeller shaft).

    For example, marine propellers, pitched blade turbine etc.

(b) Radial flow impellers: The impeller blade in radial flow impellers is parallel to the axis of the impeller. As a result, the radial-flow impeller discharges flow along the impeller radius in distinct patterns.

For example, flat blade turbine, paddle, anchor etc.

(iii) Heavy duty mixers: These mixers are mainly used for viscous and paste type materials. In case of high-viscosity materials, the mixing operation parameters changes from mixer with dominant turbulence (as in liquid agitators) to mixers with dominant viscous drag forces. Some viscous materials exhibit non-Newtonian behaviour. Therefore mixing of such material requires special heavy duty mixers such as double arm mixers, planetary mixers and dual and triple shaft mixers.

8.6.1 Double Cone Blender

Mixing is a common process step in the manufacture of products for industries such as healthcare, food, chemical, cosmetics, detergents, fertilizers and plastics. The double cone blender (DCB) is used to produce homogeneous solid-solid mixture.

Principle:

Double cone blenders are most often used to dry blending of free solids, the solid being blended in these blenders can vary in bulk density and percentage of the total mixture, matter being blended is constantly intermixed as double cone rotates. Normal cycle time is 10 min and can be more or less depending upon the complexity of material being mixed.

Construction:

The main body of this blender consists of two cone-shaped sections welded at their bases to a central cylindrical section. The axis of rotation is perpendicular to the cone axis and passes through the cylindrical section. The driving motor is located at one of the two lateral supports holding the blender body. Double cone blender is made out of stainless steel. All welding are done by Argon Arc Process. This is totally mirror polished from inside and outside. Unit is mounted on mild steel / stainless steel stand fitted with ball bearings. It is available in capacity of 20 L to 3000 L. The conical shape at both ends enables uniform mixing and easy discharge. The cone is statically balanced which protects the gear box and motor from any excessive load.

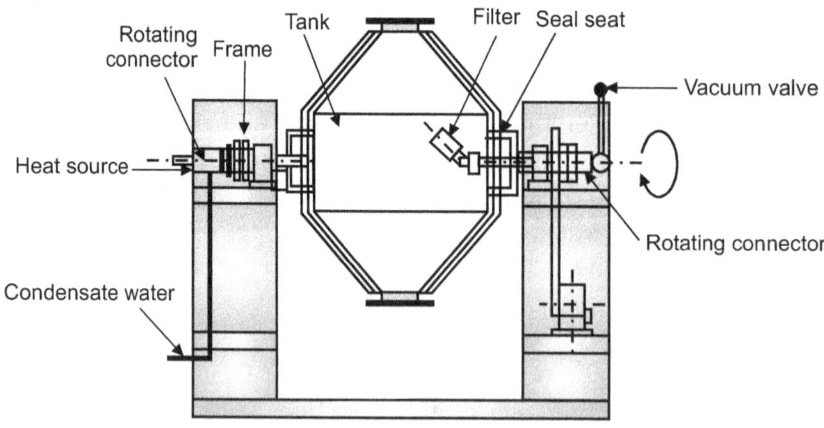

Fig. 8.1: A Double Cone Blender

The suitable size of butter fly valve at one end of the cone is provided for material discharge and hole with openable cover is provided at other end of the cone for material charging and cleaning. The driving arrangement consists of a motor through a reduction gear box and stainless steel baffles which are provided inside the blender. It has variable speed options available. Safety railing along with limit switch and platform are optional features for bigger models. Ancillary provisions include facility for incorporation of a liquid spray system to introduce liquids in spray form during the process. The unit can be equipped with an automated loading system for introducing powders and granules into the blender body by means of a vacuum unit with self-cleaning hoses. It includes a product receiving hopper with an automated self-cleaning filter; as well as a control panel for the unit. The loading/discharge can be carried out with pneumatically actuated retractable hermetic bellows.

Working:

Powdery or granular materials are fed into the double cone containers using vacuum intake system or manual feeding. The continuous rotation of the containers make the material to move in a complex and forceful manner to achieve uniform mixing. The conical shape at both ends contribute in uniform mixing and easy discharge. Depending upon the characteristic of the material, paddle type baffles can be provided on the shaft for better mixing, uniform blending and de-agglomeration. Dust free bin charging system ensures minimum material handling. The solids are introduced into the blender through the loading aperture. The mixing takes place axially, as a result of the powder bed moves through the different sections. Mixing is thorough but it depends on the rotating speed. The mixture is discharged through a hermetically closing butterfly valve which is operated manually or automatically. The blender provides efficient mixing actions when loaded at 50 % of its volume. The effective volume for optimum homogeneity is between 35-70% of gross volume.

Advantages:

(i)   DCB is an efficient and versatile mixer blender with closed container providing good product rolling and cross mixing.

(ii) The 'Slant' design (off center) and conical shape at both ends enables uniform mixing and easy discharge.

(iii) It performs mixing, uniform blending and de-agglomeration functions.

(iv) The cone is statically balanced which protects the gear box and motor from any excessive load.

(v)   Powder loading and discharge are through separate opening.

(vi) Depending upon the characteristic of the product, paddle type baffles can be provided on the shaft for better mixing.

(vii) Contact parts are made of S.S.304 or S.S.316 preventing corrosion and product contamination. It has dust free bin charging system that ensures minimum material handling.

(viii) Additional features such as spay system, loading system, receiving hopper, flame proof electrical fittings can be fitted.

Disadvantages:

(i)   DCB is not suitable for fine powders.

(ii)   Particles with wide variation in size such as fine and large particles cannot be mixed efficiently due to low shear exhibited in this equipment.

(iii) It requires more space and are not suitable for installation in rooms with low ceiling heights.

Applications:

(i)   The DCB are useful for mixing dry powder and granules for tablets and capsules formulations.

(ii)   It is used for dry granules sub lots mixing to increase the batch size at bulk lubrication stage of tablet granules.

(iii) It can be suitable for dry powder to wet mixing.

(iv)   It can be used for pharmaceutical, food, chemical, cosmetic products etc.

(v)   It is suitable for mixing highly flowable powdery and granular materials, with superior mixing quality.

(vi)   It can be suitable for the material mixing in food, essence, dye, chemical, plastic, rubber industry.

(vii) It is suitable for medical intermediate, flavouring, graphite, coffee powder, iron powder whose specific gravity is under 7 g/cm^3 that has certain fluidity with the liquid content under 10%.

8.6.2 Twin Shell Blender

There are three popular shapes of twin shell blenders (also known as a tumble blender), namely; the V-blender, the double cone blender, and the slant cone blender. Tumble type blending is most suited for products of uniform particle size and density, and where requirements for fast, thorough cleaning are desirable for sanitary applications. The V-blender is one of the most commonly used tumbler as they offer both short blending times and efficient blending.

Principle:

Tumble blenders works upon the action of gravity to cause the powder to cascade within a rotating vessel. The primary mechanism of blending in a V-blender is diffusion. Diffusion blending is characterized by small scale random motion of solid particles. Blender movements increase the mobility of the individual particles and thus promote diffusive blending. Diffusion blending occurs where the particles are distributed over a freshly developed interface. In the absence of segregating effects, the diffusive blending lead to a high degree of homogeneity.

Construction:

The V-blender is made of two hollow cylindrical shells joined at an angle of 75° to 90°. A tank formed by two V-shaped cylinders turning around a horizontal shaft ensures a perfect and quick homogenization of the components of the mix. The product enters and exits at the tip of the V easily and without dust. Liquid injection facility may be provided to obtain a granulation of the pre-mixed powder, a coating of the granules or for an automatic cleaning system. A V-blender can be provided with high-speed intensifier bars (or lump breakers) running through trunnion into the vessel, along with spray pipes for liquid addition. The intensifiers disintegrate agglomerates in the charge material or those formed during wet mixing. A schematic drawing of the V-blender with the intensifier bar is shown in Fig. 8.2. The V-blender is offered in many sizes with volume ranging from 0.25 to 100 ft^3 and can be customized with optional features such as vacuum capability, intensifier bar, spray nozzles, heating/cooling jacket, and explosion-proof motor and built-in controls. The heavy-duty models capable of blending very dense materials up to 90 - 100 kg/ft^3 are also available.

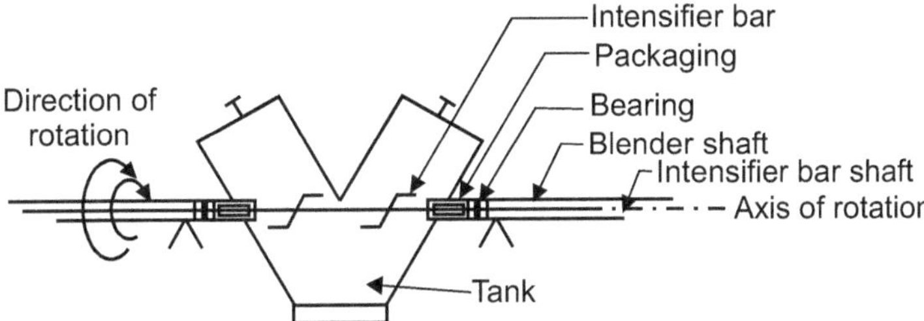

Fig. 8.2: V-Blender with Intensifier Bar

Working:

The charging of material into the V-blender is through either of the two ends or through the apex port. As the V-blender tumbles, the material continuously splits and recombines, with the mixing occurring as the material freely and randomly falls inside the vessel. The repetitive converging and diverging motion of material combined with increased frictional contact between the material and the vessel long straight inner wall surface result in gentle and homogenous blending. In case of monodisperse powders there is no mechanism involved in movement of the powders across the line of symmetry of the blender. For such materials, care must be taken to load each side of the blender equally to ensure desired homogeneity of blends. Blending efficiency is affected by the volume of the material loaded into the blender. The recommended fill-up volume for this blender is 50 to 60% of the total blender volume. For example, if the fill material in the blender is increased from 50% of the total volume to 70% of the total volume, the time required for homogenous blending may be doubled. Blender speed may also be a key to mixing efficiency. At lower blender speeds, the shear forces are low. Though higher blending speeds provide more shear, it can lead to greater dusting resulting in segregation of fines. This means that the fines become air-borne and settle on top of the powder bed once the blender has been stopped. There is also a critical speed which, if approached diminishes blending efficiency considerably. As the revolutions per minute increases, the centrifugal forces at the extreme points of the blender exceeds the gravitation forces required for blending. Consequently, the powder tends to gravitate to the outer walls of the blender shell. As the size of the blender increases, the rotational speed decreases usually in proportion to the peripheral speed of the blender extreme. V-blenders are designed to operate at 50% to 80% of the critical speed. Discharge from the V-blender is normally through the apex port which is fitted with a discharge valve.

Advantages:

(i) Twin shell blenders offers short blending times usually 5 to 15 min and the less space requirements and its efficient homogeneous mixing capability makes it a choice of blender.

(ii) Particle size reduction and attrition are minimized due to the absence of any moving blades. Hence it can be used for fragile materials.

(iii) Charging and discharging of material is easy.

(iv) The shape of blender body such as the sanitary butterfly discharge valve results in a near complete discharge of product.

(v) The absence of shaft projection eliminates product contamination.

(vi) Provision of the intensifier bars makes this blender adaptable for drying as well as wet mixing, and mixing of fines, coarse particle compositions and cohesive powders.

(vii) There is no dust generation during feeding and discharging of the product.

(viii) It is possible to control of the temperature of the product mix and can have provision of injecting a liquid to aid mixing.

(ix) It is suitable for mixing ingredients as low as 5% of the total blend size.

Disadvantages:

(i) They require high head room space for equipment installation and operation.

(ii) They are not suited for blending particles of different sizes and densities which may segregate at the time of discharge.

(iii) Provision of intensifier bars may lead to undesired particle attrition and has intensifier bar shaft sealing and cleaning problems.

(iv) The low mixing shear action limits its use for some very soft powders or granules.

Applications:

(i) V-blenders are used for the dry blending of free flowing solids in pharmaceuticals and nutraceutical industries.

(ii) General applications of V-blenders are in mixing of food products, milk powder, coffee, dry flavours, ceramics powders, pigments, pesticides and herbicides, plastic powders, animal feeds, spice blends, fertilizers, baby foods, cosmetics and polyethylene.

(iii) This type of blender is primarily used for mixing up to 10 ingredients.

8.6.3 Ribbon Mixer Blender

Ribbon blender is a light duty blender mainly used for easy to mix powder components which are pre-processed like dried granules and pre-sieved powders. It is a low shear mixer and mostly used for solid-solid mixing. Solid-liquid mixing can also be achieved when high shearing force is not desired. It occupies less head room space for large volume mixing.

Principle:

Ribbon blenders operate on the combined convection and diffusion mechanisms. Convective mixing is the macro movement of large portions of the solids. Convection mixing occurs when the solids are turned over along the horizontal axis of the agitator assembly. The diffusion mixing involves the micro mixing that occurs when individual particles are moved relative to the surrounding particles. In the ribbon blender diffusion occurs when the particles in front of the ribbon are moved in one direction while nearby particles are not moved or lag behind. Together, these two types of action result in the mixing and blending of solids.

Construction:

A ribbon blender consists of a U-shaped horizontal trough containing a double helical ribbon agitator that rotates within, Fig. 8.3. The agitator's shaft is positioned in the centre of the trough and has welded spokes on which the helical ribbons (also known as spirals) are welded. Since the ribbon agitator consists of a set of inner and outer helical ribbons, it is referred to as a "double" helical ribbon agitator. The gap between the ribbon's outer edge and the internal wall of the container ranges from 3 to 6 mm depending on the application. The internal and external ribbon spirals are pitched to move material axially, in opposing directions as well as radially. This combination promotes fast and thorough blending. The agitator shaft is located within the blender container. A spray pipe for adding liquids is mounted above the ribbons. For materials that tend to form agglomerates during mixing, high speed choppers can be provided for disintegration of the agglomerates.

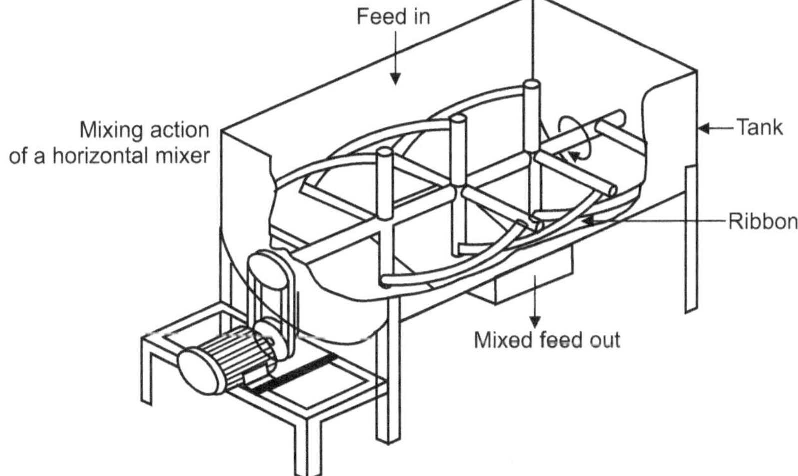

Fig. 8.3: Ribbon Mixer Blender

The ribbon blender is powered by a drive system comprised of a motor, gearbox, and couplings. These blenders are generally powered by 10 - 15 HP motor for 1000 kg of product mass to be blended. The power requirement may range from 3 - 12 kW/m^3 depending on the products to be blended. Top speeds is in the range of 300 feet/min are typical. The agitator shaft exits the blender container at either end, through the end plates bolted or welded to the container. The area where the shaft exits the container is provided with a sealing arrangement to ensure that material does not travel from the container to the outside and vice-versa. The blender assembly along with the drive system components viz. motor, gearbox, couplings and bearing supports is mounted on a supporting frame.

Working:

The feed material is charged in the blender through nozzles or feed-hoppers mounted on the top cover of the blender. The material is loaded by typically filling 40 and 70 % of the total volume of the container. This is generally up to the level of the outer ribbon's tip. The ribbon agitator is designed to operate at a peripheral speed (also known as tip speed) of approximately 100 m/min, depending on the application and the size of the equipment. During the blending operation, the outer ribbons of the agitator move the material from the ends to the center while the inner ribbons move the material from the center to ends. Radial movement is achieved by rotational motion of the ribbons. The difference in the peripheral speeds of the outer and inner ribbons results in axial movement of the material along the horizontal axis of the blender. As a result of the radial and the counter-current axial movement, homogenous blending is achieved in short time. Blending is generally achieved within 15 - 20 min of start-up with a 90 - 95 % or better homogeneity. The particle size and its bulk density have the strongest influence on the mixing efficiency of the ribbon blender. Ingredients with uniform particle size and bulk densities tend to mix faster as compared to ingredients with variation in these attributes.

After blending, the material is discharged from a discharge valve located at the bottom of the trough. The discharge can be fitted with any of various valves, viz. slide-gate, butterfly, and flush bottom, spherical and other types depending on the application. The operation of the valves can be manual or pneumatically actuated. Ribbon blenders can be designed for multiple discharge ports. In a ribbon blender the material is discharged by rotation of the ribbon agitator. It is practically difficult to achieve 100% discharge in the ribbon blender. A higher clearances between the external periphery of the outer ribbon and the container can result in unmixed spots at the trough bottom and can lead to discharge problems.

Advantages:

(i) Ribbon blender is used for solid-solid mixing with relatively fast blending cycles with reproducible product quality.

(ii) It requires very little maintenance even when subjected to frequent product changeovers.

(iii) It is a cost saving blender and is versatile in application to blend solids in combination with its ability to perform heating, cooling, coating, and other processes that makes it a very popular blender.

(iv)   Ribbon blenders can be designed to operate in both batch and continuous modes and can have huge built up capacities of 50 m^3.

(v)   It protects motor and ribbon blender from overload. When the load is too large to block and rotate, the working liquid is ejected from the fusible plug to separate the working machine and the load, so that the motor and equipment will not be damaged when starting and overloading.

(vi)   This blender has stable start load features for the operation and for effective isolation of the impact and torsional vibration of the equipment.

(vii)   When overloaded, the working liquid does not spatter.

(viii) Hydraulic lift is stable, flexible and easy to operate and maintain, guide, safe and reliable.

(ix)   It is a small vibration mixing system with low noise.

Disadvantages:

(i)   In this mixing equipment the power consumption and mixing time is very high.

(ii)   The efficiency or effectiveness of mixing is lower than other type of mixers.

(iii)   The hydraulic coupler is not loaded with the inverter in general, and cannot adjust the rotating speed of the ribbon blender effectively.

(iv)   Although the loading of hydraulic couplings is easy, it can not improve the start-up performance of the ribbon blender.

(v)   The ribbon blender cannot be cleaned during use.

Applications:

(i)   Ribbon blenders are used to blend large volumes of dry solids.

(ii)   It can blend and mix dry free flowing powders as well as wet materials.

(iii)   It is best suited for mixing of bulk drugs, formulation compositions, chemicals, and cosmetic powders.

(iv)   It used in dry blending of components in capsule formulations.

(v)   It can also be used in lubrication of dry granules in large quantity.

(vi)   It heats, cools, and dries materials during process.

(vii)   It is employed in coating solid particles with small amounts of liquids to produce formulations.

(viii) It has applications in mixing of nutraceuticals, cosmetics and veterinary formulations.

(ix)   Its other applications includes blending and mixing of abrasives, engineered plastic resins, pesticides and herbicides, animal feeds, epoxy resins, pet foods, bakery premixes, pigments, cake mixes, instant drink blends, fertilizers, plastic powders, carbon black, fire retardants, polyethylene, chemicals, gypsum, PVC compounding, leaning compounds, instant breakfast cereals, spice blends and dietary supplements.

8.6.4 Sigma Blade Mixer

The sigma blade mixer is one of the most popular mixer used for mixing and kneading high viscosity materials. It belongs to the family of double arm kneader mixers. It is commonly used mixer for mixing high viscosity materials.

Principle:

The principle involved in this mixers, wherein a very viscous materials are handled, is shearing which is produced by inter-meshing sigma shaped blades. This action promotes both lateral and transverse motion of the material. The geometry and profile of the sigma blade is designed such that the viscous mass of material is pulled, sheared, compressed, kneaded, and folded by the action of the blades against the walls of the mixer trough. The extent to which this happens depends on the action of the blades either tangential or overlapping and the speed of rotation of the blades. The helix angle of the blade can be modified depending on the required shearing.

Construction:

It consists of two mixing blades fitted horizontally in each trough of bowl. The shapes of blades resemble the Greek letter sigma (Σ) and hence are called as sigma blade mixers. The clearance between the blades and the vessel walls is as low as 2 mm. The low clearances produces high shear within the material. The blades are rotated through heavy duty drive systems consisting of a motor, gearbox, couplings, and gears. The top speed of the sigma mixer is generally limited to 60 m/min. The mixer trough has jacket for circulation of hot or cold media to maintain the required temperature conditions within the mixer. The discharge of the material from the mixer container is either by tilting of the mixer container or from bottom discharge valve or through an extruder/screw located in the lower portion between the two trough compartments.

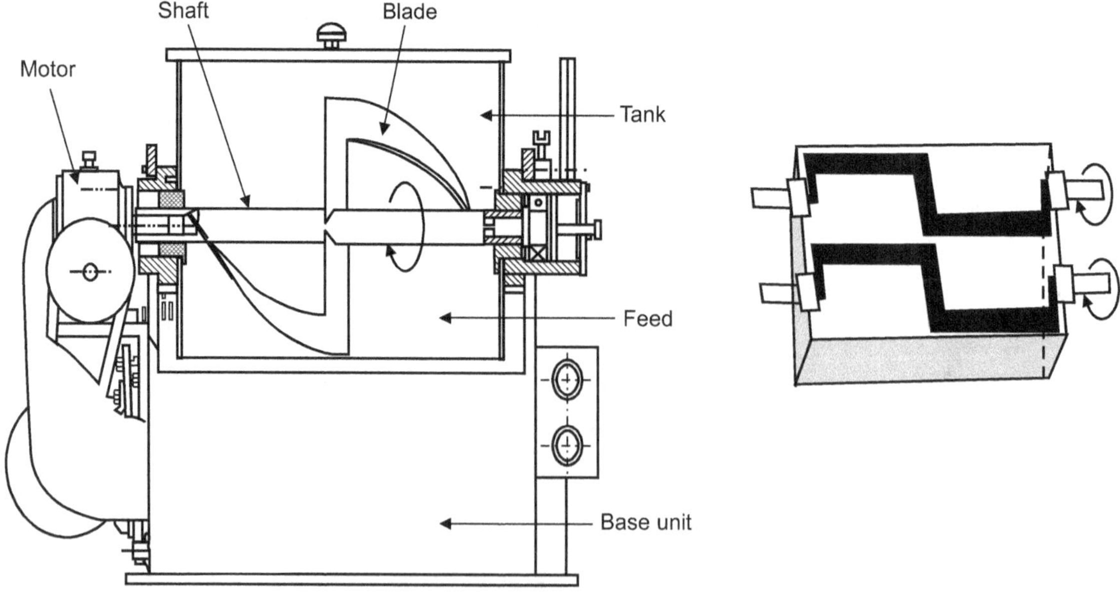

Fig. 8.4: Single and Double Blade Sigma Mixer

Working:

Powders are loaded through the top of the trough to typically 40 to 65 % of the mixer's total volumetric capacity. The entire mixing process is carried out in a closed trough because of the dust. The blades move at a different speed using the drive system that includes motor, gear reducer, couplings, gears, bearings and seals. The material moves up and down and shears between the blades and the wall of the trough. The equipment is also attached to the perforated blades to break lumps and aggregates. The discharge of the material is either by tilting the mixing vessel, through bottom discharge valve, or through a discharge screw. The homogeneous mixture is obtained within 10 to 30 min with a mixing homogeneity up to 99%.

Advantages:

(i)   The sigma blade mixer leaves less dead spot during mixing operations.

(ii)   It is ideal for mixing and kneading of highly viscous mass and sticky products.

(iii) These types of mixers and their variants can handle the highly viscous materials up to as 10 million centipoises.

(iv)   The provision of perforated blades makes it suitable for breaking lumps and aggregates.

(v)   The losses such as loss of volatile solvent during mixing can be prevented by closing the trough chamber and maintaining low temperature.

Disadvantages:

(i)   The power consumption in sigma blade mixer is very high compared to other types of mixers.

(ii)   Requires more space for installation.

(iii) It requires proper blade speed adjustments.

(iv)   There may be dead spots in the mixing tank.

Applications:

(i)   The sigma blade mixer is a commonly used mixer for high viscosity materials in preparing emulsions, syrups and ointments.

(ii)   Sigma blade mixers are used for wet granulation process in the manufacture of tablets, capsules and pill masses.

(iii) It is used for solid-liquid mixing as well as for solid-solid mixing.

(iv)   It is the best mixer employed in the mixing components of pasty, sticky, and gritty slurries with high viscosities.

(v)   Other applications of sigma blade mixer include mixing of adhesives, chemicals, chewing gum, food and confectionery products, hot-melts, inks and pigment products, soaps and detergents, sugar pastes etc.

8.6.5 Planetary Mixer

Planetary mixer is high shear mixer and is available in variable speed drive. It is suitable for mixing of ointments, inks, sauces, pastes and foam used in the pharmaceutical, food, chemical and allied industries.

Principle:

The principle of planetary mixer is based on rotation of planetary blades on their own axis while they travel around the center of the mixing bowl which ensures complete and effective mixing. The mixing blades revolve in opposite direction to sweep the entire circumference of the vessel as well as rotate around its own axis. Highest level of mixing is achieved in short intervals.

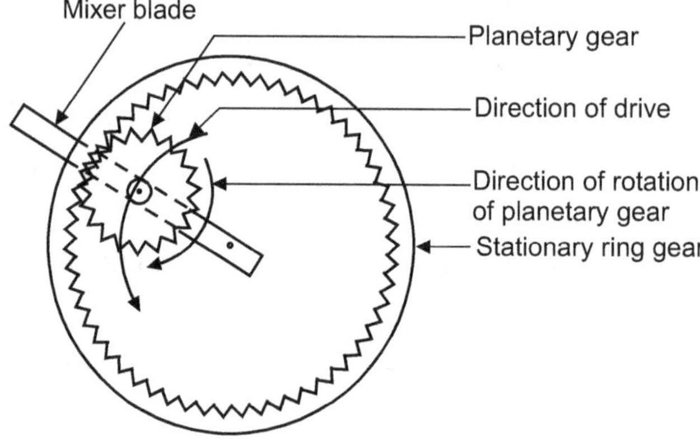

Fig. 8.5: Schematic of Planetary Mixer Principle

Construction:

Planetary mixer bowl, all its contact parts and beater are made up of stainless steel (SS304) or (SS316) materials, as per requirements. The mixer bowl is divided in to an upper cylindrical section and a lower hemispherical section. The mixing elements (beaters) used for mixing are shaped to match the lower curved surface of the bowl. The most commonly used beaters are the batter, wire whip, and hook type. Planetary mixers are provided with high speed emulsifier in the centre of the bowl. Scrapers with teflon edges may be provided to wipe any material which may stick onto the internal surface of the bowl. Single planetary mixers are constructed in a range of sizes.

There are multiple bowls and beater designs with the same mixer assembly. For small size mixers the lifting and lowering of the bowl is through a manual arrangement. In case of larger units bowl is lowered beneath the motor along with the beater using a motorized or hydraulically operated mechanical arrangement. There is a facility for the movement of bowl away from the machine using a suitable trolley with wheels. The single planetary mixers are available in small sizes to production size units with capacities of 50 - 300 L. The mixer motor may range upto 1.0 HP for smaller sizes to about 10 – 15 HP for the 300 L, depending on the material to be mixed.

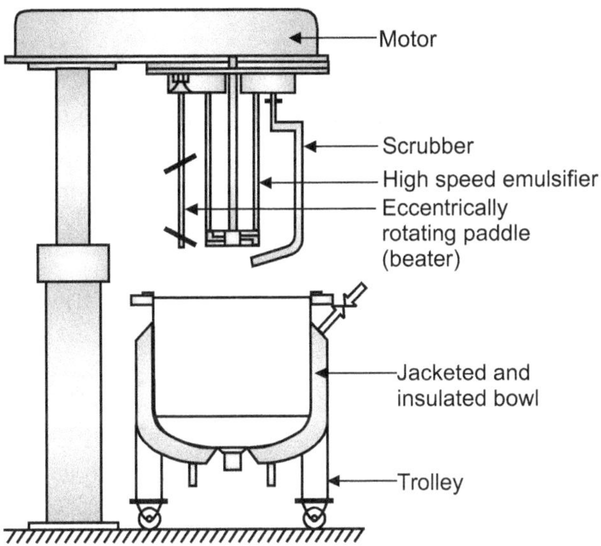

Fig. 8.6: Planetary Mixer

Working:

The planetary mixer works on homogenous mixing action. The material to be mixed is loaded in to the bowl. The planetary motion of the beater enables faster and better mixing of material at a considerably short time. The operation at slow speed is suitable for dry mixing with less dust generation and faster speed for kneading operation during wet granulation. The bowl is secured to a semi-circular frame at the time of mixing. Beaters can be intermittently cleaned completely by removing from vessel or by rotating the blades in the vessel loaded with solvent. After the mixing is completed, the bowl is lowered and can be easily detached and removed from the mixer assembly. The mixed contents are discharged either by hand scooping, or through a bottom discharge valve or by hydraulically operated automatic discharge systems.

Advantages:

(i)　There are virtually no dead spaces in the mixing bowl.

(ii)　Single planetary mixers are relatively inexpensive and versatile in applications,

(iii)　Portable mixing bowl with top mounted agitator has a dual advantage of material transfer with no risk of packing contamination.

(iv)　The product quality is better and more homogeneous.

(v)　The noise and vibration levels are low due to use of insulating materials and strong and solid construction.

(vi)　Security cover or bars and sensor technology reduces occupational labour accidents.

(vii)　It exhibit higher level of hygienic products and mixer is easy to clean.

(viii)　The sturdy equipment has long durability as it is made-up of high quality stainless steel.

(ix)　Being a compact equipment, it requires less space.

Disadvantages:

(i)   The equipment generates heat which may be unsuitable for proper mixing.

(ii)   When handling high viscosity materials the energy required is more.

(iii)   As this equipment consists of moving parts maintenance is required.

(iv)   As labour requirement is more, the process cost is also high.

Applications:

(i)   The single planetary mixer has common applications in the pharmaceutical, chemical and cosmetic industries.

(ii)   Planetary mixers are used for wet/dry solid-solid materials mixing.

(iii)   It is used in manufacturing of starch paste heated with steam or thermal fluid in electrically heating jacket with or without a flush bottom valve for discharge.

(iv)   It is used for dry powder to wet phase mixing for wet granulation.

(v)   The single planetary mixer is used for mixing of light pastes, gels, and dough.

(vi)   This mixer is commonly used in food and bakery industry due to its simple construction and operation.

(vii)   These mixers are designed for intensive mixing, dispersing and kneading of adhesives, sealants, light caulks, pastes, coatings, granulations, and similar products of medium to high viscosity.

8.6.6 Propellers

A propeller is a device consisting of a rotating shaft with propeller blades attached to it and used for mixing relatively low viscosity dispersions, liquids (low viscosity) and maintaining contents in suspension. It rotates at a very high speed (up to 8000 r.p.m.) and thus mixing operation is rapid. They are much smaller in diameter than paddle and turbine mixers.

Principle:

A propeller transmits power by converting rotational motion into thrust. A pressure difference is produced between the forward and rear surfaces of the airfoil-shaped blade, and a fluid is accelerated behind the blade. The thrust from the propeller is transmitted to move the liquid through by the main shaft and finally by the propeller itself.

Construction:

The system consists of vessel fitted with propeller. The vessel is made-up of stainless steel 316L grade resistant to acids, alkalis and abrasion having curved or flat-bottom. It has 1.5:1 height to width ratio. The vessel is covered with cooling jacket for better temperature control. Propellers consist of number of blades attached to the shaft. Generally, 3-6 bladed design is most commonly used for mixing liquids, Fig. 8.7. Blades may have right or left handed orientation. Two or more propellers are used for large and deep tanks. The size of propeller is small and may be increased up to 0.5 m depending upon the depth size of the tank. Typically the diameter of the propeller is within the range 0.13 - 0.67 of the tank diameter. Small size propellers can rotate up to 30000 r.p.m. and produce longitudinal movement. Radial agitators consist of propellers that are similar to marine propellers. They consist of two to four blades that move in a screw like motion propelling the material to be agitated parallel to the shaft. A propeller agitator is shaped with blades tapering towards the shaft to minimize centrifugal force and produce maximum axial flow. Propeller agitators are popular for simple mixing applications.

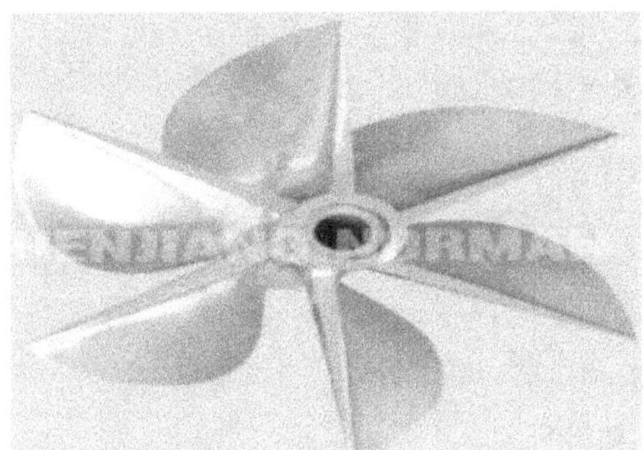 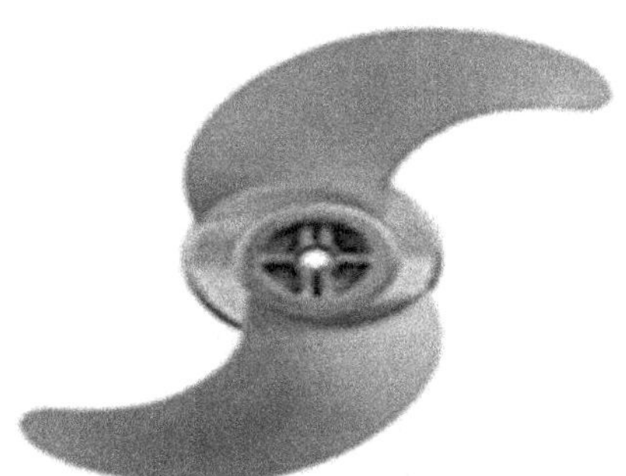

Fig. 8.7: Marine and Cutter Type Propeller Blades

Ideal properties of propellers:

(i)   They need to provide a wide range of operating speeds and hence shearing rates.

(ii) They must ensure complete (homogeneous) mixing.

(iii) They should be economical in use

(iv) They must provide effective mixing in dispersion of solids in the production of pharmaceutical suspensions without changing particles size.

(v)   They must allow for different mounting typos such as off-centre and side-entry.

(vi) They must be easy to clean after use.

Working:

The liquids to be mixed are transferred to the mixing vessel through pumping. When propeller is started a vortex is formed due to centrifugal force imparted to the liquid by the propeller blades, Fig. 8.8. This action causes liquid bulk to back-up around the sides of the vessel and create a depression at the center around the shaft. The liquid flow patterns achieved by propellers are axial and may be directed towards the top or towards the bottom of the vessel depending up on whether the drive is rotated clockwise or anticlockwise. As the speed of rotation is increased air may be sucked into the fluid by the formation of a vortex. The vortex formation is suppressed to considerable levels by fitting baffles in vertical position into the vessel. Vertical propeller mixer consists of three blades of suitable size depending upon the diameter of vessel. Horizontal or inclined propeller or marine propellers can also be used on side-entry mixers. Propellers are mounted on the impeller shaft inclined at an angle to the vessel axis to improve the mixing. It provide good blending capability in small batches of low to medium viscosity liquids.

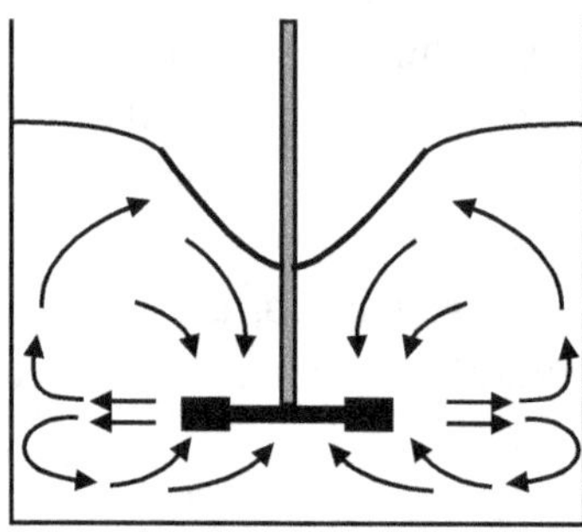

Fig. 8.8: Vortex Formation

Advantages:

(i)   Propellers are used when high mixing capability is required.

(ii)   They are very effective for mixing liquids having maximum viscosity of 2 Pa.s or slurry with up to 10% solids of fine particle size.

(iii)   They are effective in mixing gas-liquid dispersions at laboratory scale.

(iv)   Propellers increases the homogeneity of materials,

(v)   Can be used in two different patterns for drying and pressing

Disadvantages:

(i)   Propellers are not effective with liquids of viscosity greater than 5 Pa.s. For example, glycerin and castor oil.

(ii)   Need to be operated at high speed to avoid solid settlings in reactor vessels.

(iii)   They need to be operated at low speeds if drying is an additional objective.

(iv)   Vortex causes frothing and possible oxidation.

Applications:

(i)   Propellers are used when huge quantities of liquids and dispersions are to be mixed.

(ii)   These are useful for mixing liquids having a viscosity of about 2 Pa.s.

(iii)   These can handle corrosive materials with glass lining.

8.6.7 Turbine Mixer

Turbine mixer is another type of process agitator. They are used as an alternative to propellers for mixing low viscosity liquids and typically for the effective mixing of medium viscosity liquids. The velocity of mixing using turbine systems is low compared to propellers.

Principle:

Turbine mixer agitators can create a turbulent movement of the fluids due to the combination of centrifugal and rotational motion. These combined motions causes effective mixing of low to medium viscosity fluids.

Construction:

A turbine consists of a circular disc to which a number of short blades are attached. Compared to propellers the diameter of turbines is approximately 0.13-0.67 to that of the diameter of the vessel, with 0.33:1 being most typical. There is a wide range of turbine designs, Fig. 8.9. The blades may be straight, pitched, curved or disk type. Turbine rotates at a lower speeds usually 50 – 200 r.p.m. than the propellers. Flat blade turbines produce radial and tangential flow but as the speed increases radial flow dominates. Pitched blade turbine produces axial flow. Near the impeller zone of rapid currents, high turbulence and intense shear is observed. Shear produced by turbines can be further enhanced using a diffuser ring. The diffuser ring is a stationary perforated ring which surrounds the turbine.

Working:

A mixer is filled through with an opening at its top. Usually it is a pan or drum within which mixing blades revolve about the vertical axis. The variable speed drill with turbine mixer whip air into the material mixture. The air in mixture yield bubbles contributing mixing. The top entry turbine mixer is fitted with various impellers and turbines to suit heat and mass transfer in solids, suspensions and liquids. This type of mixer does not damage product. Top entry high shear causes uniform emulsification and homogenization. The mixing blades revolve about the vertical axis.

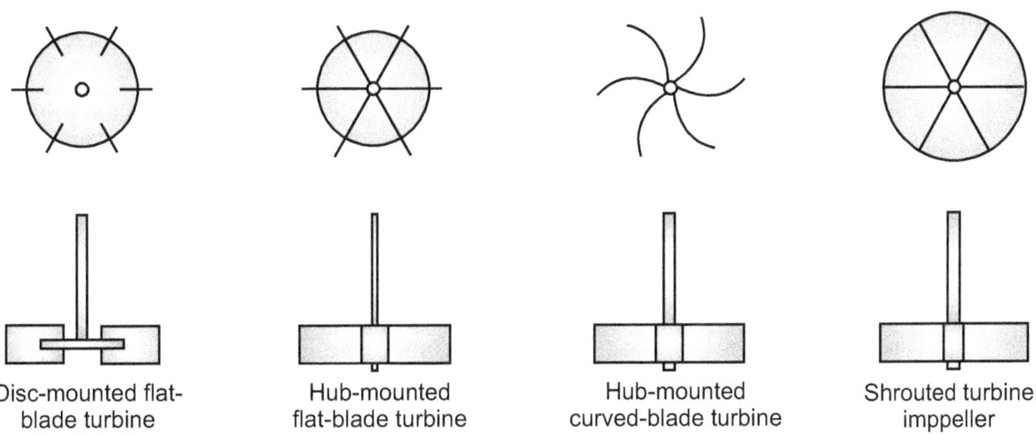

| Disc-mounted flat-blade turbine | Hub-mounted flat-blade turbine | Hub-mounted curved-blade turbine | Shrouted turbine imppeller |

Fig. 8.9: Types of Turbine Design

Advantages:

(i) Turbines are used in emulsification as they generate higher shearing forces than propellers even at low pumping rates.

(ii) They are effective in mixing high viscous solutions with a wide range of viscosities up to 7.0 Pa.s.

(iii) They are highly suitable for making dispersion containing 60% solids.

(iv) Turbines are suitable for liquids of large volume and high viscosity with the additional provision of baffles in the tank.

(v) As they generate high radial flow efficiency of mixing is high.

(vi) In low viscous materials of large volumes turbine create a strong currents which spread throughout the tank destroying stagnant pockets.

Disadvantages:

(i) They are not preferred for solvents with high viscosity such as more than 20 cP.

(ii) There is possibility of air entrapment that may cause oxidation of material being mixed.

Applications:

(i) Highly used in chemical reactions and extraction operations. For example, liquid and gas reactions.

(ii) Used in preparing emulsions, suspensions and syrups.

8.6.8 Paddles

Paddles are used as impellers in mixing liquids. It consists of flat blades attached to a vertical shaft and rotates at speed lower than 100 r.p.m. A variety of paddle mixers having different shapes and sizes, depending on the nature and viscosity of the product are available for use in industries. Paddle is one of the most primary types of agitators with blades that reach up to the tank walls.

Principle:

Paddle agitators work with producing a uniform laminar flow of liquids. Paddles push the liquid radially and tangentially with almost no axial action unless blades are pitched. The large surface area of blades in relation to the container helps them to rotate in the proximity of walls of the container and effectively mix the viscous liquids or semi-solids.

Construction:

A paddle consists of a central hub with long flat blades attached to it vertically. Two blades or four blades are very common, Fig. 8.10. Sometimes blades are pitched and may be dish or hemispherical in shape and have a large surface area in relation to the tank in which they are used. A paddle rotates at a low speed of 100 r.p.m. In deep tanks several paddles are attached one above the other on the same shaft. At very low speeds it gives mild agitation in unbaffled tank but as for high speeds baffles are necessary.

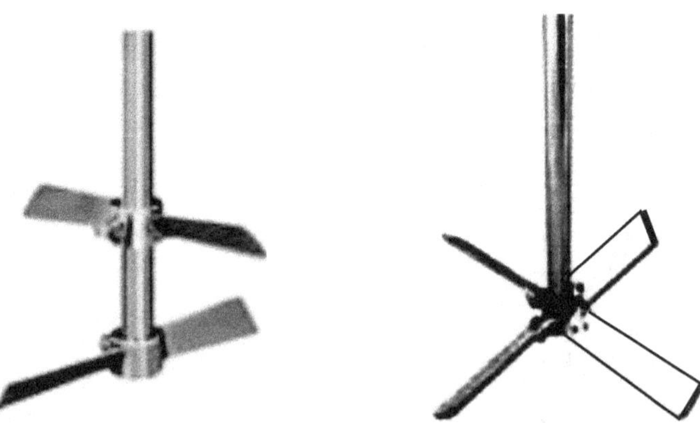

Fig. 8.10: A Paddle with Single And Double Blade Attachment

Working:

The material to be mixed is charged from the top of the trough. If required, liquid spraying arrangement can be provided. The normal filling level is slightly above the shafts. Thus, there is surplus space in the mixer trough to provide air around the particles so that they can move freely. The random movement in the trough gives 98 - 99% mixing homogeneity. The peripheral speed of paddles is about 100 r.p.m.

Advantages:

(i)　As paddle-impellers mixes liquids with low speed the possibility of vortex formation is least.

(ii)　These are heavy duty mixers suitable for slow operation.

(iii)　They can mix systems effectively with 2 or 4 blades.

Disadvantages:

(i)　Mixing of the suspensions is poor, thus, baffled tanks are required.

(ii)　As they are heavy duty mixers power consumption is very high.

(iii)　They are not efficient for mixing variety of materials with different consistencies.

Applications:

(i)　Paddles are used in the manufacture of antacid suspensions and antidiarrheal mixtures such as bismuth-kaolin mixture.

(ii)　They are used in the mixing of solids, slurries, crystals forming phases during super saturated cooling.

8.6.9 Silverson Emulsifier Mixer

Silverson mixer has been the leader in high shear mixing for over 60 years. The Silverson high speed shear mixer is used for mixing liquid/liquid or liquid/solid mixtures at speeds upto 8000 r.p.m. The mixer body is raised or lowered electrically. It stops automatically at the higher and lower limits of movement. It has several accessories with the mixer, which can be interchanged depending on mixing conditions required and material being mixed.

Principle:

The principle of Silverson mixer is based upon shearing force. It produces intense shearing forces and turbulence by use of high speed rotors. Circulation of material takes place through the head by the suction produced in the inlet at the bottom of the head. Circulation of the material ensures rapid breakdown of the dispersed liquid into smaller globules.

Construction:

It consists of long supporting columns and a central portion, Fig. 8.11. Central portion consists of a shaft which is connected to motor at one end and other to the head. Head carries turbine blades. Blades are surrounded by a mesh, which is further enclosed by a cover having openings. It consists of following other accessories:

(i)　**General purpose disintegrating head:** Suitable for general mixing or disintegration of solids.

(ii) Square hole high shear screen: High shear screen suitable for emulsion and fine colloid suspension preparation.

(iii) Emulsor screen: Lower shear screen suitable for liquid/liquid and emulsion preparations.

(iv) Axial flow head: Used in addition to one of the above screens to force liquid flow upwards This can reduce aeration or help maintain large suspensions, but high mixing speeds can cause liquid to be ejected from the mixing vessel.

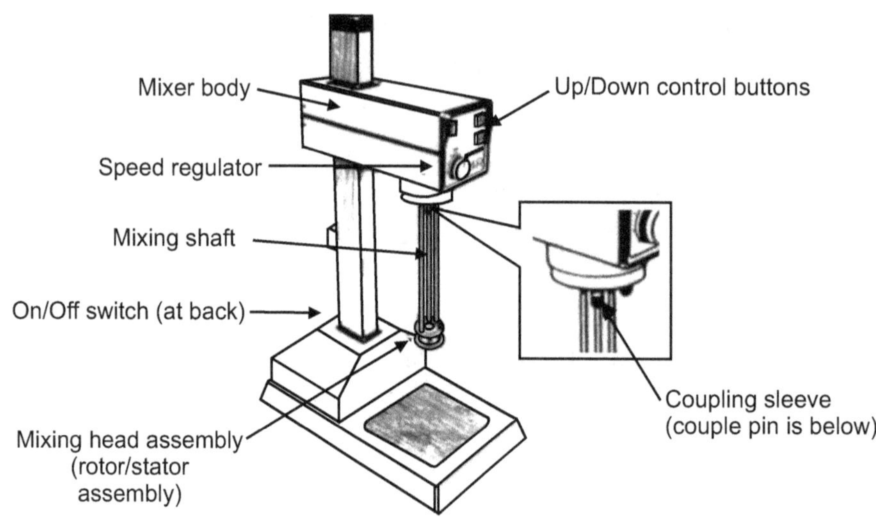

Fig. 8.11: Silverson High Shear Mixer

Working:

The precision-machined Silverson work head generates exceptionally high shear rates in a three stage process that rapidly homogenizes the product to the required uniformity.

(i) The high-speed rotation of the rotor blades within the precision-machined mixing work head exerts a powerful suction, drawing liquid and solid materials into the rotor/stator assembly, Fig. 8.12 (a).

(ii) The centrifugal force drives the material towards the periphery of the work head where they are subjected to a milling action in the precision-machined clearance between the ends of the rotor blades and the inner wall of the stator, Fig. 8.12 (b).

(iii) Finally the intense hydraulic shear wherein the materials are forced at high velocity out through the perforations in the stator, then through the machine outlet and along the pipe work. At the same time, fresh materials are continually drawn into the work head, maintaining the mixing and pumping cycle, Fig. 8.12 (c and d).

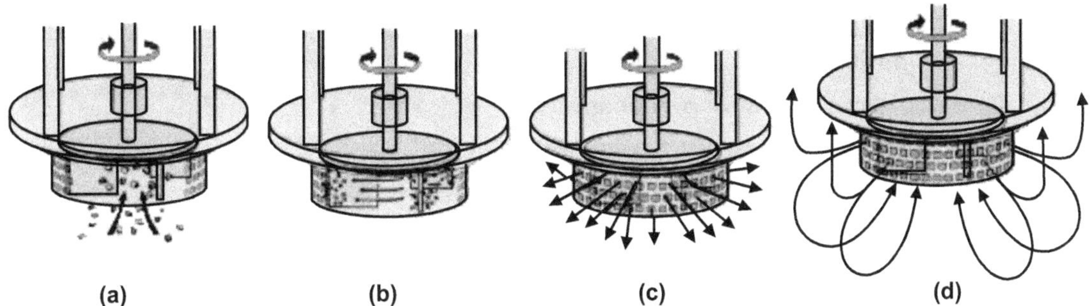

(a)   (b)   (c)   (d)

Fig. 8.12: Working of Silverson Mixer

Advantages:

(i)   It is efficient and rapid in operation and is capable of reducing mixing times by up to 90%.

(ii) It is speedy, versatile, self-pumping, aeration-free and efficient shear mixer.

(iii) It is capable of producing a fine droplet or particle size, typically in the range of 2 - 5 microns.

(iv) Being proficient it reduces operating costs.

(v)   The product to pass through the homogenizer at a much faster rate, normally in a single pass.

(vi) Being versatile it allows performing the widest range of mixing applications.

Disadvantages:

(i)   It requires feed to be premixed and of uniform and fine globule or particle size.

(ii) It may face a problem of mesh clogging.

(iii) It requires more power.

Applications:

(i)   It is used to mix, emulsify, homogenize, solubilize, suspend, disperse and disintegrate solids.

(ii) It is used for homogenization of vast variety of products such as creams and ointments, lotions, sauces and flavour emulsions.

(iii) A homogeneous product is rapidly produced when blending liquids are of similar or greatly varying viscosities, eliminating problems of stratification.

(iv) It is used to prepare emulsions in the range of 0.5 to 5 microns.

(v)   Silverson mixers can disintegrate matter of animal, vegetable, mineral or synthetic origin in a single operation.

(vi) It is used to uniformly mill both solid and semi-solid materials into either solution or fine suspension.

(vii) It is also used in rapid gelling. For example, solubilizing and dispersing gums, alginates, CMC, carbopols etc., resulting in an agglomerate-free solution within minutes.

REVIEW QUESTIONS

1. What is mixing? What are its objectives?
2. Give applications of mixing in pharmacy.
3. What is difference between mixing and agitation?
4. What are types of mixture?
5. Enlist and explain various factors affecting mixing of pharmaceutical materials.
6. Differentiate between liquid mixing and solid mixing.
7. Discuss various mechanisms involved in mixing.
8. Discuss mixing of liquid.
9. Discuss mixing of solids.
10. Discuss mixing of semi-solids.
11. Classify mixing equipments based upon principle mechanism involved. Comment on criterion for selection equipments for mixing.
12. Discuss principle, construction, working, advantages, disadvantages and applications of double cone blender.
13. Discuss principle, construction, working, advantages, disadvantages and applications of V-blender.
14. Discuss principle, construction, working, advantages, disadvantages and applications of ribbon blender.
15. Discuss principle, construction, working, advantages, disadvantages and applications of sigma blade mixer.
16. Discuss principle, construction, working, advantages, disadvantages and applications of planetary mixer.
17. What is difference between propellers, paddles and turbines?
18. Short note on propellers used in pharmaceutical practice.
19. Discuss principle, construction, working, advantages, disadvantages and applications of paddles.
20. Discuss principle, construction, working, advantages, disadvantages and applications of turbines.
21. What is blending? How it is different from mixing?

✍ ✍ ✍

Chapter ... **9**

FILTRATION

9.0 INTRODUCTION

Filtration is a unique unit mechanical or physical process of separating suspended and colloidal particles from fluids (liquids or gases) by interposing a medium through which only the fluid can pass. It is a process that removes particles from suspension in water. Removal takes place by a number of mechanisms that include straining, flocculation, coagulation, sedimentation and surface capture. Filters can be categorized by the main method of capture, for example, exclusion of particles at the surface of the filter media (straining), or deposition within the media (in-depth filtration).

When the proportion of solids in a liquid is less, the term clarification is used. It is a common operation which is widely employed in the production of sterile products, bulk drugs, and in liquid oral formulation. The suspension of solid and liquid to be filtered is known as the "slurry". The porous medium used to retain the solids is described as the filter medium; the accumulation of solids on the filter is referred to as the filter cake, while the clear liquid passing through the filter is the filtrate. The porous medium used to retain the solids is known as filter medium. The accumulated solids on the filter are referred as filter cake and the clear liquid passing through the filter is filtrate. The pores of the filter medium are smaller than the size of particles to be separated. Therefore, solids are trapped on the surface of the filter medium. After a particular point of time, the resistance offered by the filter cake is high that stops the filtration.

Filtration is also used to describe some biological processes, especially in water treatment and sewage treatment in which undesirable constituents are removed by absorption into a biological film grown on or in the filter medium as in slow sand filtration.

Water Filtration Process:

During filtration in a conventional down-flow depth filter, waste water containing suspended matter is applied to the top of the filter bed. As the water passes through the filter bed, the suspended matter in the wastewater is removed by a variety of removal mechanisms. With passage of time, as material accumulates within the interstices of the granular medium, the head-loss through the filter starts to build up beyond the initial value. After some period of time, the operating head-loss or effluent turbidity reaches a predetermined head loss or turbidity value. The filter must be cleaned (backwashed) to remove the material (suspended solids) that has accumulated within the granular filter bed.

Backwashing is accomplished by reversing the flow through the filter. A sufficient flow of wash water is applied until the granular filtering medium is fluidized (expanded), causing the particles of the filtering medium to abrade against each other.

Classification of Filtration Process:

    (a)   Depth filtration:

        (i)   Slow sand filtration.

        (ii)   Rapid porous and compressible medium filtration.

        (iii) Intermittent porous medium filtration.

        (iv) Recirculating porous medium filtration.

    (b)   Surface filtration:

        (i)   Laboratory filters used for TSS test.

        (ii)   Diatomaceous earth filtration.

        (ii)   Cloth or screen filtration.

    (c)   Membrane flirtation:

Mechanisms of Filtration:

The mechanisms whereby particles are retained by the filter medium are of significance only in the early stages of liquid filtration. Once a preliminary layer of particles has been deposited, the filtration is effected by the filter cake. The filter medium serves only as a support.

    (a) Straining: The simplest filtration procedure is "straining", in which, like sieving, the pores are smaller than the particles. These particles are retained on the filter medium as a bed.

    (b) Entanglement: If the filter medium consists of a cloth with a nap or a porous felt, then particles become entangled in the mass of fibers. Usually the particles are smaller than the pores, so that it is possible that impingement is involved.

    (c) Attractive forces: In certain circumstances, particles may collect on a filter medium as a result of attractive forces. The ultimate in this method is the electrostatic precipitator, where large potential differences are used to remove the particles from air streams. In practice, the filtration process may combine various mechanisms, but the solids removal is effected normally by a straining mechanism once the first complete layers of solids has begun to form the cake on the filter medium.

9.1 OBJECTIVES

The main learning objective of filtration is to separate solids from liquid or gas medium. The other objectives include:

    (i)   To eliminate the contaminant particles so as to recover dispersing fluid.

    (ii)   To recover solid particles by eliminating the dispersing fluid.

    (iii) To produce high-quality solvents and solids.

(iv)   To purify air and pharmaceutically useful gases by removing particulate matter.

(v)   To sterilize thermolabile parentral products.

9.2 APPLICATIONS

(i)   **Water Purification:** Purification of water for pharmaceutical use is the most important application of filtration. Water used in pharmaceutical industries for various applications has to comply with different standards specified in official pharmacopoeias. These standards are namely; purified water, Water For Injection and Sterile Water For Injection. To produce water complying with these standards potable water is required initially to be filtered. Filtration is commonly used for the removal of residual biological floc in settled effluents from secondary treatment before disinfection to remove residual precipitates from the metal salt or lime precipitation or phosphate.

(ii)   **Pharmaceutical Industry:** Filtration, as a physical operation is very important in chemistry for the separation of materials of different chemical composition. This is one of the most important techniques used by chemists to purify compounds. Various enzymes, amino acids, antibiotics, pharmaceutical intermediates, bulk drugs, medicine, blood products, antibiotics, calcium phytate, chinese inositol, growth derived sand, organic phosphorus, glucoamylase etc. are purified by using filtration. Filtration may be simultaneously combined with other unit operations to process the feed stream, as in the bio-filter, which is a combined filter and biological digestion device.

(iii)   **Biopharmaceutical Industry:** The separation process of filtration is widely used in the biopharmaceutical industry to remove contaminants such salts, particulate matter, micro-organisms etc. from liquids, air, and gases.

(iv)   **Chemical Industry:** Filtration is used for separation and purification of dyes, pesticides, silicic acid, glycerin, white carbon, sodium carbonate, additives, basic chemicals, chemical filler, pigment, white alumina, manganese, caustic soda, soda ash, and alkali salts mud, saponins, and graphite etc.

(v)   **Food Industry:** Wine filter press, yeast, fruit juice filter press, edible oil, vegetable oil, soy sauce, sugar mills, rice wine, white wine, fruit juices, soft drinks, beer, yeast, citric acid, vegetable protein, plant density sweetener, glucose etc are filtered to remove unwanted matter.

(vi)   **Environmental Engineering:** Filtration is used for separation and purification of chemical waste water, mining waste water, domestic waste water, leather waste water and salt mud waste water.

(v)   **Clay Industry:** Filtration is used for separation and purification of kaolin, bentonite, activated clay, clay and electronic ceramics clay.

(vi) Heating, ventilation and air conditioning (HVAC): Filtration is used for obtaining high quality air from poor quality air that contain micro-organisms and particulate matter such as dust and smoke; volatile organic compounds and allergens responsible for respiratory illnesses and allergy, asthma and sick-building symptoms. Ideally, these triggers are eliminated or reduced significantly by the air filters in a building's HVAC system. Advances in air filtration have led to the development of systems that provide superior air with reduced energy costs and help commercial and institutional buildings to achieve green-building milestones.

(vii) Making new food and beverage products: Bacteria and spoilage organisms in milk are easily removed by micro filters with pore sizes ranging from 0.1 to 20 microns. Ultra filtration units with pores ranging from 0.01-0.2 microns have been shown to affect the appearance and sensory properties of fluid milk because of the protein molecules that can be retained and then added back.

(viii) Cane and beet sugar industries: Ultra filtration/micro filtration process in cane sugar production acts as a pre-treatment prior to other separation technologies by removing impurities from the raw juice, including starch, dextran, gums, waxes, proteins and polysaccharides.

9.3 THEORIES OF FILTERATION

The flow of any liquid through any porous medium offers a resistance to its flow. The rate of filtration in such cases is expressed as;

$$\text{Filtration rate } = \frac{\text{Driving force}}{\text{Resistance by filter medium}} \qquad \text{... (9.1)}$$

The net driving force in filtration is pressure above the medium minus pressure below the medium. The resistance offered by filter medium is not constant over the period of filtration as it goes on increasing with time due to particle deposition on filter medium. Rate is expressed as volume of filtrate per unit time as dv/dt.

Depending on dispersing (fluid) medium filtration theory is divided in two parts.

9.3.1 Gas Filtration Theory

Gas filtration includes filtration of aerosol and lyosol. Membrane filters and nucleopore filters are used for gas filtration which works on three mechanisms.

(i) Diffusion deposition: In this mechanism the path followed by individual small particles do not coincide with the streamlines of the fluid because of Brownian motion. With decreasing particle size the intensity of Brownian motion increases and thus as a consequence, the intensity of diffusion deposition also increases.

(ii) Direct interception: This mechanism involves finite size particles. These particles are intercepted as they approach the collecting surface to a distance equal to its radius. A special case of this mechanism is the so-called 'sieve effect', or 'sieve mechanism'.

(iii) Inertial deposition: The presence of a body in the flowing fluid results in a curvature of the streamlines in the neighborhood of the body. Because of their inertia, the individual particles do not follow the curved streamlines but are projected against the body and may deposit there. It is obvious that the intensity of this mechanism increases with increasing particle size and velocity of flow.

(iv) Gravitational deposition: Individual particles have a certain sedimentation velocity due to gravity. As a consequence, the particles deviate from the streamlines of the fluid and, owing to this deviation; the particles may touch a fiber.

(v) Electrostatic deposition: Both the particles and the fibers in the filter may carry electric charges. Deposition of particles on the fibers may take place because of the forces acting between charges or induced forces.

9.3.2 Liquid Filtration Theory

The term filtration covers all processes in which a liquid containing suspended solid is freed of some or the entire solid when the suspension is drawn through a porous medium. Filtration is of two types namely; 'Cake filtration' where the proportion of solids in suspension is large and most of the particles are collected in the filter cake which can subsequently be detached from the medium and 'Deep bed filtration' where the proportion of solids is very small. For example, in water filtration, the particles are often considered as smaller than the pores of the filter medium and penetrate at a considerable depth for being captured.

Kozeny-Carman Equation:

In filtration because the particles forming the cake are small and the flow through bed is slow, streamline conditions are almost invariably obtained, and therefore at any instant it may be represented as Fig. 9.1.

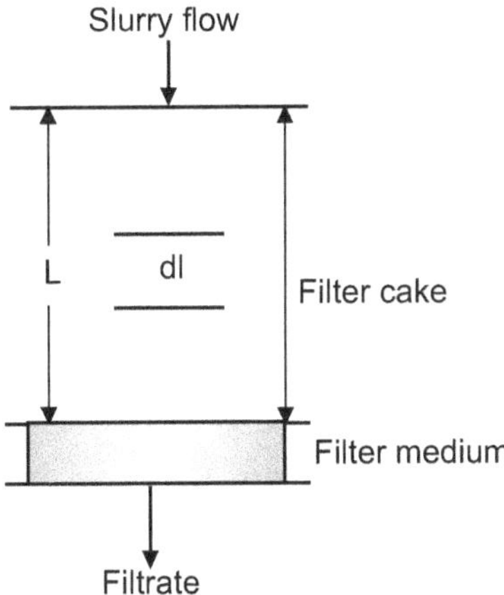

Fig. 9.1: Schematic of Filtration

This is explained by Kozeny-Carman equation:

$$U = \frac{1}{A}\frac{dv}{dt} = \frac{\Delta P}{r\mu\,(l + L)} \qquad \qquad ...\,(9.2)$$

where,   U = Flow rate

$$A = \text{Filter area}$$
$$v = \text{Total volume of filtrate delivered}$$
$$t = \text{Filtration time}$$
$$\Delta P = \text{Pressure drop across cake and medium}$$
$$r = \text{Specific cake resistance}$$
$$\mu = \text{Filtrate viscosity}$$
$$l = \text{Cake thickness and}$$
$$L = \text{Thickness of cake equivalent to medium resistance}$$

Kozeny-Carman equation has certain limitations that it does not take into account the depth of the granular bed which is lesser than the actual path travelled by the fluid. The actual path is not straight throughout the bed, but it is sinuous or tortuous.

Poiseulle's Law:

This law considers that filtration is similar to the streamline flow of a liquid under pressure through capillaries. It can be expressed as;

$$\frac{1}{dv}\frac{A}{dt} = \frac{\Delta P}{\mu \, (R_m + R_c)} \qquad \qquad ...\,(9.3)$$

$$\text{Cake resistance } (R_m) = \frac{\sigma W}{A} \qquad \qquad ...\,(9.4)$$

$$\text{Specific cake resistance } (\sigma) = \sigma'\Delta P^s \qquad \qquad ...\,(9.5)$$

The filter resistance is much less than the cake resistance i.e. $R_c << R_m$. Therefore, on rearranging equation (9.2):

$$\frac{1}{dv}\frac{A}{dt} = \frac{\Delta P}{\sigma \, (\sigma' \, \Delta P^s \times WA)} \qquad \qquad ...\,(9.6)$$

Where,
$$V = \text{Filtrate volume (L)}$$
$$A = \text{Filter area (m}^2)$$
$$t = \text{Time (h)}$$
$$\Delta P = \text{Pressure driving force (N)}$$
$$\mu = \text{Broth viscosity (Pa.s) m}^2/\text{h}$$
$$W = \text{Mass of filter (kg)}$$
$$R = \text{Resistance (m}^{-1})$$
$$\sigma = \text{Specific cake resistance (m/kg)}$$
$$S = \text{Compressibility factor}$$

Darcy's Equation:

When using Poiseulle equation for filtration it is considered that capillaries in filter medium are highly irregular and non-uniform. In order to approximate the flow rate the height of cake is taken as length of capillaries and a correction factors is introduced for the radius of capillaries. This makes flow rate more simplified and is expressed as

$$U = \frac{KA\,\Delta P}{\eta L} \qquad \qquad \ldots (9.7)$$

Where,

U	=	Flow rate (L/sec)
K	=	Permeability coefficient of the cake (m^2)
A	=	Surface area of filter medium (m^2)
ΔP	=	Pressure difference across the filter, Pa
r	=	Capillary radius in filter bed (m)
L	=	Capillary length (m)
H	=	Viscosity of liquid (Pa.s)

The permeability coefficient (K) in eq. 9.7 depends on porosity, specific surface area and compressibility of cake. This coefficient may be defined as the flow rate of a liquid of unit viscosity across unit area of cake with unit thickness under the unit pressure gradient.

9.4 FACTORS INFLUENCING FILTRATION

The most important factors on which the filtration depends are:

(i)   Proportion of solids in the slurry.

(ii)   Properties of the liquid namely density, viscosity, corrosiveness etc.

(iii)   Properties of the solid such as particle shape, size, size distribution and compressibility.

(iv)   The properties of filter medium especially resistance and initial layers of cake formed.

The following are the factors that influences rate of filtration :

(i)   **Permeability Coefficient:** According to Darcy's equation permeability coefficient (K) represents the resistance of both the filter medium and the filter cake. As the thickness of the cake increase, the rate of filtration decreases. Also the surface area of the particles, the porosity of the cake, and rigidity or compressibility of the particles could also affect the permeability of the cake.

(ii)   **Area of Filter Medium:** The total volume of filtrate flowing through the filter is proportional to the area of the filter. The area can be increased by using larger filters. For example, in the rotary drum filter, the continuous removal of the filter cake gives an infinite area for filtration.

(iii)   **Pressure Drop:** The rate of filtration is proportional to the pressure difference across both the filter medium and filter cake. The pressure drop can be achieved in a number of ways:

Gravity: A pressure difference could be obtained by maintaining a sufficient head of slurry above the filter medium. The pressure developed will depend on the density of the slurry.

Vacuum: The pressure below the filter medium may be reduced below atmospheric pressure by connecting the filtrate receiver to a vacuum pump and creating a pressure difference across the filter.

Pressure: The simplest method is to pump the slurry onto the filter under pressure.

Centrifugal force: Application of higher centrifugal force on slurry increases rate of filtration.

(iv) Viscosity of Filtrate: It is considered that an increase in the viscosity of the filtrate increases the resistance of flow, so that the rate of filtration is inversely proportional to the viscosity of the fluid. This problem can be overcome by two methods:

Temperature: The rate of filtration may be increased by raising the temperature of the liquid, which lowers its viscosity. However, it is not practicable if thermolabile materials are involved or if the filtrate is volatile.

Dilution: Dilution is another alternative but the rate must be doubled.

(v) Thickness of Filter Cake: The rate of flow of the filtrate through the filter cake is inversely proportional to thickness of the cake. Preliminary decantation may be useful to decrease the amount of the solids that ultimately help to increase filtration rate.

(vi) Particle Size of Solids: Generally the larger the particle size the higher the filtration rate ($Kg/m^2/h$). A small average particle size, a narrow distribution range has a high filtration rate.

(vii) Ratio of Slimes to Coarser Particles: The slimes (or extreme fines) in a slurry affect filtration rates to a vastly greater extent than their percentage. Particularly, difficult slurry is one that contains relatively coarse particles and a number of very fine or slimy particles with little or no intermediate size.

(viii) Flocculation/Dispersion of Fine Solids: Flocculation is generally desirable for slurries of fine solids which are in a dispersed state and generally filter poorly. The wide variety of polyelectrolyte flocculants provides space for a substantial improvement in filtration rates. Effective use of flocculants, especially polyelectrolytes, on moderately high concentration slurry requires strong agitation to get good solids-flocculant contact. A minimum of further agitation and minimum aging are important. Some slurry may be so viscous as to create filtering problems and a dispersant may be a better way to gain fluidity than dilution.

(ix) Slurry Age: Sometimes processes involve detention times which provide a conditioning effect modifying filter performance. Samples stored for longer time for testing involve a risk that excessive aging may have some effect on filtration.

(x) Agitation Speed: Some slurry, particularly with a wide particle size range tends to classify in the test slurry container or the filter tube. Increasing the agitation speed (or stirring) to a point that the coarse and fine particles are always thoroughly mixed may be desirable. A too high speed could limit cake thickness; prevent coarser particles from forming in the cake or cause delicate flocs to break down.

(xi) Cycle Time: Cycle time of the filter drum speed is generally expressed in seconds or minutes per revolution. Generally the faster the drum speed the higher the output. However, under these conditions, the cake is thinner and sometimes wetter, so discharge may deteriorate. At all times, a dischargeable cake must be produced.

(x) Cake Compression: Cake compression is normally achieved as an adjunct to the filtration step to reduce cake moistures of compressible cakes.

(xi) Type of Filter Medium: Filtering characteristics of fabrics depend mostly on the type of yarn and weave. Yarns can be mono-filament, multi-filament, spun from staple fiber, or a combination of the latter two. A high twist can make a multi-filament perform more like a mono-filament. Permeability and porosity are prime qualities in cloth selection. The Frazier permeability rating, expressed as cfm/sq ft, is a measure of air flow at one-half inch water pressure through a dry cloth, and is comparable to per cent open area. Porosity and particle retention may not be accurately indicated by permeability; there being no direct measure of porosity.

(xii) Filter Cloth Condition: Cloth conditioning refers to the reduction of pore size or open area due to entrapment of fine solids in the interstices.

(xiii) Filter Aids: Filter aids like diatomaceous earth, perlite, powdered coal, and fly-ash or paper pulp may be added to the slurry to increase its filtration rate and cake porosity.

(xiv) Solid Concentration in Slurry: In general, the greater the percentage of suspended solids in a given slurry, the higher the cake filter rate in $Kg/m^2/h$ and the lower the filter rate in $m^3/m^2/h$. Where maximum solids capacity is desired it is advisable to consider thickening the slurry by gravity. In some applications involving thickening with sludge recycle, particle size is actually increased and both cake and filtrate rates can increase.

(xv) Filter Thickening: Filter thickening normally occurs in a continuous filter rotating in a tank containing slurry wherein the solids in the filter tank increase in concentration and shift to a coarser size distribution. While an equilibrium concentration and size distribution is usually obtained, it may sometimes be necessary to dilute the pulp.

(xvi) Slurry pH: The slurry pH and particle dispersion are closely related. The change in pH can be one of the most effective methods to achieve flocculation and thus the improved filterability.

9.5 FILTER AID

The "Filter Aids" is a group of inert materials that can be used in filtration pretreatment. Usually, the resistance to flow due to the filter medium itself is very low, but will increase as a layer of solids builds-up, blocking the pores of the medium and forming a solid cake. The filter aid is used to prevent the medium from becoming blocked and to form an open, porous cake, so reducing the resistance to flow of the filtrate.

There are two objectives related to the addition of filter aids. One is to form a layer of second medium which protects the basic medium of the system. This is commonly referred to as "precoat". The second objective of filter aids is to improve the flow rate by decreasing cake compressibility and increasing cake permeability. This type of usage is termed as "admix" or "body feed". Filtration without filter aid, with precoat, and with precoat and body feed is shown in Fig. 9.2. The particles must be inert, insoluble, incompressible, and irregular shaped. The common filter aids are diatomaceous earth (Kieselguhr, DE), perlite, cellulose and others.

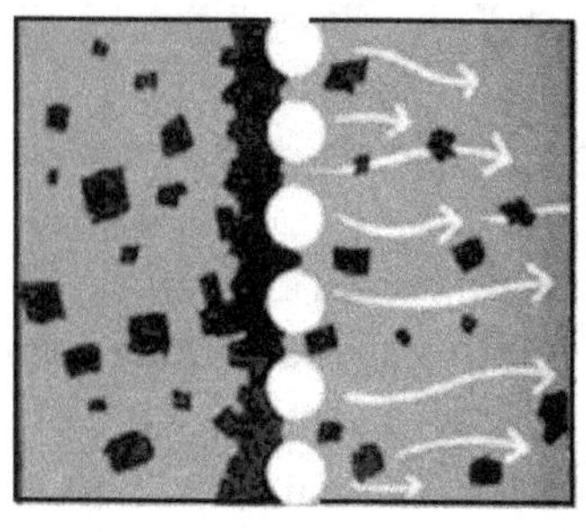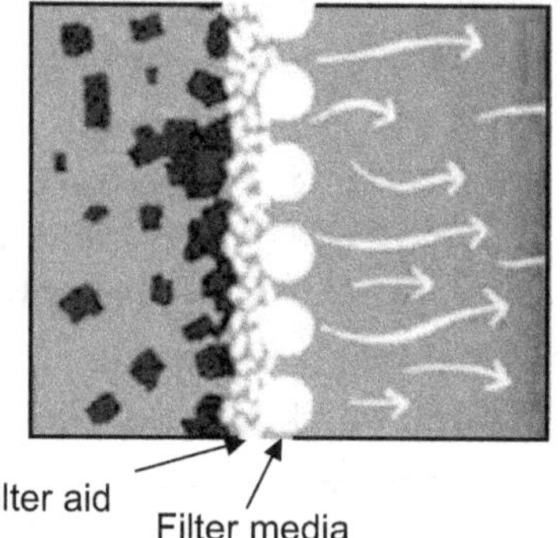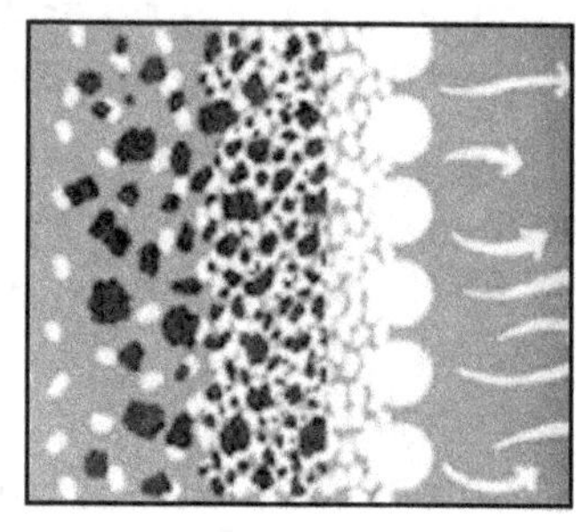

(a) Filtration without filter aid;   **(b) Filtration with "precoat"**   **(c) Filtration with "admix" and "precoat"**

Fig. 9.2: Mechanism of Filtration with Filter Aids

(i)   **Diatomaceous earth:** Diatomaceous earth (DE) is the skeleton of ancient diatoms. They are mined from ancient seabed, processed, and classified to make different grade of filter aids. DE is the most commonly used filter aid today. However, the crystalline type DE is a suspicious carcinogen and inhalation needs to be avoided during handling. There are different grades of commercial DE. A finer grade may be employed to increase the clarity of filtrate. The smaller the filter aid particle size, the smaller the process particles can be removed. However, the filtration rate is lower. There is always a balance between initial filtrate clarity and filtration rate. The particle size capture by various filter aids may also vary because of liquid viscosity, surface charge etc.

(ii)   **Perlite:** Perlite is another important mineral filter aid. It is a particular variety of naturally occurring glassy volcanic rock, characterized by onion like, splintery breakage planes. After crushing and heating, this rock expands in an explosive fashion to about ten times its original volume. Diatomaceous earth and perlite are silica based minerals.

(iii) **Cellulose and others:** There are several other special materials used as filter aids, including asbestos, cellulose, agricultural fibers, saw dust, rice hull ash, paper fibers etc. Cellulose can be used for filtration system that cannot tolerate silica. The filterability of cellulose is much worse than DE or perlite but cellulose can be incinerated as well as providing better cake integrity. Calcined rice hull ash and fibers from used newspapers are relatively new filter aids. They are used for wastewater sludge dewatering.

9.5.1 Problems in Filtration

There are three major types of filter problems. They can be caused by chemical treatment before the filter, control of filter flow rate, and backwashing of filters.

(i)   **Chemical addition before filtration:** Coagulation and flocculation stages of the water treatment must be monitored continuously. Adjustments in the amount of coagulant added must be made frequently to prevent the filter from becoming overloaded with suspended material. This overload may cause the filter to prematurely reach its maximum head loss. If there is early turbidity breakthrough in the filter effluent, more coagulant may have to be added to the coagulation process. There may be a need for better mixing during the coagulation or the addition of more filter aid. If there is a rapid increase in filter head loss, too much coagulant may be clogging the filter. Less coagulant or less filter aid should be used.

(ii)   Control of filtration flow rate: When a filter is subjected to rapid changes in flow rate it causes filter media to be dirtier. When a feed flow changes, the filter flow also has to change to run the process smoothly. If there is an increase in feed rate, the flow rate should be increased gradually to reduce the impact on the filter. Addition of filter aids may also reduce the impact on the filter medium. This problem can be avoided by keeping one filter in reserve to accept this additional flow. Many plants are not operated continuously, and the start-up at the beginning causes a gush to the filter(s). The filters should be backwashed before putting them back into operation or operated to waste until the effluent meets the standards.

(iii) Backwashing of Filters: Backwashing of the filters is the single most important operation in the maintenance of the filters. If the filter is not backwashed effectively, problems may occur that may be impossible to correct without totally replacing the filter media. These problems could be caused by improper backwashing procedures:

9.6 FILTER MEDIA

The surface upon which solids are deposited on or in a filter is called the "Filter medium". Filters are used in several different industries, including pharmaceutical, food and beverage, cosmetic and chemical. Without efficient filters, the end products would be of poor quality and the safety element would not be there. The types of filter media and their characteristics are given in Table 9.1.

9.6.1 Properties of Ideal Filter Medium

(i)   It must be capable of delivering a clear filtrate at a suitable production rate.

(ii) It must withstand the mechanical stresses without rupturing or being compressed.

(iii) No chemical or physical interactions with the components of the filtrate should occur.

(iv) It must retain the solids without plugging at the start of filtration.

(v)   For sterile filtration the pore size must not exceed the dimension of bacteria or spores.

9.6.2 Classification of Filter Media

The list of some of the main types of filter media that are used to keep products clear, consistent and uncontaminated is given below.

(i)   Woven filters: Woven filters include wire screens and fabrics of cotton, wool, and nylon. Wire screens, for example, stainless steel are durable, resistance to plugging and easily cleaned. Cotton is a common filter, however, Nylon is superior for pharmaceutical use, since it is unaffected by mold, fungus or bacteria and has negligible absorption properties. Bag filter is common examples of this type. Bag filters come in several different varieties, and are best suited for situations where large solids must be removed from a liquid. In this scenario, the liquid would flow through the bag and the solids would get caught inside. Bag filters may be made from a variety of different materials, and are usually available in different lengths and micron ratings to suit whatever job you need it for.

(ii) Non-woven filters: Filter paper is a common example of non-woven filter medium since it offers controlled porosity, limited absorption characteristic, and low cost. A panel filter is non-woven type filter. It is industrial filter that may come in a variety of different shapes and sizes, depending on the application. In the majority of cases, panel filters are plain and are found inside ventilation or air conditioning units.

(iii) Membrane filters: Membrane filters are basic tools for micro-filtration, useful in the preparation of sterile solutions. These filters are made by casting of various esters of cellulose, or from nylon, Teflon, polyvinyl chloride. The filter is a thin membrane with millions of pores per square centimetre of filter surface. A cartridge filter is cylindrical in shape, but occasionally it looks flat. Cartridge filters use a barrier/sift method to remove sediment and harmful solids from liquid. Some cartridge filters are designed to remove microscopic elements and some are designed to stop larger particles from getting into the finished product. Membrane filters are cartridge units and are economical and available in pore size of 100 μm to even less than 0.2 μm. They can be either surface cartridges or depth type cartridges. Surface cartridges are corrugated and resin treated papers and used in hydraulic lines.

For example, ceramic cartridges and porcelain filter candles. They can be reused after cleaning. Depth type cartridges are made-up of cotton, asbestos or cellulose. These are disposable items, since cleaning is not feasible.

(iv) Porous plates: These include perforated metal or rubber plates, natural porous materials such as stone, porcelain or ceramics, and sintered glass. Sintered glass, sintered metal, earthenware and porous plastics are used for fabrication. These are used for its convenience and effectiveness.

(v) Hydraulic Filters: Hydraulic filters are industrial filters that are designed to purify petroleum-based liquids such as oils. These types of filters are often found in a different hydraulic system to prevent a breakdown caused by oil impurities. Hydraulic filters can also be used to purify water-based liquids.

(vi) Strainers: Strainers often become part of the manufacturing process when the process contains solids that are too large to be caught up in other types of filter media. Strainers consist of baskets that can be removed and cleaned out regularly to prevent them from being stucked inside. Some strainers can be cleaned without interrupting the system, while others cause some disruption each time when they are cleaned.

(vii) Air Filters: Air filters are an important part of most industrial processes, as they remove dust, dirt and other particles from the air. Most air filters consist of a mesh that catches the particles when air is forced through. If the air is to be protected from gases and odors as well as particles, a high efficiency particulate air filter is used.

(viii) Gas Filters: Gas filters are a type of industrial filters that helps to remove contaminants or particulates from a dry or liquid gas stream. Depending on the situation, the contaminants may be solid or liquid. Some of the different elements and accessories for gas filters include gas filter separators, coalescers and gas scrubbers.

Table 9.1: Type of filter media, characteristics and their application

Type of filter media	Characteristics	Application
Metal fiber media (non-woven metal fiber).	Excellent durability, corrosion and abrasion resistance.	Polymer and gas industry.
Multilayer sintered mesh.	It can be reused.	Gas industry.
Stainless steel (plain, twill and Dutch type)	Water proof inside and plastic woven cloth outside.	Oil, chemical, food, pharmaceutical and aviation industry.
Anthracite filter media.	It has high efficiency.	Water purification.
Filter media treated by graphite.	Made-up of fiber glass.	Used in cement and steel industry. Used as filter cloth for air filter.
Activated carbon fabric (non-woven type)	Little air current resistance, strong strength.	Used in air conditioner as auto air filter or carbon air filter.
Aramide filter fabric	Easiness of cake peeling, high stability, anti-distortion.	Used in one dressing, chemical and brewing industry, equipped in filter presses, vacuum filters etc.
Autoroll filter media	It has metal structure, saves energy and work stably.	Used in air filtrate.
Air filter	Pocket type of filter.	Air conditioning and electronic industry, food industry, applied to the pre-filtration of coarse efficiency.

9.7 EQUIPMENTS USED IN FILTRATION

Filtration equipment is used to filter, thicken, or clarify a mixture of different elements. There are several different ways to classify equipment.

9.7.1 Types of Equipments

Below is the description of various types of filtration equipments:

(i) Sedimentation equipment: These equipments use a gravitational force or chemical process to cause particles to settle to the bottom. Equipments that use flocculation and gravity sedimentation are included in this category.

Flocculation: Flocculation is the formation of a cake or aggregate, usually through a chemical process, although a magnetic field may be used for particles containing iron. Flocculation is an important process in the treatment of waste water.

Gravity sedimentation: Gravity sedimentation is used to reduce the solids concentration of the material to be processed. It can be either a clarification or a thickening process. In gravity sedimentation, the heavier particles sink to the bottom under the force of gravity. The rate of settling varies depending on the difference in density between the liquid phase and the solids and the size of the solid particles.

(ii) Gravity filtration equipment: Gravity filtration equipment uses the hydrostatic pressure of a pre-filter column above the filter surface to generate the flow of the filtrate. Common products include bag filters, gravity nutsches, and sand filters. Bag filters are used mainly as collection equipment. They use bag-shaped woven-fabric or felt filters. Bag filters are not recommended for process filtration. A gravity nutsche is a tank with a perforated or porous false bottom. They may or may not have a separate filter medium. The hydrostatic head of the slurry in the tank provides the filtration driving force. The sand filter is the most common type of gravity filters used. It is constructed of a tank containing layers of gravel and sand or pulverized anthracite. The size of the bed particle decreases from bottom to top of the bed. This granular bed forms the filter media. Sand filters are clarifying equipment that forms a cake on the surface. They are used almost exclusively for water conditioning.

(iii) Vacuum filtration equipment: Vacuum filtration is a category of liquid-solid separation equipment and this type of filtration equipment has many different types. Vacuum filters are available in batch (vacuum nutsches and vacuum leaf filters) and continuous (drum filters, disk filters and horizontal filters) operating cycles. Continuous vacuum filters are widely used in the process industry. The three main classes of continuous vacuum filters are drum, disk, and horizontal filters. All of these vacuum filters have the following common features:

(i)   A filtering surface that moves from a point where a cake is deposited under a vacuum to a point of solids removal, where the cake is discharged through mechanical or pneumatic means, and then back to the point of slurry application.

(ii) A valve to regulate pressure below the surface.

(iii) An apparently continuous operating cycle that is actually a series of closely spaced batch cycles.

For example, disc filters, horizontal belt filters, rotary drum filters, rotary drum pre-coat filters, table filters, tilting pan filters, tray filters, and vacuum nutsches.

(iv) Pressure filtration equipment: Pressure filters operate at super atmospheric pressures at the filtering surface. The media is fed to the machine by diaphragm, plunger, screw and centrifugal pumps, blow cases and streams from pressure reactors. Most pressure filters are batch or semi-continuous machines. Rotary drum pressure filters have continuous operating cycles and are more expensive and less flexible than batch machines. For example, automatic pressure filters, candle filters, filter presses, horizontal plate pressure filters, polishing filters, and vertical pressure leaf filters.

(v) Thickening equipment: Thickening equipments (Thickeners) are used to separate solids from liquids by means of gravity sedimentation. Most thickeners are larger, continuous operation pieces of equipment. They are used for heavy duty applications such as coal, iron ore taconites, copper pyrite, phosphates, and other beneficiation processes. Thickeners are a category of industrial filtration equipment that includes conventional thickeners, high-rate thickeners, lamella thickeners, and tray thickeners

(vi) Clarifying equipment: Clarifying equipments (Clarifiers) encompass conventional clarifiers, sludge-basket clarifiers, suction clarifiers, and reverse osmosis (RO) clarifiers. The primary end product of clarifiers is a clarified liquid. They are virtually identical in design to thickeners, but have a lighter duty drive mechanism. They are generally used for industrial and residential waste. For example, conventional clarifiers, reverse osmosis equipment, sludge-blanket, suction, and other clarifiers.

(vii) Centrifugal separators: Centrifugal separators uses centrifugal force to separate solid particles from a liquid solution. They include both centrifuges and hydrocyclones. A centrifuge is a device for separating particles from a solution according to their size, shape, density, viscosity of the medium and rotor speed. A hydrocyclone uses centrifugal force to separate particulate elements of different sizes, shapes, and densities

9.7.2 Plate and Frame Filter Press

Principle:

The mechanism of this filter is surface filtration. The slurry enters the frame by pressure and flows through the filter medium. The filtrate is collected on the plates and sent to the outlet. A number of frames and plates are used so that surface area increases and consequently large volumes of slurry can be processed simultaneously with or without washing.

Construction:

The construction of a plate and frame filter press is shown in the Fig. 9.3. The filter press is made of two types of units, plates and frames.

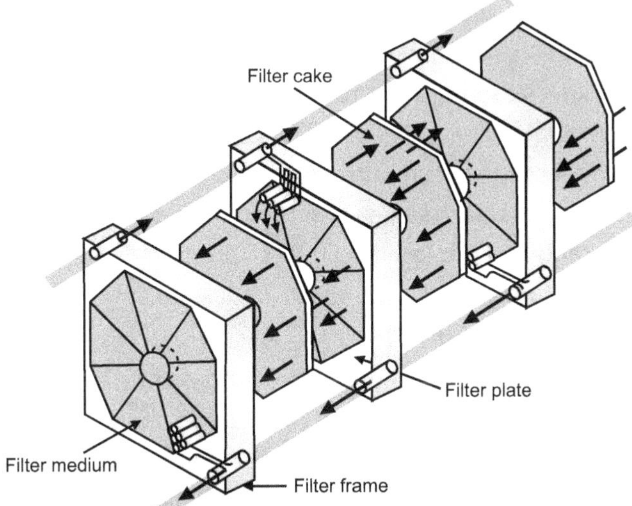

Fig. 9.3: Frame and Press Filter

The components of this filter are as follows.

(i)   **Frame:** It maintains the slurry reservoir and has inlet (eye) for slurry.

(ii) **Filter medium:** It is for solid retention.

(iii) **Plate:** This equipment along with section-supports the filter medium, receives the filtrate and has outlet (eye).

(iv) Assembly of plate and frame filter press.

Plate and frame are usually made of aluminium alloy. Sometimes these are also coated for protection against corrosive chemicals and made suitable for steam sterilization. Frame contains an open space inside wherein the slurry reservoir is maintained for filtration and an inlet to receive the slurry. The plate has a studded or grooved surface to support the filter cloth and an outlet. The filter medium (usually cloth) is fitted between plate and frame. Frames of different thicknesses are available and frame with optimum thickness is chosen. Selection is mainly based upon the thickness of the cake formed during filtration. Plate, filter medium, frame, filter medium and plate are arranged in the sequence as shown in Fig. 9.3 and clamped in a supporting structure. A number of plates and frames are used to have a large surface area. These filtration units are operated in parallel. Channels for the slurry inlet and filtrate outlet can be arranged by fitting inlet to the plates and frames, these join together to form a channel. In some types, only one inlet channel is formed, while each plate is having individual outlets controlled by valves.

Working:

The working of the frame and plate process can be described in two steps, namely filtration and washing of the cake (if desirable). The working of a plate and frame press is shown in Fig. 9.4. Slurry enters the frame from the feed channel and passes through the filter medium on to the surface of the plate. The solids form a filter cake and remain in the frame. The thickness of the cake is usually half the frame thickness as filtration occurs on each side of the frame. Thus, two filter cakes are formed, which meet eventually in the centre of the frame. The optimum thickness of filter cake for any slurry depends on the solid content in the slurry and the resistance of the filter cake. The filtrate drains between the projections on the surface of the plate and escapes from the outlet. With the time resistance of the cake increases and the filtration rate decreases. It is advisable to stop the process at a certain point rather than continuing at very low flow rates. On completion of filtration the press is emptied and the cycle is restarted.

Washing: Generally washing of the filter cake is necessary and for that the ordinary plate and frame press is not suitable. The cake built-up at the centre in the frame brings flow to a standstill. Thus, water washing of cake using the same channels used for the filtrate is inefficient. A modification of the plate and frame press is another option. In modified form an additional channel is included for washing, Fig. 9.3 (d). In half the wash plate there is a connection from the wash water channel to the surface of the plate.

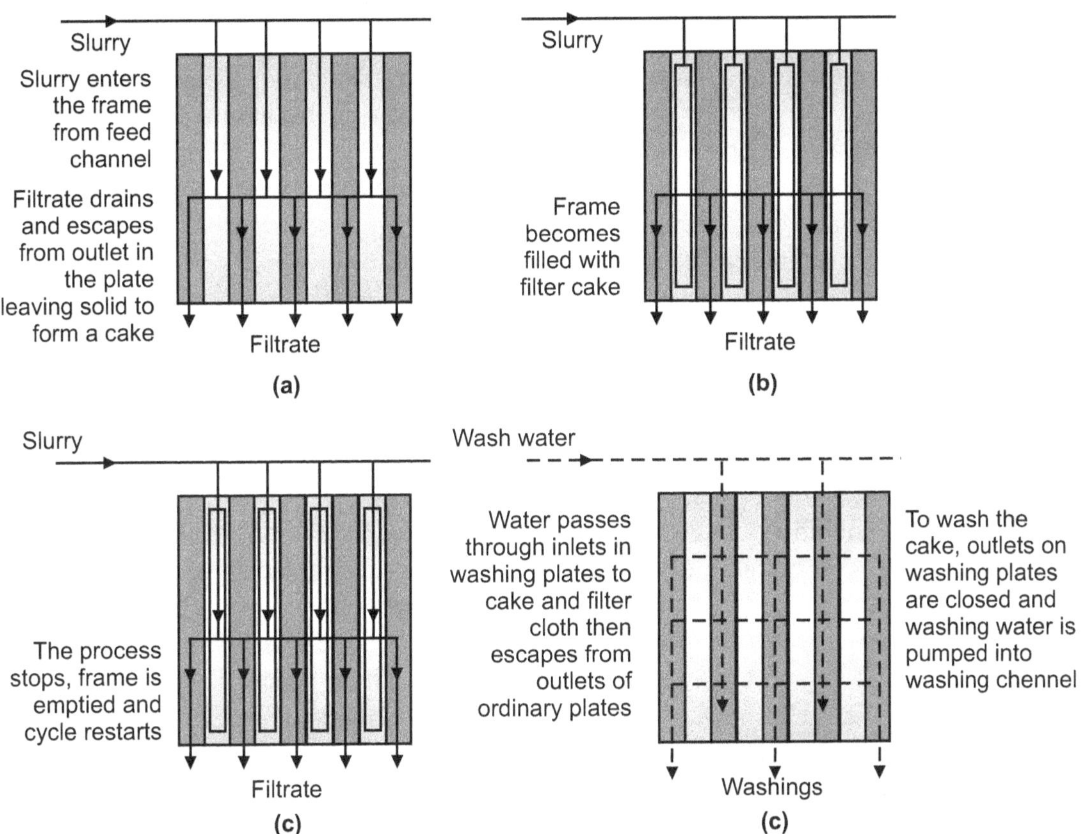

Fig. 9.4: Filtration Operation with Wash Water Facility

The steps of the filtration are as follows:

(i)   Slurry enters the plates and filtration proceeds in the ordinary way until the frames are filled with cake.

(ii) To wash the filter cake, the outlets of the washing plates are closed.

(iii) Wash water is pumped into the washing channel. The water enters through the inlets on to the surface of the washing plates.

(iv) Water passes through the filter cloth and enters frame which contains the cake. The water washes the cake, passes through the filter cloth and enters the plate down the surface.

Finally washed water escapes through the outlet of that plate.

Thus, provision of special washing plates makes it possible for the wash-water to flow over the entire surface of washing plate that makes the uniform resistance of cake to the flow and the entire cake is washed efficiently. The water wash is efficient only when the frames are full with filter cake. If the cake does not fill the frame completely the wash water causes the cake to break on the washing plate side of the frame and the washing will be less effective. It is essential to allow the frames become completely filled with the cake. This helps in emptying the frames as well as in washing the cake correctly.

Special Provisions:

A provision of glass tube (sight glass) to observe contamination can be made at the outlet on each plate. This permits the inspection of quality of the filtrate. The filtrate goes through the control valve to an outlet channel. The filtration process from each plate can be seen. In the case of a broken cloth, the faulty plate can be isolated and filtration can be continued with one plate less. A provision of filter sheets composed of asbestos and cellulose capable of retaining bacteria can be used for sterile filtration with whole filter press and filter medium previously sterilized. Usually steam is passed through the assembled unit for sterilization. The examples include collection of precipitated antitoxin, removal of precipitated proteins from insulin liquors and removal of cell broth from the fermentation medium. Heating/cooling coils can be incorporated in the press for the filtration of viscous liquids.

Advantages:

(i)   Simple in operation, convenient in maintenance, and safe in operation with multiple safety devices. Variety of materials such as cast iron (for handling common substances), bronze (for smaller units), stainless steel (to avoid contamination), hard rubber or plastics (to avoid metal) and wood (for lightness) can be used.

(ii)   It provides a large filtering area in a relatively small floor space.

(iii)   It is versatile equipment whose capacity can be varied according to the thickness and the number of frames used. Surface area can be increased by employing chambers up to 60.

(iv)   This press has sturdy construction that makes use of pressure difference of 2000 kilopascals to be used.

(v)   Cake washing is very efficient.

(vi)   Operation and maintenance is low as it has no moving parts and the filter cloths can be easily renewable.

(vii)   The presence of all external joints makes plate to be isolated in case of if any leaks and the contamination of the filtrate can be avoided.

(viii) It produces dry cake in the form of slab.

Applications:

(i)   Filter presses are used in a huge variety of different applications, from dewatering of slurries to purification. At the same time, filter press technology is widely established for ultrafine dewatering as well as filtrate recovery.

(ii)   Solid-liquid separation in alcohol, chemical, metallurgy, pharmaceutical, light industry, coal mining, food-stuff, textile, environmental protection, energy source and other industries.

Disadvantages:

(i)   It is a batch filter so there is a good deal of 'down-time', which is non-productive.

(ii)   The filter press is an expensive. The emptying time, the labour involved and the wear and tear of the cloth results in high cost process.

(iii) The operation is critical as the frames should be full otherwise inefficient washing results in difficulty to remove cake.

(iv) The filter press is used for slurries containing less than 5% solids. So high costs make it imperative that this filter press is used for expensive materials such as collection of precipitated antitoxin and removal of precipitated proteins from insulin liquors.

9.7.3 Filter Leaf

The filter leaf is the simplest form of filter consisting of a frame that encloses a drainage screen or grooved plate and the whole unit being covered with filter cloth. The outlet for the filtrate connects to the inside of the frame. The frame used may be of circular, square or rectangular shape. There are two types of filter leaf namely; vertical and horizontal.

Construction:

The filter leaf is a versatile piece of equipment. The slurry is pumped under pressure into a vessel that is fitted with a stack of vertical leaves that serve as filter elements. Each leaf has a centrally located neck at its bottom which is inserted into a manifold that collects the filtrate. The leaf is constructed with ribs on both sides to allow free flow of filtrate towards the neck and is covered with coarse mesh screens that support the finer woven metal screens or filter cloth that retain the cake, Fig. 9.5 (enlarged section).

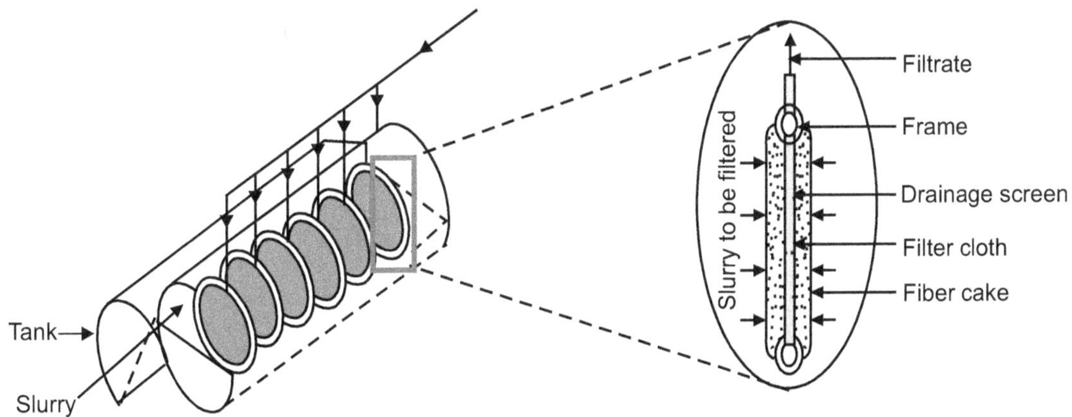

Fig. 9.5: Filter Leaf

The space between the leaves may vary from 30-100 mm depending on the cake formation properties and the ability of the vacuum to hold a thick and heavy cake to the vertical leaf surface. The space is set by the filtrate necks of the leaves at the bottom end and with spacers at the top end brackets. For fast filtering slurries the space may be doubled by removing every second plate so consequently the cake space doubles but the filtration area is reduced to half.

The Vessel:

There are two types of vessel configuration namely vertical vessels and horizontal vessels. The leaves inside horizontal tanks, Fig. 9.5, may be positioned either along the tank axis or perpendicular to the axis. The leaves are graduated to fit to the circular contour of the tank to reduce the slurry heel volume that surrounds the leaves. The vessels are fitted with highly secured cake discharge openings to ensure safe sealing of the tank under pressure. For wet cakes the vessel normally has a small outlet fitted with a valve while for dry cakes the opening is large and the closure locks up electrically or hydraulically with a bayonet wedge. The head cover of vertical vessels is often pivoted to swung away to allow the upwards removal of the leaves in the stack. In vertical leaf filter cakes depart easily while in horizontal leaf filter it is necessary to incorporate means to assist discharge. For such cakes that do not discharge readily a special mechanism that vibrates the entire stack such as oscillating high impact jet headers is provided. The headers also serve to wash the filtering medium and dislodge particles that clog the metal screen or cloth. The largest leaf filters in horizontal vessels have a filtration area of 300 m^2 and in vertical vessels is 100 m^2, both designed for an operating pressure of 6 bars.

Selection Criteria:

Vertical leaf filters are best selected when minimum floor space for large filtration areas is required. If, the liquids are volatile and may not be subjected to vacuum, there is a risk of environmental hazard from toxic, flammable or volatile cakes, high filtrate clarity is required for polishing applications, handling saturated brines that require elevated temperatures the tank may be steam jacketed and the cake may be discharged either dry or as a thickened slurry. They should be selected with care if, the cake is thick and heavy and the pressure is not sufficient to hold it on the leaf. Coarse mesh screens are used and the filtration step must be preceded with a precoat to retain cakes with fine particles. The precoating with a thin layer of diatomite or perlite is not a simple operation and should be avoided whenever possible.

Working:

The operation of a vertical pressure leaf filter is labour intensive and requires a complex manipulation of valves so installations are in most cases fully automated.

(i) **Precoating:** The precoating stage is done when the contaminants are gelatinous and sticky and the precoat layer forms a barrier that avoids cloth blinding. Likewise the interface between the precoat and the cloth departs readily so the cake discharges leaving a clean cloth. In addition, it is done when a clear filtrate is required immediately after the filtration cycle commences otherwise recirculation must be employed until a clear filtrate is obtained.

(ii) **Filtration:** Once the precoating stage is completed the process slurry is pumped into the filter, the forming cake is retained on the leaves and the filtrate flows to further processing. When the solids are fine and slow to filter, a filter-aid is added to the feed slurry in order to enhance cake permeability. The addition of filter-aid increases the solids concentration in the feed so it occupies additional volume between the leaves and increases the amount of cake for disposal. Similarly, for all those applications when the cake is the product, precoat and filter-aid may not be used since they mix and discharge together with the cake.

(iii) Heel Removal: Once the filtration cycle is completed air or gas is blown into the vessel and the slurry heel that surrounds the leaves is pushed and displaced downwards until it reaches the lowest part of the leaf stack. At this point the remaining heel slurry is evacuated back to the feed tank by a special dip pipe that is located at the very bottom of the vessel so that the vessel is empty from slurry.

(iv) Cake Drying: The air then continues to pass through the cake until the captive moisture is reduced to a minimum and the cake is in practical terms considered to be dry.

(v) Cake Discharge: At this stage the air pressure is released, the cake outlet is opened and the leaf stack is vibrated to discharge the cake. The cake outlet opening must be interlocked with a pressure sensor to avoid opening under pressure. On some filters the cloth or mesh screen may be backwashed with water after cake discharge to dislodge and remove any cake residue that adhered to the medium

Advantages:

(i)   The cloth or woven mesh screens that cover the leaves of horizontal tanks may be accessed easily once the stack is pulled out of the vessel.

(ii)   If there is cake bridges between the leaves manually washing of the medium with high impact jets is possible.

(iii) Filter leaf is mechanically simple since there are no complex components in it.

(iv)   The method has the advantage that the slurry can be filtered from any vessel and the cake can be washed simply by immersing the filter, in a vessel of water.

(v)   A number of leaves can be connected to provide a larger area for filtration.

(vi)   Labour costs for operating the filter are comparatively moderate.

(vii) The special feature of the leaf filter is the high efficiency of washing.

Disadvantages:

(i)   High headroom is required for dismantling the leaves on vertical vessels.

(ii)   Large floor space is required for discharging the cake on horizontal vessels.

(iii) The emptying of the vessel in between cake filtration, washing and drying requires close monitoring of the pressure inside the vessel to ensure that the cake holds on to the candles.

(iv)   The operation of a vertical pressure leaf filter is labour intensive and requires a complex manipulation of valves.

Applications:

(i)   The vertical pressure leaf filter is used for the polishing slurries with very low solid content of 1- 5% or for cake filtration with a solid concentration of 20 - 25%.

(ii) The vertical leaf filters are suitable for handling flammable, toxic and corrosive materials since they are autoclaved and designed for hazardous environments when high pressure and safe operation are required.

(iii) The vertical leaf filters may be readily jacketed for applications whenever hot or cold temperatures are to be maintained.

9.7.4 Rotary Filter

In large scale filtration when continuous operation is desirable and it is necessary to filter slurries containing a high proportion of solids. Rotary drum filter, patented in 1872, is one of the oldest filters used in the industrial liquid-solids separation. A rotary drum filter is one which is continuous in operation and has a system to remove the cake formed and in addition it can handle concentrated slurries too. It offers a wide range of industrial processing applications and provides a flexible application of dewatering, washing and/or clarification.

Construction:

The rotary drum filter usually consists of 16 - 20 filter units. It has the shape of longitudinal segments of the periphery of a cylinder, Fig. 9.6. Each filter unit is rectangular in shape with a curved profile and are joined to form a drum. Each unit has a perforated metal surface to the outer part of the drum and is covered with filter cloth. Appropriate connections are again made from each unit through a rotating valve at the centre of the drum. Rotary filters may be up to 2 m in diameter and 3.5 m in length, giving areas of the order of 20 m^2. The drum is suspended on an axial over a trough containing liquid/solids slurry with approximately 50-80% of the screen area immersed in the slurry. One form is the rotary disc filter, in which the sector shaped filter leaves form a disc with the outlet from the each leaf connected to the vacuum system, compressed air, and the appropriate receivers, in the correct sequence, by means of special rotating valve.

Special attachments may be included for special purposes; for example if the cake shrinks and cracks as it dries out, cake compression rollers can be fitted. These compress the cake to a homogenous mass to improve the efficiency of washing as the cake passes through the washing zone, or to aid drainage of wash water as the cake passes to the drying zone. Where the solids of the slurry are such that the filter cloth becomes blocked with the particles, a pre coat filter may be used. This is variant in which a precoat of filter aid is deposited on the drum prior to the filtration process. The scraper knife then removes the solid filtered from the slurry together with a small amount of the precoat. The knife moves slowly to avoid precoat removal.

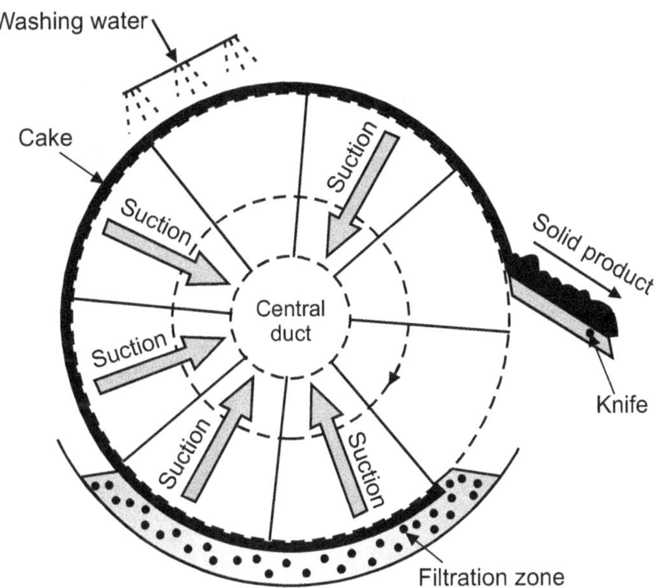

Fig. 9.6: Rotary Drum Filter

An alternative discharge method can be used, for example, a string discharge rotary filter, Fig. 9.7. The string discharge filter is operated by means of a number of loops of string which pass the drum, and cause the cake to form over the strings. The strings are in contact with the surface of the drum-up to the cake removal zone, where they leave the surface and pass over additional small rollers before returning to again contact the drum.

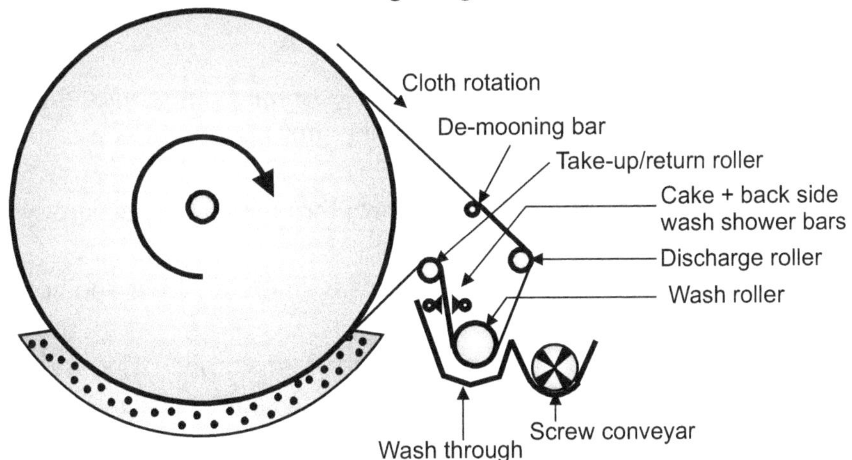

Fig. 9.7: String Discharge Rotary Drum Filter

Working:

The basic operating zones in rotary filter are given Table 9.2. As the drum rotates into and out of the trough, the slurry is sucked on the surface of the cloth and rotated out of the liquid/solids suspension as a cake. When the cake is rotating out, it is dewatered in the drying zone.

Table 9.2: Various zones in rotary drum filter

Zone	Position	Service	Connected to
Pick-up	Slurry trough	Vacuum	Filtrate receiver
Drainage	--	Vacuum	Filtrate receiver
Washing	Wash sprays	Vacuum	Wash water receiver
Drying	--	Vacuum	Wash receiver
Cake removal	Scraper knife	Compressed air	Filter cake conveyor

The cake is dry because the vacuum drum is continuously sucking the cake and taking the water out of it. At the final step of the separation, the cake is discharged as solid product and the drum rotates continuously to another separation cycle. In case of string discharge filter the strings of filter lift the filter cake of the filter medium, and the cake is broken by the sharp bend, over the discharge roller so that it is easily collected while the strings return to the drum.

Advantages:

(i)   The rotary filter is automatic and continuous in operation with very low labour costs.

(ii)   These filters have a large filter area and thus the high output capacity.

(iii)   Variation of the speed of rotation enables the cake thickness to be controlled,

For example, for solids that form an impermeable cake, the thickness may be limited to less than 5 mm and for coarse solids forming a porous cake the thickness may be 100 mm or more.

Disadvantages:

(i)   This filter has ancillary components such as vacuum pumps, vacuum receivers and traps, slurry pumps and agitators with many moving parts it is a complex piece of equipment.

(ii)   The cake tends to crack due to the air drawn through by the vacuum system so that washing and drying are not efficient.

(iii)   Being a vacuum filter the pressure difference is limited to 1 bar and hot filtrates may boil.

(iv)   The rotary filter is suitable only for straight forward slurries, being less satisfactory if the solids formed an impermeable cake or will not separate cleanly from the cloth.

Applications:

(i)   The rotary filter is most suitable for continuous operation on large quantities of slurry.

(ii)   It is used in the collection of calcium carbonate, magnesium carbonate and starch.

(iii)   It is especially useful for filtering the fermentation liquor in the manufacture of antibiotics where the mould is difficult to filter by ordinary methods because it forms a felt-like cake.

(iv)   It is useful for the slurry that contains considerable amount of solids (15-30%).

9.7.5 Membrane Filters

A membrane is a thin layer of semi-permeable material that separates substances when a driving force is applied across the membrane. It works on the principle of physical separation. These are used for removal of bacteria, micro-organisms, particulates, and natural organic material, which can impart colour, tastes, and odours to water and react with disinfectants to form disinfection byproducts. Advancements are made in membrane production and module design with the view to reduce capital and operating costs. The membrane processes includes:

(i)   Microfiltration

(ii)   Ultrafiltration

(iii)   Nanofiltration

(iv)   Reverse osmosis

Construction:

Membrane filters are plastic membranes based on cellulose acetate, cellulose nitrate or mixed cellulose esters with pore sizes in the micron or submicron range. They are very thin about 120 μ and must be handled carefully. They act like a sieve trapping particulate matter on their surface. Several grades of filters are available with pore sizes ranging from 0.010 ± 0.002 μ to 5.0 ± 1.2 μ. Type codes VF and SM are given by Millipore Filter Corp. for these two extreme ranges respectively.

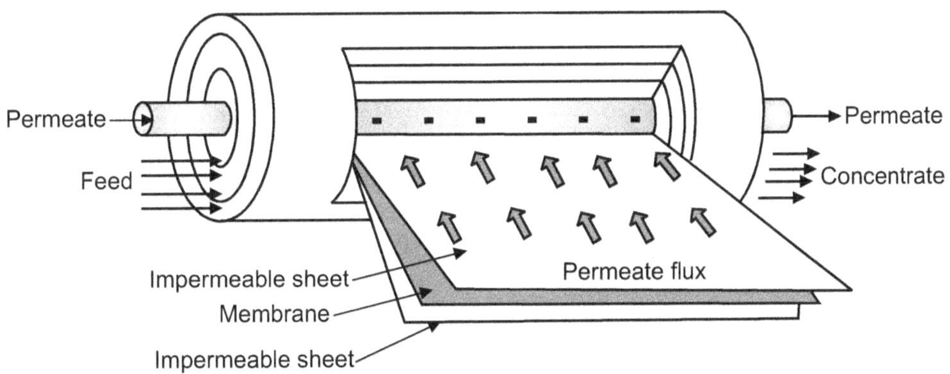

Fig. 9.8: Spiral Wound Membrane Filter

Filters with pore sizes from 0.010 to 0.10 μ can remove virus particles from water or air. Filters with pore sizes from 0.30 to 0.65 μ are employed for removing bacteria. Filters with the larger pore sizes, *viz.* 0.8, 1.2 and 3.0 to 5.0 μ are employed, for example, in aerosol, radio activity and particle sizing applications. Membrane filters are manufactured as flat sheet stock or as hollow fibers and formed into several different types of membrane modules. Module construction involves potting or sealing the membrane material into an assembly, such as with hollow-fiber module. These types of modules are designed for long-term use over the course of a number of years. Spiral-wound modules, Fig. 9.8, are also manufactured for long-term use.

Working:

The membrane separation process is based on the presence of semi-permeable membranes. The principle is membrane acts as a very specific filter that will let water flow through, while it catches suspended solids and other substances. During use membrane filters are supported on a rigid base of perforated metal, plastic or coarse sintered glass as in the case of fibrous pad filters. If the solution to be filtered contains a considerable quantity of suspended matter, preliminary filtration through a suitable depth filter avoids clogging of the membrane filter during sterile filtration. They are brittle when dry and can be stored indefinitely in the dry state but are fairly tough when wet.

(i)   Microfiltration (MF): Microfiltration is defined as a membrane separation process using membranes with a pore size of approximately 0.03 to 10 µ, a molecular weight cut-off (MWCO) of greater than 10,00,000 Daltons and a relatively low feed water operating pressure of approximately 100 to 400 kPa (15 to 60 psi). Sand, silt, clays, Giardia lamblia and Crypotosporidium cysts, algae, and some bacterial species are removed by MF. This filter is not an absolute barrier to viruses but when used in combination with disinfectant it appears to control them. There is a growing emphasis on limiting the concentrations and number of chemicals that are applied during water treatment. By physically removing the pathogens, membrane filtration can significantly reduce chemical addition, such as chlorination. It can also be used to remove natural synthetic organic matter to reduce fouling potential. The pretreatment helps to increase removal of organic material. MF can also be used as a pretreatment to reverse osmosis (RO) or Nano-filteration (NF) to reduce bad odor as well as to remove hardness from ground water.

(ii)   Ultrafiltration (UF): The ultra filters has a pore size of approximately 0.002 to 0.1 µ, with a MWCO of approximately 10,000 to 100,000 Daltons, and an operating pressure of approximately 200 to 700 kPa (30 to 100 psi). It removes all microbiological species such as partial removal of bacteria, as well as humic materials and some viruses but is not an absolute barrier to viruses. Disinfection can provide a second barrier to contamination and is therefore recommended. The primary advantages of low-pressure UF membrane processes are :

(i)   No need for chemicals (coagulants, flocculants, disinfectants, pH adjustment).

(ii)   Size-exclusive filtration.

(iii)   Constant quality of the treated water in terms of particle and microbial removal.

(iv)   The process and plant are compact.

(v)   Simple and automatic, however, fouling can cause difficulties in membrane technology for water treatment.

(iii) Nanofiltration: Nanofiltration membranes have a nominal pore size of approximately 0.001 µ and a MWCO of 1,000 to 100,000 Daltons. Pushing liquid through these very small size membrane pores requires a higher operation pressure. Operating pressures are usually near to 600 kPa and can be as high as 1,000 kPa. NF can apparently remove all cysts, bacteria, viruses, and humic materials. They provide an excellent protection from disinfection by-product (DBP) formation (if the disinfectant residual is added) and remove alkalinity. NF also removes hardness from water, which accounts for NF membranes sometimes being called "softening membranes." Hard water treated by NF needs pretreatment to avoid precipitation of hardness ions on the membrane.

Reverse Osmosis (RO):

Reverse osmosis can effectively remove nearly all inorganic contaminants from water. It can effectively remove radium, natural organic substances, pesticides, cysts, bacteria and viruses. It is particularly effective when used in series with multiple units. Disinfection is also recommended to ensure the safety of water. Advantages of this filter include removal of nearly all contaminant ions and most dissolved non-ions. It is relatively insensitive to flow and total dissolved solids. It operates immediately without any minimum break-in period. It is possible to concentrate effluents with low solid. It is capable of removing bacteria and particles. The operational simplicity and automation features allow for less supervision.

Limitations:

(i)   High capital and operating costs.

(ii)   Managing the wastewater (brine solution) is a potential problem.

(iii) High level of pretreatment is required in some cases.

(iv)   Membranes are prone to fouling.

(v)   Produces the most waste water at between 25-50 % of the feed.

Advantages:

(i)   Filtration rate is rapid.

(ii)   They are disposable and hence no cross contamination take place.

(iii) No bacterial growth through the filter takes place during prolonged filtration.

(iv)   Adsorption is negligible they yield no fibres or alkali into the filtrate.

Disadvantages:

(i)   Ordinary types are less resistant to solvents like chloroform.

(ii)   They may clog though rarely.

Applications:

(i)   It allows the isolation and categorization of micro-organisms.

(ii)   It is used in removal of ammonium ions from potable water.

(iii) **Dairy industry:** MF is a valuable part in the manufacture of dairy ingredients. It has applications in milk, whey and clarified cheese brine.

(iv)   **Starch and sweetener industry:** It can be used to increase in the performance of the products for example, clarification of corn syrups such as dextrose and fructose, the concentration of rinse water from starch, the enrichment of dextrose, the depyrogenation of dextrose syrup and the division/concentration of maceration water.

(v)   **Sugar industry:** MF can be used to clarify unprocessed juice without using primary clarifiers. It can be used to clarify, divide and concentrate various sugar solutions in the production process.

(vi) **Chemical industry:** MF can be used in many chemical processes to desalinate diafilter and purify dyes, pigments and optical brighteners, to clean the waste water and rinse water currents, for the concentration and dehydration of minerals such as kaolin clay, titanium dioxide and calcium carbonate, the clarification of caustic agents and the production of polymers or the recuperation of metals.

(vii) **Pharmaceutical industry:** It is used in the harvesting of cells or the recuperation of biomass in the process of fermentation during manufacturing of antibiotics. MF improves production as well as reduces labor and maintenance costs. It is used in the industrial production lines for enzymes in concentrating them prior to other processes.

9.7.6 Cartridge Filters

Cartridge filters are fabric or polymer-based filters designed primarily to remove particulate material from fluids. They are usually rigid or semi-rigid and manufactured by affixing the fabric or polymer to a central core. Pre-formed cartridge filters of all sizes are one of the simplest and most commonly-found means of removing particulate material from water supplies.

Principle:

The main principle of this filter is physical filtration. These systems work by pushing water from the reservoir into the cylinder. A cylinder collects the larger debris and the secondary filter catches anything that the first one may have missed. The water passes through the polyester filters, and dirt gets stuck on the screen allowing for clean water to pass by. The liquid to be filtered is imported and clear liquid flows to the discharge port. Drainage inlet filter size, structure and size of the filter depends on the design flow and the filter medium characteristics of the liquid.

Construction:

It is designed to remove solid particulate material from the water. These may be constructed in a number of different ways and from various materials, including pleated paper or fiber, plastics such as polypropylene or nylon, cellulose, membrane, fiber glass, ceramics etc. It is characterized by a composite structure of the filter cartridge, saving the volume of the cylinder. It is easy to clean and maintain and can be designed to a pressure upto 5 M.Pa and 280 °C temperature. The shell is made of carbon steel or stainless steel. Filter cartridge housings consists of single cartridges up to hundreds of cartridges, Fig. 9.9.

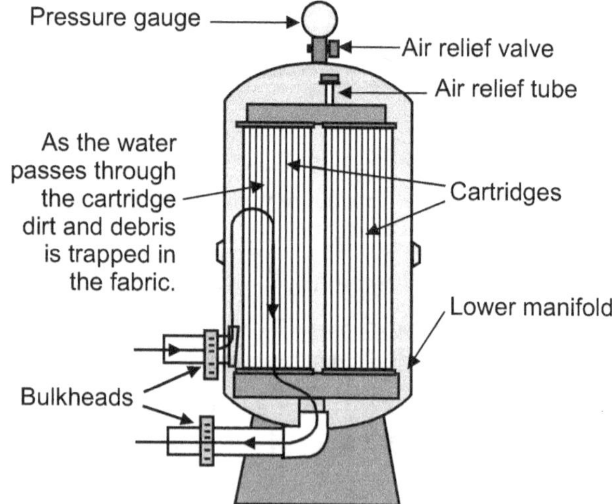

Fig. 9.9: Cartridge Filter

The housing is sized based on the flow rate, viscosity of liquid, filtration efficiency required and allowable clean differential pressure drop. Cartridge filter is used in chemical industry to filter 50 – 150 μ particles of the media. These filters are rated by the maximum size of particle they allow to pass through. A "nominal" rating means that a stated percentage of pores in the filter are smaller than a specified size. An "absolute" rating states the maximum pore size that may be found anywhere on the filter. These filters are often installed in series in descending order of pore size to maximize removal efficiency and protect downstream filters or other treatment processes.

Working:

When the liquid through the cylinder enters into the basket, the solid impurity particles are blocked in the filter basket, and clean fluid through the filter basket is discharged from the filter outlet. For cleaning, the bottom of the head plung is unscrewed to drain the fluid after removing flange cover. After cleaning the components are reloaded. Therefore, the use of maintenance is very convenient. Solid material suspended in the water gets trapped on the cartridge filter. The filter is rated to remove particles of a certain size. A typical choice would be a 20 μ filter followed by a 5 and / or 1 μ filter, but the exact choice depends on the quality of the supply and the substance(s) that need to be removed. The filter should be clearly marked with its size rating.

Advantages:

(i)   Cartridge filters are relatively cheap, compact and requiring minimal maintenance other than changing the cartridge.

(ii) These filters are disposable and easily replaceable.

(iii) Cartridge filter systems are modular and can theoretically accommodate any flow rate by increasing or decreasing the number of filter or filter arrays.

(iv) Being cheaper they are suitable in their use in smaller water systems.

(v)   These filters are of high quality with reasonable structure.

(vi) They have higher flow rates.

(vii) They are easy to maintain and assemble with high filter accuracy.

(viii) They require low maintenance and oversight.

Disadvantages:

(i)   As cartridge filters are not backwashed, they are simply replaced once they become dirty or block.

(ii) The use of coagulants or a pre-coat with a cartridge filter is not usually recommended.

(iii) Cartridge filtration for water treatment is limited by two source namely; water quality and system size.

Applications:

(i)   It is used in the chemical and petrochemical production of weak corrosive materials, such as: water, oil, ammonia, hydrocarbons and so on.

(ii) In the chemical production of corrosive materials, such as: caustic soda, soda ash, concentrated sulphuric acid, carbonic acid, uronic acid and so on.

(iii) In the case of the cooling of low-temperature materials, such as: liquid methane, liquid ammonia, liquid oxygen and various refrigerants.

(iv) In food production of the health requirements materials, such as: beer, beverages, dairy products, syrup and so on.

(v) In pharmaceutical production of tissue culture media, enzymes, aqueous solutions, chemical and reagent purification, immunological and cosmetic products.

(vi) It can be used to remove general debris such as leaves or sediment, or chemical precipitates that have been encouraged to form in the water (for example by oxidation) to enable their removal.

9.7.7 Meta Filter

Metafilter is the commonest filter used in the pharmaceutical industry.

Principle:

Meta filter is a type of pressure filter. Pressure filters feed the product to the filter at a pressure greater than that which would arise from gravity alone. Meta filter functions as a strainer (service filtration) for the separation of particles. The metal rings contain semi circular projections, which are arranged as a nest to form channels on the edges. This channel offers resistance (strainer) to the flow of solids (forced particles). The clear liquid is collected into a receiver from the top.

Construction:

The metafilter, in its simplest form, consists of a grooved drainage rod on which is packed a series of metal rings. These rings are usually of stainless steel and are about 15 mm inside diameter, 22 mm outer diameter and 0.8 mm in thickness. These rings have a number of semicircular projections on one surface and when they are packed on the rod, the opening between the rings is about 0.2 mm, Fig. 9.10. The height of the projections and the shape of the section of the ring are such as that when the rings are packed together, all the same way up, and tightened on the drainage rod with a nut, channels are formed that taper from about 250 μm down to 25 μm. One or more of these packs is mounted in a vessel, and the filter may be operated by pumping in the slurry under pressure or, occasionally, by the application of reduced pressure to the outlet side.

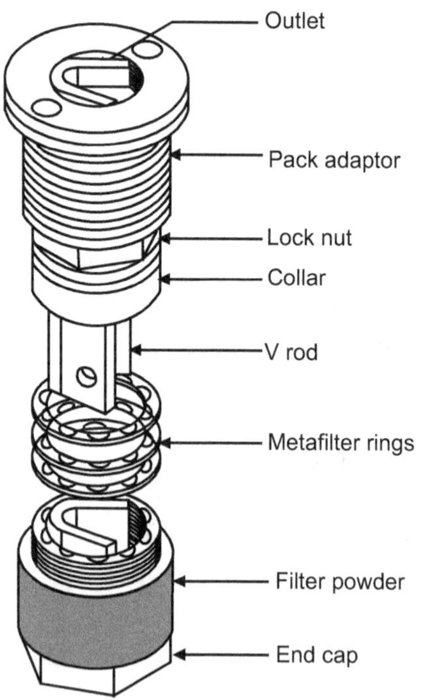

Fig. 9.10: Meta filter

In this form, the metafilter can be used as a strainer for coarse particles, but for finer particles a bed of a suitable material such kieselguhr is first built up. The pack of rings, therefore, serves essentially as a base on which the true filter medium is supported.

Working:

Meta filters are placed in a vessel and may be operated by pumping the slurry under pressure or occasionally by the application of reduced pressure to the outlet side. The slurry passes through the channels formed on the edges between the rings. The clear liquid rises-up and collected from the outlet into the receiver. When vacuum is applied, liquid flows from outside to inside. In this form a metafilter can only be used as strainer for coarse particles. But for separation of finer particles, a bed of suitable materials such as Kieselguhr is used. In this way the pack of rings acts as a base on which the true filter medium is supported.

Advantages:

(i)   The metafilter is sturdy having enough strength to handle high pressures with no danger of bursting the filter medium.

(ii) As it has no filter medium as such, the running costs are low and are very economical.

(iii) This filter provides excellent resistance to corrosion and avoid contamination of the most sensitive product.

(iv) It is sustainable to filter off very fine particles.

(v)   It can be used to sterilize some liquids by filtration.

(vi) It also can be used to remove larger particles simply by building up a bed of coarse substances, or even by using the Meta filter candle itself if the particles are sufficiently large.

(vii) Removal of the cake is effectively carried out by back flushing with water.

Applications:

(i)   The small surface of the metafilter restricts the amount of the solids that can be collected. This, together with the ability to separate very fine particles, means that the metafilter is used almost exclusively for clarification purposes.

(ii) The strength of the metafilter permits the use of high pressures (15 bars) making it suitable for viscous liquids.

(iii) It can be constructed with appropriate corrosion resistant materials.

(iv) Specific examples of pharmaceutical uses include the clarification of syrups, elixirs, injection solutions, and of products such as insulin liquors.

REVIEW QUESTIONS

1. What is filtration? Classify and explain filtration processes.
2. Discuss in detail mechanisms of filtration.
3. What are objectives of filtration? Discuss various applications of filtration?
4. Discuss in detail theories of filtration.
5. Discuss factors influencing filtration.
6. Discuss Darcy's equation to estimate rate of filtration.
7. What are filter aids? Discuss their functions and elaborate upon various filter aids used in filtration.
8. What are filter media? Give its ideal properties. Discuss various filter media along with their characteristics.
9. Classify filtration equipments along with principle concept involved giving examples of each.
10. Discuss principle, construction, working, advantages, disadvantages and applications of Frame and Plate filter press.
11. Discuss stepwise operation of a Frame and Plate filter.
12. Discuss principle, construction, working, advantages, disadvantages and applications of filter leaf.
13. Discuss stepwise operation of a vertical pressure filter leaf.
14. Discuss principle, construction, working, advantages, disadvantages and applications of rotary drum filter.
15. Write short note on string discharge rotary filter.
16. Discuss various membrane filtration methods.
17. Discuss principle, construction, working, advantages, disadvantages and applications of cartridge filter.
18. Discuss principle, construction, working, advantages, disadvantages and applications of meta filter.
19. Discuss principle, construction, working, advantages, disadvantages and applications of membrane filter.

✍ ✍ ✍

Chapter ... 10

CENTRIFUGATION

10.0 INTRODUCTION

Centrifugation is the use of the centrifugal forces generated in a spinning rotor to separate particles, living components such as cells, viruses, sub-cellular organelles, macromolecules such as proteins and nucleic acids and macromolecular complexes such as ribonucleoproteins and lipoproteins. The three main methods of separation by centrifugation are differential pelleting, rate-zonal centrifugation and isopycnic centrifugation. The first two methods separate particles primarily on the basis of size. The latter method isopycnic centrifugation separates particles on the basis of their density. The choice of centrifugation method depends on the nature of the particles and often when more than one separation technique is required. For example, membrane fractionation often involves first making an enriched fraction from a cell homogenate by differential pelleting followed by isopycnic centrifugation to obtain purified fractions.

Centrifugation is one of the most important and widely applied research techniques in biochemistry, cellular and molecular biology and in evaluation of suspensions and emulsions in pharmacy and medicine. Centrifugation, clearly, plays an important role in the pharmaceutical industry in the production of bulk drugs, biological products, and determination of molecular weight of colloids and in the evaluation of suspensions and emulsions.

The earth's gravitational force is sufficient to separate many types of particles over time. A tube of anticoagulated whole blood left standing on a bench top will eventually separate into plasma, red blood cell and white blood cell fractions. However, the length of time required precludes this manner of separation for most applications. In practice, centrifugal force is necessary to separate most particles. In addition, the potential degradation of biological compounds during prolonged storage means faster separation techniques are needed. The rate of separation in a suspension of particles by way of gravitational force mainly depends on the particle size and density. Particles of higher density or larger size typically travel at a faster rate and at some point will be separated from particles less dense or smaller. This sedimentation of particles, including cells, can be explained by the Stokes equation, which describes the movement of a sphere in a gravitational field. Equation (10.1) calculates the velocity of sedimentation utilizing five parameters.

$$V = \frac{d^2 (\rho - \rho_o)\, g}{18\, \eta} \qquad \dots (10.1)$$

Where, $\qquad\qquad$ V = Sedimentation rate or velocity of settling the sphere d = Diameter of the sphere

p = Particle density

L = Medium density

n = Viscosity of medium

g = Gravitational force

10.1 OBJECTIVES

Centrifugation is a technique of separating substances which involves the application of centrifugal force. The particles are separated from a solution according to their size, shape, density, viscosity of the medium and rotor speed. Separation is achieved by spinning a vessel containing material at high speed; the centrifugal force pushes heavier materials to the outside of the vessel. A centrifuge is a laboratory device used for the separation of immiscible fluids, gas or liquid.

10.2 PRINCIPLE

Centrifugation is used to separate all types of particle based upon their sedimentation properties. The sedimentation properties of particles depend on a number of different factors including size, density and shape. However, both density and shape vary significantly depending on the composition of the solution in which the particles are suspended. Particles are separated primarily on the basis of either their density (isopycnic separations) or size (differential pelleting and rate-zonal separations). The density affect sedimentation to a much lesser extent than size. In centrifugation it is important to differentiate between the speed of centrifugation (r.p.m.) and the relative centrifugal force (RCF or G) since these are often confused.

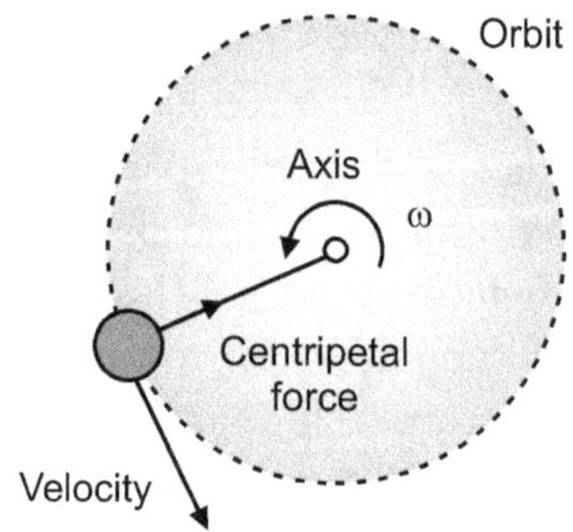

Fig. 10.1: Principle of Centrifugation

The centrifugal force generated by a centrifuge can easily be calculated from the equation

$$RCF = 11.18 \times R \times \left(\frac{r.p.m.}{1000}\right)^2 \qquad \ldots (10.2)$$

where, R is the distance from the centre of rotation in centimeters; that is, the centrifugal force increases as the particles move down the centrifuge tube. As a general rule, the greater the centrifugal force the shorter the separation time. However, centrifugation also generates hydrostatic forces within the solution and so excessive centrifugal forces can disrupt some biological particles such as ribosomes.

The other very important aspect in optimizing centrifugal separations is the choice of rotor. Centrifuge rotors can be divided up into five different types and of these the most frequently used are fixed-angle and swinging bucket rotors.

As a general guide, fixed-angle rotors are used for efficient pelleting and isopycnic centrifugation of macro-molecules, while swinging bucket rotors are primarily used for isopycnic gradients for cells and organelles and rate-zonal centrifugation. The other three types of rotor are vertical rotors that can be used for gradient separations where no pelleting occurs, zonal rotors that are used for large-scale gradient separations, and analytical rotors where instead of tubes the samples are centrifuged in sector-shaped cells with transparent sides. The efficiency of rotors for pelleting particles is expressed in terms of their k-factors with the most efficient rotors having the smallest k-factors.

Applications of Principle:

High centrifugal force is required if the particles in suspensions are very small. To separate such small particles from suspensions the centrifuge is designed to be small in size that can operate at very high speed of rotation. If a large amount of material is to be separated and a low centrifugal effect is sufficient to separate the suspension then the diameter of the centrifuge is increased and speed is kept low.

10.3 APPLICATIONS

(i) Bulk drugs production:

In the synthetic chemical reactions the product formed is crystal. The crystallized drugs are separated from the mother liquor by the process of centrifugation.

For example, traces of mother liquor are separated from aspirin crystals by use of centrifugal force.

(ii) Production of biological products:

During manufacturing most of the biological products are either proteinaceous or macromolecules which remain as colloidal dispersion in water. A normal filtration method is not suitable to separate these colloid particles and thus in those cases centrifugal methods are used. The examples include:

- (a) Insulin purification from other precipitates of protein materials by centrifugation.
- (b) Blood cell separation from plasma by centrifugal method.
- (c) Bacterial enzymes are separated from bacterial culture medium by sedimenting the bacterial cells by centrifugation.
- (d) Dirt and water are separated from olive oil and fish-liver oils.
  - (i) It has application in the field of medicine such as DNA/ RNA separation.
  - (ii) In purification of mammalian cells, fractionation of sub-cellular organelles and fractionation of membrane vesicles.
  - (iii) Used in diagnostic laboratories for blood and urine test.

(iii) Stability testing of dispersed system:

Suspensions and emulsions have problems of sedimentation and creaming, respectively over the storage periods. These problems are not observed immediately after the preparation of a suspension or emulsion. To investigate the stability of these preparations rates of sedimentation and creaming in suspension or emulsion, respectively, is determined using a centrifuge by rotating at 200 to 3000 r.p.m. The absence of sedimentation and creaming is indication of stability of those preparations.

(iv) Determination of molecular weight of colloids:

Polymers, proteins and such macromolecules often exist in colloidal dispersions. The molecular weights of those substances can be determined by ultra-centrifugation. The larger molecules gets arranged at periphery and the lighter molecules near the center.

(v) Other applications:

(i)   Centrifugation is used to separate skim milk from whole milk and to separate two miscible substances.

(ii)   Separating particles from an air-flow using cyclonic separation.

(iii) Separation of urine components and blood components in forensic and research laboratories.

(iv)   Aids in separation of proteins using purification techniques such as salting out, for example, ammonium sulfate precipitation.

(v)   The other medical applications include the separation of blood cells from blood (plasma), and the removal of fibrinogen (serum). They are also used to determine the haematocrit and to separate urinary components.

(vi)   Centrifugation is used to analyze the hydrodynamic properties of macromolecules

10.4 EQUIPMENTS USED FOR CENTRIFUGATION

There are two types of centrifugal techniques for separating particles, differential centrifugation and density gradient centrifugation. Density gradient centrifugation can further be divided into rate-zonal and isopycnic centrifugation. An industrial centrifuge is a machine used for fluid/particle separation. Industrial centrifuges can be classified into 3 main types as given the Table 10.1.

Table 10.1: Classification of Industrial Centrifuges

Type	Principle	Examples
Filtration centrifuge	Using perforated baskets, which perform a filtration-type operation (work like a spin- dryer)	Perforated basket centrifuge
Sedimentation centrifuge	With a solid walled vessel, where particles sediment towards the wall under the influence of the centrifugal force.	Tubular bowl centrifuge
Continuous centrifuge	A continuous process or very high capacity is required	Continuous flow centrifuge

10.4.1 Perforated Basket Centrifuge

There are three types of perforated basket centrifuge namely; batch type (top-driven or bottom-driven), semi-continuous type and continuous type.

Principle:

Centrifugal force generates a pressure which forces the liquid through the caked solids, the filter cloth, the backing screen, and the basket perforations. The filter cloth retains the solid particles inside the rotating basket.

(A) Batch Type Top Driven Centrifuge:

This centrifuge is used for chemical and pharmaceutical manufacturing for separation purpose due to easy discharge from the bottom. This centrifuge is used when concentration of slurry is high.

Construction:

This centrifuge consists of a rotating basket suspended on a vertical shaft and driven by a motor from top. This centrifuge is called as top driven or bottom discharge basket centrifuge, Fig. 10.2. The sides of the basket are perforated and are also covered with a screen on the side. Surrounding the basket is a stationary casing that collects the filtrate. The basket diameter is ranging from 20 to 48 inch with 1800 to 800 r.p.m. speed of rotation. The larger is the diameter lowest is the speed. The basket is made-up of stainless steel covered with Monel. The size of perforations may be 3 mm but for very fine particles basket is lined with fine mesh or cloth supported on coarse gauge. Unbalanced basket cause strain and vibrations. The machine picks its top speed in short time to avoid longer operation at critical speed which is undesirable for cake and its removal.

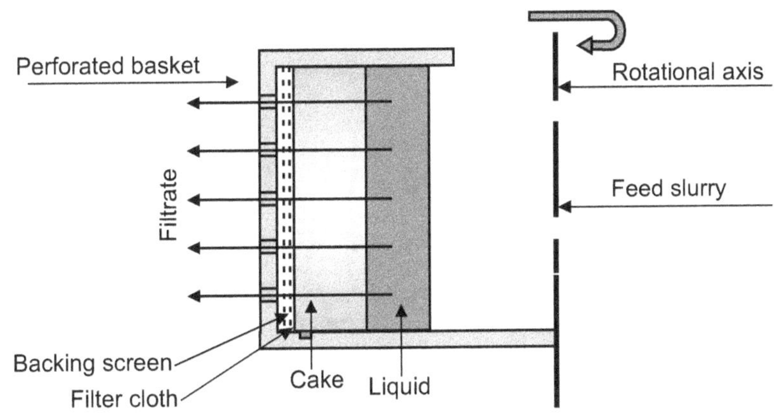

Fig. 10.2: Vertical Basket Top Driven Centrifuge

Working:

   (i) **Feeding:** The slurry is introduced to the rotating basket having a filter cloth. The filter cloth captures the solids. Centrifugal force drives the liquid through the caked solids and the mother liquor is discharged through perforations in the basket circumference.

(ii) **Washing:** A wash liquid is introduced and is driven through the caked solids. The plug flow action of the wash liquid purifies the solids and removes residual mother liquor.

(iii) **Spinning:** Residual liquor is driven from the caked solids and is discharged through the basket perforations to achieve maximum cake dryness.

(iv) **Scraping:** A scraper knife advances into the rotating basket to discharge the solids to downstream equipment. The solids are discharged through openings in the basket bottom.

(v) **Residual heel removal:** After scraping, a 6-10 mm layer remains inside the rotating basket. With the scraper in an advanced position, high pressure nitrogen or air is used to dislodge this residual heel. This step can be performed after several centrifuge cycles, or after each cycle.

(B) Batch Type Bottom Driven Centrifuge:

Construction:

Batch type under driven centrifuge consists of a rotating basket placed on a vertical shaft and driven by a motor from bottom called as under driven or top discharge basket centrifuge, Fig. 10.3. The sides of the basket are perforated and are also covered with a screen on the inside. Surrounding the basket is a stationary casing that collects the filtrate.

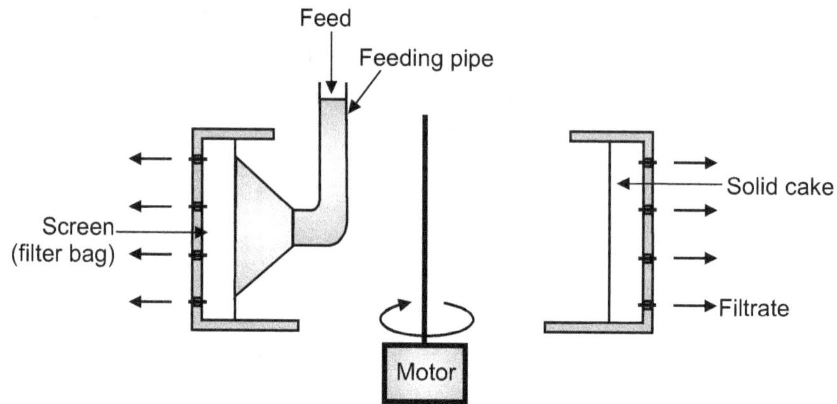

Fig. 10.3: Vertical Basket Bottom Driven Centrifuge

Working:

When the basket rotates, the product enters centrally is thrown outside by centrifugal force and held by filter cloth. The filtrate is forced through the cloth and is removed through liquid outlet. The solid material is remained on the cloth. The cake can be washed-off by water to get filtrate. The stepwise operation is given below.

(a) **Feeding:** The slurry is introduced to the rotating basket having a filter bag. The filter bag captures the solids. Centrifugal force drives the liquid through the caked solids and the mother liquor is discharged through perforations in the basket circumference.

(b) Washing: A wash liquid is introduced and is driven through the caked solids. The plug flow action of the wash liquid purifies the solids and removes residual mother liquor.

(c) Spinning: Residual liquor is driven from the caked solids and is discharged through the basket perforations to achieve maximum cake dryness.

(d) Solids Discharge: The filter bag containing the solids is removed from the basket and the filter bag inverts to discharge the solids into a receiver, or the solids are removed manually by scooping them from the filter bag.

Advantages:

(i)　Initial cost is considerably high but after it is cheaper to use.

(ii)　Perforated basket centrifuge is a rapid in operation.

(iii)　The centrifuge is very compact and hence can be accommodated in small floor place.

(iv)　It can handle concentrated slurries-up to paste like consistency.

(v)　The final product has very low moisture content.

(vi)　The dispersed solids are separated as cake.

Disadvantages:

(i)　Being this centrifuge involves number of steps the entire cycle is complex,

(ii)　It is a batch process and speed is required to be controlled thus involves considerable labor costs.

(iii)　Lengthy operation results in to formation of hard cake due to the continuous, application of centrifugal force. This makes cake removal a difficult task.

(iv)　Being it has moving components there is considerable wear and tear of the equipment.

Applications:

(i)　It is applicable when very fine particles are to be separated from the mixture.

(ii)　These centrifuges are used to separate crystals from mother-liquor.

(iii)　Liquids can be clarified by removing unwanted solid dirt from oils.

(iv)　Sugar crystals are separated using perforated centrifuge.

(v)　Used for removing precipitated proteins from insulin.

(vi)　It is extensively used for separating crystalline drugs such as aspirin and sulfamethaxazole from mother liquor.

10.4.2 Non-Perforated Basket Centrifuge

This is a sedimentation centrifuge. This type of centrifuge is used when resistance to flow of liquid offered by cake is high. The non-perforated basket centrifuge is used in separation of suspension whose solid content is higher. The principle involved in separation of solid particles in this machine is density difference as they move away from axis of rotation. It consists of a simple drum-shaped basket or bowl, usually rotating around a vertical axis. The solids accumulate and compress as effect of the centrifugal force, but they are not dewatered. The residual liquid is drained out when the rotation of the bowl is stopped. The layer of solids is removed manually by scraping. Unloading can be achieved semi-automatically first by use of a skimmer pipe to remove the residual liquid and then by lowering a knife blade into the solid and so cutting it out from the bowl. This allows avoiding the switching-off of the machine.

The separation is based on the difference in the densities of solid and liquid phases without a porous barrier.

Construction:

It consists of a metallic basket. The basket is suspended on vertical shaft and is driven by a motor using a suitable power system. The basket contains a non-perforated side-wall that retains solid phase on its sides during centrifugation, Fig. 10.4. The liquid that remains at the top is removed by a skimming tube.

Working:

The suspension is fed continuously into the basket. During centrifugation, solid phase is retained on the sides of the basket, while liquid remains on the top. The liquid is removed over a weir or through a skimming tube. When a

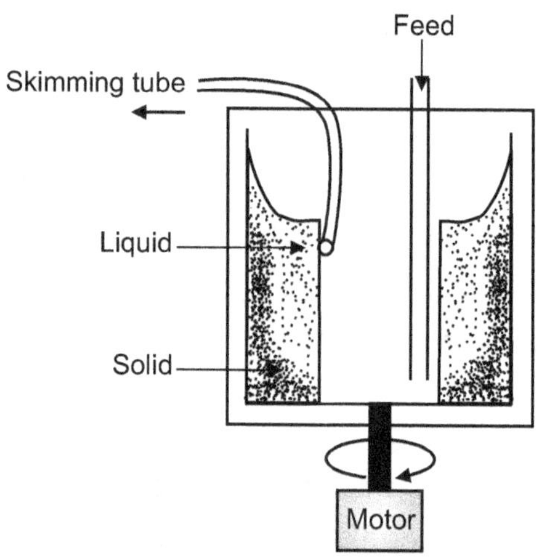

Fig. 10.4: Non-Perforated Basket Centrifuge

suitable depth of solids has been deposited on the walls of the basket, the operation is stopped. The solids are then scraped-off by hand or using a scraper blade.

Applications:

(i)   Non-perforated basket centrifuge is useful when the deposited solids offer high resistance to the flow of liquid.

(ii) It allows avoiding the switching-off of the machine.

10.4.3 Semi-Continuous Centrifuge

Principle:

Semi-continuous centrifuge is a filtration centrifuge. The separation is done on the basis of difference in the densities of the solid and liquid. This separation occurs through a perforated wall. The bowl contains a perforated side-wall, Fig. 10.5. During centrifugation, the liquid phase passes through the perforated wall, while solid phase retains in the bowl. The solid is washed and removed by cutting the sediment using a blade.

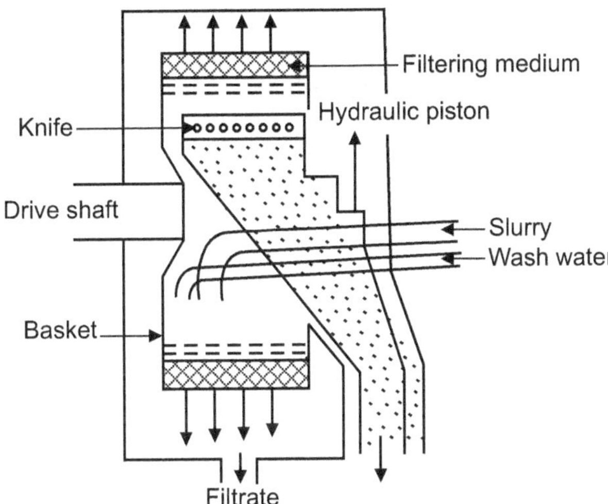

Fig. 10.5: Semi-Continuous Centrifuge

Construction:

It consists of a rotating basket placed on a horizontal shaft and driven by a motor from side. The side of the basket is perforated. Surrounding the basket is a stationary casing that collects the filtrate. Slurry is introduced through a pipe that enters the basket through the center. To wash the crystal the wash-pipe is also introduced through the center of the basket. The layer of cake is removed by a chute fitted with a knife. The knife cuts down the cake within the basket. The knife-chute assembly is raised with the help of a hydraulic apparatus.

Working:

The basket is rotated horizontally by a motor. The slurry is introduced through the slurry entry pipe. The liquid passes out through the perforated side. The crystals remain within the basket. When the cake height is about 2 - 3 inches the slurry entry is stopped by a "feeler-diaphragm valve assembly". The basket rotates at a predetermined time then the cake is washed with water. The basket is rotated for another predetermined time. After that the hydraulic apparatus raise the knife-chute assembly to cut the cake. The cake is collected through the chute.

Advantages:

(i)   It is a short-cycle centrifuge.

(ii) It work automatically reducing labor cost.

(iii) It can be batch operated when solids can be drained fast from the bowl.

Disadvantage:

(i)   It has problems during drain discharge.

(ii) Its high speed considerably breaks crystals.

(iii) Many moving parts are involved making the construction and functioning more complicated.

Applications:

The semi-continuous type centrifuge has following applications :

(i)   Crystals can be separated from mother-liquor.

(ii)   Liquids can be clarified by removing unwanted solid dirt from oils.

(iii) It is used to purify mononuclear cells from human peripheral blood.

10.4.4 Super Centrifuge

Principle:

It is a solid bowl type continuous centrifuge used for separating two immiscible liquid phases. It is a sedimentation type of centrifuge in which during centrifugation the heavier liquid is thrown against the wall of the bowl while the lighter liquid remains as an inner layer. The two layers are simultaneously separated.

Construction:

It consists of a long, hollow, cylindrical bowl with a diameter between 15 - 50 cm which rotates at high-speed to generate a settling acceleration of up to about 18,000 g (where, g is the acceleration due to gravity) for industrial models and 65,000 g for laboratory models. The bowl is suspended from a flexible spindle at the top and the bottom is fitted loosely in a bush, Fig. 10.6. It is rotated on its vertical axis. Feed is introduced through the bottom through a nozzle. Two liquid outlets are provided at different heights. Inside the bowl there are three baffles (not shown in the figure) to catch the liquid and force it to travel at the same speed of rotation as the bowl wall.

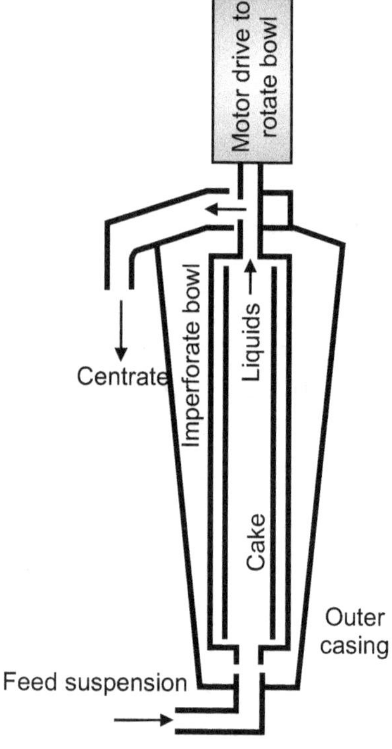

Fig. 10.6: Super-centrifuge

Working:

The centrifuge is allowed to rotate on its vertical axis at about 2000 r.p.m. The feed is introduced at the bottom through the bowl neck using a nozzle under pressure. A distributor disperses the feed to prevent travel too far along the bowl length. During centrifugation, two liquid phases separate based on their densities. The heavier liquid moves towards periphery and the lighter liquid forms an inner layer. Both the liquids climb-up to the top of the vertical bowl. These two layers are simultaneously separated and removed from different heights through modified outlets. The centrate discharges from the top of the bowl by overflowing into a collecting cover.

Application:

   (i)   Super centrifuge is used for separating liquid phases of emulsions in foods and pharmaceuticals.

10.4.5 Continuous Centrifuges

Continuous centrifuges constitute the second and third-generations. In second-generation centrifuges there is continuous discharge of both liquid and solids from the basket and are the pusher and conical screen types. The examples of third-generation centrifuges include the screen decanter, baffle ring, screen baffle and siphon centrifuges.

Conical screen centrifuges: These centrifuges are available in a wide variety of designs. A first classification of these is the angle of the screen (a) wide-angle (slip discharge and guide channel centrifuges) and (b) small-angle screens. Small-angle screen centrifuges are subdivided according to the method of solids discharge used: vibration (vibration centrifuge); oscillation (oscillating and tumbler centrifuges); metering (worm or scroll screen centrifuges); and pushing (pusher conical screen centrifuge). Conical screen centrifuges may rotate about either the vertical or the horizontal axis.

Pusher centrifuge: They consists of a rotating perforated drum lined with a slot screen and a push plate reciprocating with a frequency of about 1 Hz, with a variable advance of between 30 and 60 mm. At first sight, the mechanical design of a tumbler appears complicated, but the construction is simple in comparison with other types of continuous centrifuge. This is reflected in low capital and running costs and its applications, which have covered freely filtering materials such as iron ore, coal fines and coarser crystalline materials. Although the shape of the drum is conical like that of a conical basket centrifuge, the tumbler typically enables longer residence times.

The geometry and complex motions of many continuous centrifuges make them extremely difficult to formulate. The third-generation represents improvements in process technique being built-in into the continuous centrifuges. In the screen decanter centrifuge, sedimentation and filtration are combined to reduce the total time for separation and limiting their application to easily filterable products.

In the baffle ring centrifuge, the particles bounce against rotating rings to effect a further release of liquid. In the screen baffle centrifuge, the particles bounce against screens. Applications of both the ring and screen baffle machines are limited to granular particles. The siphon centrifuge is an adaptation of peeler and pendulum machines. The siphoning action downstream of the filter medium increases the pressure difference across the basket, leading to an increase in capacity.

REVIEW QUESTIONS

1. What is centrifugation? Write about parameters involved in velocity of sedimentation.

2. What is objective of centrifugation? Discuss principle of centrifugation and its applications.

3. Write about pharmaceutical and other applications of centrifugation.

4. Classify equipments used for centrifugation.

5. Discuss principle, types, construction, working along with advantages, disadvantages and applications of perforated basket centrifuge.

6. Discuss principle, construction, working and applications of non-perforated basket centrifuge.

7. Discuss principle, construction, working along with advantages, disadvantages and applications of semi-continuous centrifuge.

8. Discuss principle, construction, working and applications of super centrifuge.

9. Write note on continuous centrifuges.

✍ ✍ ✍

Chapter ...**11**

MATERIALS OF PHARMACEUTICAL PLANT CONSTRUCTION, CORROSION AND ITS PREVENTION

11.0 INTRODUCTION

A number of equipments have been used in the manufacture of pharmaceuticals, bulk drugs, antibiotics, biological products etc. A wide variety of materials are used in making number of equipments. At the dawn of the new millennium, the pharmaceutical and biotechnology industries are seeking ways to leave behind the currently-used troublesome materials of construction and to accelerate conversion to problem-freeing, leading-edge, improved material. Throughout this century, the materials of processing equipment construction used in these industries include stainless steel and glass that imposed constant and increasing problems such as rouging, pitting, corrosion, metallic-poisoning, aggravated compliance issues, cost and environmentally adverse cleaning protocols, and inadvertent fracture etc. The development of increasingly sophisticated pharmaceutical manufacturing products and processes are being limited by what can be synthesized, manufactured and stored in glass-lined or, particularly, stainless steel components.

Equipment made with wetted surfaces of fluoropolymers, especially Teflon® PFA HP, represents the most functional 21st century material of construction for pharmaceutical and biotechnological research and manufacturing. The non-polar, high service temperature, chemically inert, hydrophobic nature of a fluoropolymer surface provides non-interactive, essentially "force field"-like containment for pharmaceutical and biotechnological process fluid streams. These attributes promise reduced production cost and lessened downtime for regulatory compliance procedures, plus synthesis and process design freedoms. Proven service in the chemical and microelectronics industry for a quarter century give ready evidence of high purity, non-wetting and non-corrosive performance, and a supply of ample equipment for adoption by the pharmaceutical and biotechnology industries. Moreover, fluoropolymer fabricators with similar years of experience can provide desired specialty items. And new fluoropolymer resin offerings from DuPont and other fluoropolymer resin suppliers further enhance the adaptability of this material to satisfy ongoing industries' needs.

Pharmaceutical and biotechnology industries confront major challenges such as increased competition, industry consolidation and globalization, high research and development costs, pervasive government guidelines, and extremely demanding manufacturing and distribution requirements.

Objectives:

(i)   To study physical, chemical and mechanical properties of materials used in construction pharmaceutical plants.

(ii) To study new materials of plant construction for more productive pharmaceutical and biotechnology industry.

(iii) To understand corrosion, its mechanisms and types and to know about methods of corrosion prevention.

(iv) To compare the material science of the current materials of construction stainless steel and glass with that of the increasingly adopted material of construction.

(v)   To compare biochemical and microbiological impact on materials of plant construction.

In building a process plant, there are many materials of construction options available to consider. In addition to the applications that dictate what materials are to be needed previous experiences, continuity and plant standards can also play a crucial role in this decision. Common building materials used for process industry include carbon steel, stainless steel, steel alloys, graphite, glass, titanium, plastic, monel, and many more.

11.1 FACTORS AFFECTING MATERIALS SELECTED FOR PHARMACEUTICAL PLANT CONSTRUCTION

There are several variables that influence the decision of selecting the best material of construction for any plant. In some cases, the root cause of metal corrosion is selection of materials that are inherently incompatible with the environment. In other cases, corrosion is a result of mechanical design, where incompatible metals are joined together or components meet in a manner that results in narrow spaces between the components. Corrosion can also be the result of faulty manufacturing processes that result in microstructures that render an alloy susceptible to corrosion. The three major variables are corrosion resistance, cost and expected operating life. There are other minor variables such as compatibility of material of construction with existing plant installations, plant operating conditions, ease of maintenance, and cleaning requirements to name a few. While these are less critical, they are still important to keep in mind as you establish the criteria for particular plant. The selection of a material for the construction of equipment depends on the following factors:

11.1.1 Chemical Factors

Whenever a chemical substance is placed in a container or equipment the chemical is exposed to the material of construction of the container or equipment. Therefore, the material of construction may contaminate the product or the product may destroy the material of construction.

(a) Contamination of product: Iron contamination may change the colour of the products (like gelatin capsule shells), catalyze some reactions that may enhance the rate of decomposition of the product. Leaching of glass may make aqueous product alkaline. This alkaline medium may catalyze the decomposition of the product. Heavy metals such as lead inactivate penicillin.

(b) Destruction of material of construction: The products may be corrosive in nature. They may react with the material of construction and may destroy it. The life of the equipment is reduced. Extreme pH, strong acids, strong alkalis, powerful oxidizing agents, tannins etc. reacts with the materials. It is important to know what chemicals are to be processed. Selection should be done consciously and while selecting appropriate materials that comply with the chemical composition of process it should be ensured that it will perform to the expectations.

(c) Chemical inertness: Aggressive reaction environments tend to dissolve metals from unlined mild steel or alloy reactors. Extractable metals, such as chromium, nickel, molybdenum, and copper, can leach into and contaminate product, producing undesired catalytic effects that can cause harmful fluctuations in the process reactions. These metals can compromise product quality, negatively affect product yield, and in some cases even cause runaway reactions.

11.1.2 Physical Factors

(a) Strength: The material should have sufficient physical strength to withstand the required pressure and stresses. Iron and steel posses these properties. Tablet punching machine, die, upper and lower punches are made of stainless steel to withstand the very high pressure. Glass though has strength but is brittle. Aerosol container must withstand very high pressure, so tin plate container coated with some polymers (lacquered) are used. Plastic materials are weak so they are used in some packaging materials, like blister packs.

(b) Mass: For transportation purpose light weight packaging materials are used. Plastic, aluminium and paper packaging materials are used for packing pharmaceutical products.

(i) Wear properties: When there is a possibility of friction between two surfaces the softer surface wears off and these materials contaminate the products.

For example, during milling and grinding the grinding surfaces may wear off and contaminate the powder. When pharmaceutical products of very high purity are required ceramic and iron grinding surfaces are not used.

(ii) Thermal conductivity: In evaporators, dryers, stills and heat exchangers the materials employed have very good thermal conductivity. In this case iron, copper or graphite tubes are used for effective heat transfer.

(iii) Thermal expansion: If the material has very high thermal expansion coefficient then as temperature increases the shape of the equipment changes. This produces uneven stresses and may cause fractures. In such cases materials used should be able to maintain the shape and dimensions of the equipment at the working temperature conditions.

(iv) **Ease of fabrication:** During fabrication of equipment, the materials undergo various processes such as casting, welding, forging and mechanization etc. For example glass and plastic may be easily moulded in to containers of different shape and sizes. Glass can be used as lining material for reaction vessels.

(v) **Cleaning:** Some materials of construction can pose housekeeping issues when it comes to ease of cleaning. A smooth and polished surface makes cleaning easier. Glass with an anti-adhesive and nonporous surface resists the build-up of viscous or sticky products.

Borosilicate glass is a popular choice for processes where ease of cleaning is critical. Upon completion of an operation the equipment is cleaned thoroughly to avoid contamination of the previous product in to the next product. Glass and stainless steel surfaces generally being smooth and polished are easy to clean.

(vi) **Sterilization:** The ideal feature of glass, the transparency, allows us to see when equipment needs to be cleaned without the need for interrupting the process and performing an internal inspection. In the production of parenteral, ophthalmic and bulk drug products all the equipment are required to be sterilized. This is generally done by introducing steam under high pressure. The materials must withstand this high temperature (121°C) and pressure (15 lb/inch^2). If rubber materials are being used it should be vulcanized to withstand the high temperature.

(vii) **Transparency:** Unlike most plastic and metal materials, glass equipment provides transparency to give an unobstructed view of what is going on inside system, enhancing the observation of process. In reactors and fermenters a visual port is provided to observe the progress of the process going on inside the chamber. For this purpose borosilicate glass is often used. In parenteral and ophthalmic containers the particles, if any, are observed from with polarized light. The walls of the containers must be transparent to see through it. In this case glass is the most preferred material of choice. For photosensitive substances, brown coated glass is also available to offer extra protection. If there is concern over potential mechanical stresses inflicted on the glass, Sectrans coating is applied. This coating covers the glass surface and provides protection against scratches, blows and splintering.

11.1.3 Economic Factors

Owner's budget is very important. Initial cost of the equipment depends on the material used. Several materials may be suitable for construction from physical and chemical point of view, but from all the materials only the cheapest material is chosen for construction of the equipment. Materials those require lower maintenance cost are used because in long run it is economical. Thus, capital expenditures need to be taken into consideration to ensure that the cost do not exceed the financial limits.

11.1.4 Expected Operating Life

Although operational life is less critical, they are still important to keep in mind as we establish the criteria for the plant. It is important to know how long we plan to keep the system in operation. Whether it's a continuous or batch process, how frequently it is run, and how many years of service we hope to get out of it are all questions that need to be accounted for when determining type of system components to employ.

11.2 CORROSION

Corrosion is defined as the reaction of a metallic material with its surrounding environmental components, which causes a measurable change to the metal and can result in a functional failure of the metallic component or of a complete system.

Classification of Corrosion:

According to the environment, corrosion can be classified as;

(i) **Dry corrosion:** It involves the direct attack of gases and vapor on the metals through chemical reactions. As a result an oxide layer is formed over the surface.

(ii) **Wet corrosion:** This corrosion involves purely electrochemical reaction that occurs when the metal is exposed to an aqueous solution of acid and alkali.

For example, $\quad Zn + 2HCl \rightarrow ZnCl_2 + H_2$ $\hfill$ ... (11.1)

11.3 THEORY OF CORROSION

11.3.1 Corrosion Reaction on Single Metal

Corrosion is a natural process, which converts a refined metal to a more chemically-stable form, such as its oxide, hydroxide, or sulfide. The mechanisms of corrosion are same at microscopic level and various microstructures, composition, and mechanical design issues leads to different manifestations of corrosion. For example, a single piece of metal, Fe, when comes in contact with acid, HCl, small galvanic cells may be set-up on the surface. Each galvanic cell consists of anode and cathode regions. The interaction taking place at these two regions is as follows.

Reaction at anode:

Fe on the iron liberates two electrons to the metal and itself becomes Fe^{++} ion. Since Fe^{++} ion is soluble in water it is released in the medium. This causes corrosion of iron surface.

Reaction at cathode:

The released electron is conducted through the metal piece to the cathode region. Two electrons are supplied to two protons (H^+) to form two atoms of hydrogen. Hydrogen atoms being unstable, two H atoms combine to form a stable molecule H_2. In the absence of acid, water itself dissociates to generate H^+ ion.

$$2H^+ + 2e^- \rightarrow H_2 \qquad\qquad ... (11.2)$$

Hydrogen (H_2) forms bubbles on the metal surface. If the rate of hydrogen formation is very slow then a film of H_2 bubbles will be formed that will slow down the cathode reaction, hence the rate of corrosion will slow down. If the rate of hydrogen production is very high then hydrogen molecules cannot form the film on the surface. So the corrosion proceeds rapidly.

11.3.2 Corrosion Reactions between Metals

As is known corrosion of metals is an electrochemical reaction involving changes in metal as well as environment in contact with the metal. If two metals come in contact with a common aqueous medium then one metal will form anode and the other will form cathode. Now, if both the metals are connected with a wire the reaction will proceed. Anode metal will be corroded and hydrogen will form at the cathode.

For example, if zinc and a copper plate are immersed in an acidic medium then zinc will form anode and will be corroded while hydrogen will be formed at copper plate.

Anode reaction: $\quad\quad\quad\quad\quad\quad Zn \rightarrow Zn^{++} + 2e^-$ $\quad\quad\quad\quad\quad$ ... (11.3)

Cathode reaction: $\quad\quad 2H^+ + 2e^- \rightarrow H_2$ $\quad\quad\quad\quad\quad\quad$ ... (11.4)

So anode will be corroded and hydrogen will be evolved at cathode.

11.3.3 Corrosion Involving Oxygen

The oxygen dissolved in the electrolyte can react with accumulated hydrogen to form water. Depletion (reduction) of hydrogen layer allows corrosion to proceed.

At cathode: $\quad\quad\quad\quad\quad O_2 + 2H_2 \rightarrow 2H_2O$ $\quad\quad\quad\quad\quad\quad$ ... (11.5)

The above reaction takes place in acid medium. When the medium is alkaline or neutral oxygen is absorbed. The presence of moisture also promotes corrosion.

FACTORS INFLUENCING CORROSION:

(a) **The pH of the solution:** Iron dissolves rapidly in acidic pH. Aluminium and zinc dissolves both in acidic and alkaline pH. Noble metals such as gold and platinum are not affected by pH.

(b) **Oxidizing agents:** Oxidizing agents may accelerate the corrosion of one class of materials whereas retard another class.

For example, O_2 reacts with H_2 to form water. When H_2 is removed corrosion is accelerated. The presence of Cu in NaCl solution also follows this mechanism. Oxidizing agents forms a surface oxide (like Aluminium oxide) and makes the surface more resistant to chemical attack.

(c) **Velocity:** When corrosive medium moves at a high velocity along the metallic surface, the rate of corrosion increases. This is due to rapid formation and washing away of corrosion products to expose new surfaces for corrosion reaction. The corrosion is rapid in the bends in the pipes, propellers, agitators and pumps. Due to high velocity the accumulation of insoluble films on the surface is prevented.

(d) **Surface films:** Thin oxide films are formed on the surface of stainless (rusting). These films absorb moisture and increase the rate of corrosion.

For example, zinc oxide forms porous films. Fluid medium can enter inside the surface and thus corrosion continues. Nonporous films of chromium oxide or iron oxide prevent corrosion. Grease films protect the surface from direct contact with corrosive substances.

11.4 TYPES OF CORROSION

The corrosion when generally confined to a metal surface as a whole, it is known as general corrosion. This corrosion occurs uniformly over the entire exposed surface area, for example, swelling, cracking, softening of plastic materials. Whereas localized fluid corrosion includes inter-granular, pitting, stress, fretting corrosion and corrosion fatigue. Metabolic action of micro-organisms either directly or indirectly causes deterioration of a metal called biological fluid corrosion, Fig. 11.1.

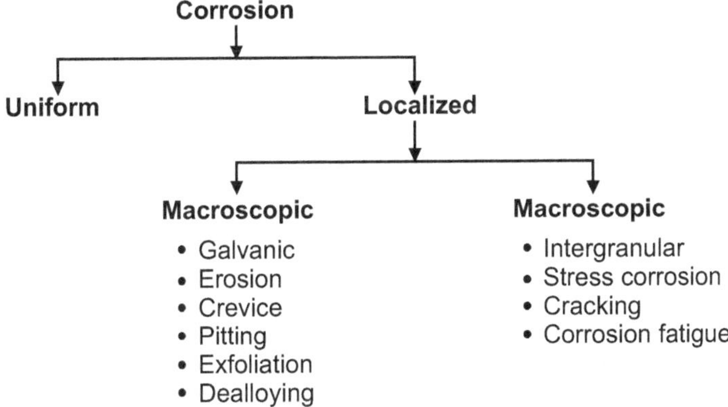

Fig. 11.1: Macroscopic and Microscopic Forms of Corrosion

We know the basics of corrosion, fundamental chemical reactions and environments in which corrosion can occur. The schematic of various types of corrosion is given in Fig. 11.2.

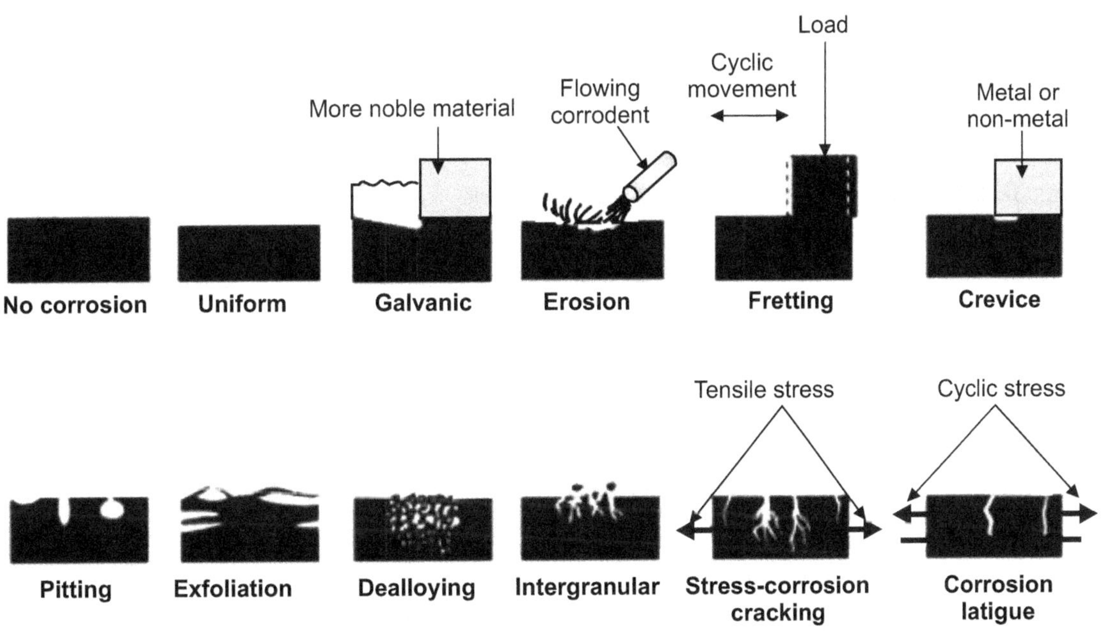

Fig. 11.2: Schematic of Common Types of Corrosion

As corrosion most often occurs in aqueous environments, the different types of corrosion a metal can experience in such conditions is described below.

11.4.1 Uniform Corrosion

Uniform corrosion is the most common type of corrosion and is due to the uniform attack across the surface of a metal. The driving force for this type of corrosion is the electrochemical activity of the metal in the environment to which the metal is exposed. It is most simple to identify as the extent of the attack is judged easily, and the resulting impact on material performance is fairly evaluated due to an ability to consistently reproduce and test the phenomenon. This type of corrosion typically occurs over relatively large areas of an exposed material's surface. Rust on a steel structure or the green thin layer (patina) on a copper roof are examples of uniform corrosion.

11.4.2 Galvanic Corrosion

Galvanic corrosion, or dissimilar metal corrosion, occurs when two different metals are located together in a corrosive electrolyte. Galvanic corrosion is the degradation of one metal near a joint or juncture that occurs when two electrochemically dissimilar metals are in electrical contact in an electrolytic environment; for example, when copper is in contact with steel in a saltwater environment. However, even when these three conditions are satisfied, there are many other factors that affect the potential for, and the amount of, corrosion, such as temperature and surface finish of the metals. The driving force for the corrosion reaction is the difference in electrode potentials between the two metals. A galvanic couple forms between the two metals, where one metal becomes the anode and the other the cathode. The anode, or sacrificial metal, corrodes and deteriorates faster than it would alone, while the cathode deteriorates more slowly than it would otherwise.

Large engineered systems employing many types of metal in their construction, including various fastener types and materials, are susceptible to galvanic corrosion if care is not exercised during the design phase. Choosing metals that are as close together as practicable on the galvanic series help to reduce the risk of galvanic corrosion. In areas where corrosion is a concern, stainless steel products offer value and protection against these threats. Stainless' favourable chemical composition makes it resistant to many common corrosives while remaining significantly more affordable than specialty alloys such as titanium and Inconel[®] alloys.

11.4.3 Flow-Assisted or Erosion Corrosion

Flow-assisted corrosion (FAC) or erosion corrosion results when a protective layer of oxide on a metal surface is dissolved or removed by wind or water, exposing the underlying metal for further corrosion and deterioration. It leads to erosion-assisted corrosion, impingement and cavitations.

11.4.4 Fretting Corrosion

Fretting corrosion occurs as a result of repeated wearing, weight and/or vibration on an uneven, rough surface. Corrosion, resulting in pits and grooves, occurs on the surface. Fretting corrosion is often found in rotation and impact machinery, bolted assemblies and bearings, as well as to surfaces exposed to vibration during transportation.

11.4.5 Crevice Corrosion

Crevice corrosion is also a localized form of corrosion and usually results from a stagnant micro-environment in which there is a difference in the concentration of ions between two areas of a metal. Crevice corrosion occurs in shielded areas such as those under washers, bolt heads, gaskets etc. where oxygen is restricted. It also occurs in crevices between components and also under polymer coatings and adhesives. These smaller areas allow for a corrosive agent to enter but do not allow enough circulation within, depleting the oxygen content, which prevents re-passivation. As a stagnant solution builds, pH shifts away from neutral. This growing imbalance between the crevice (microenvironment) and the external surface (bulk environment) contributes to higher rates of corrosion. The driving force for the corrosion is the difference between the oxygen concentration inside the crevice and outside the crevice. Crevice corrosion can often occur at lower temperatures than pitting. Proper joint design helps to minimize crevice corrosion.

11.4.6 Pitting Corrosion

Pitting is one of the most destructive types of corrosion as it can be hard to predict, detect and characterize. Pitting is a localized form of corrosion, in which either a local anodic point, or more commonly a cathodic point, forms a small corrosion cell with the surrounding normal surface. Pitting occurs in metals that are normally passive, when the passive layer breaks down. Once a pit has initiated, it grows into a "hole" or "cavity" that takes on one of a variety of different shapes, Fig. 11.3. Pits typically penetrate from the surface downward in a vertical direction. Pitting corrosion can be caused by a local break or damage to the protective oxide film or a protective coating; it can also be caused by non-uniformities in the metal structure itself. Pitting is dangerous because it can lead to failure of the structure with a relatively low overall loss of metal. Examples of passive metals are aluminum and stainless steel. Pitting is a problem if it leads to weakening or perforation of the metal. In applications where appearance is important pitting is a problem.

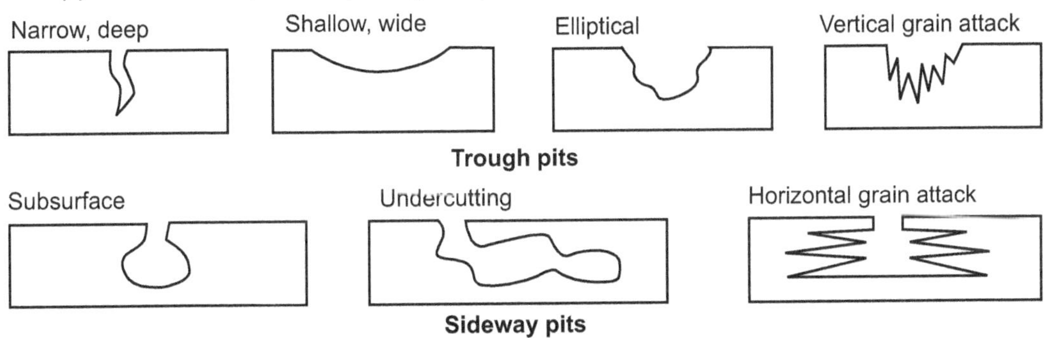

Fig. 11.3: Types of Pitting Corrosion

11.5 EXFOLIATION CORROSION

Exfoliation corrosion is a more severe form of intergranular corrosion that can occur along aluminum grain boundaries in the fuselage empennage and wing skins of aircraft. These grain boundaries in both aluminum sheet and plate are oriented in layers parallel to the surface of the material, due to the rolling process. The delamination of these thin layers of the aluminum, with white corrosion products between the layers, characterizes exfoliation corrosion. Exfoliation corrosion is often found next to fasteners where an electrically insulating sealant or a sacrificial cadmium plating has broken down, permitting a galvanic action between the dissimilar metals. Where fasteners are involved, exfoliation corrosion extends outward from the fastener hole, either from the entire circumference of the hole, or in one direction from a segment of the hole. In severe cases, the surface bulges outward, but in less severe cases, there may be no telltale blisters, and you can only detect the exfoliation corrosion by nondestructive inspection methods that are not always very effective.

11.5.1 Dealloying

De-alloying, or selective leaching, is the selective corrosion of a specific element in an alloy. This results in the formation of a porous structure that is not strong enough to support the applied mechanical loads. The specific type of corrosion that occurs depends on the several factors including metal composition, metal microstructure, environment, component geometry, stress on the component, contact between metals, and the manner in which components are joined together. The common examples are dezincification of brass alloys used for plumbing, where the zinc is leached out of the alloy forming unstabilized brass. The result of corrosion in such cases is a deteriorated and porous copper.

11.5.2 Intergranular Corrosion

Intergranular corrosion is a chemical or electrochemical attack on the grain boundaries of the affected metal. It often occurs due to impurities in the metal, which tend to be present in higher contents near grain boundaries. These boundaries can be more vulnerable to corrosion than the bulk of the metal. The result is that the metal grains fall away and the metal is weakened. The close microstructure of a metal reveals that the grains are formed during solidification of the alloy as well as at the grain boundaries between them. Intergranular corrosion can be caused by impurities present at these grain boundaries or by the depletion or enrichment of an alloying element at the grain boundaries. It occurs along or adjacent to these grains, seriously affecting the mechanical properties of the metal while the bulk of the metal remains intact. An example of intergranular corrosion is carbide precipitation, a chemical reaction that can occur when a metal is subjected to very high temperatures (800 °F - 1650 °F) and/or localized hot work such as welding. Austenitic stainless steels and precipitation strengthened aluminum alloys are examples of metals that can suffer from intergranular corrosion if the alloys are not properly processed and if they are exposed to corrosive environments. In stainless steels, during these reactions, carbon consumes the chromium forming carbides and causes the level of chromium remaining in the alloy to drop below the 11% needed to sustain the spontaneously-forming passive oxide layer. The SS 304L and 316L are enhanced versions of 304 and 316 stainless steel that contain lower levels of carbon providing best corrosion resistance to carbide precipitation.

11.5.3 Stress Corrosion Cracking

Stress corrosion cracking (SCC) is a result of the combination of tensile stress and a corrosive environment, often at elevated temperatures. In most cases, the stress or environment by themselves are insufficient to cause degradation of the metal. That is, if the stress is below the metal's yield strength the metal would not corrode in the specific environment. It is net result of external stress such as actual tensile loads on the metal or expansion/contraction due to rapid temperature changes. It may also be result of residual stress imparted during the manufacturing process such as cold forming, welding, machining, grinding etc. In stress corrosion, the majority of the surface usually remains intact; however, fine cracks appear in the microstructure, making the corrosion hard to detect. The cracks typically have a brittle appearance and form and spread in a direction perpendicular to the location of the stress. Selecting proper materials for a given environment can mitigate the potential for catastrophic failure due to SCC.

11.5.4 Fatigue or Environmental Cracking Corrosion

Environmental cracking is a corrosion process that can result from a combination of environmental conditions affecting the metal. Chemical, temperature and stress-related conditions can result in the following types of environmental corrosion:

(i)   Stress corrosion cracking.

(ii) Corrosion fatigue.

(iii) Hydrogen-induced cracking.

(iv) Liquid metal embrittlement.

11.5.5 High-Temperature Corrosion

Fuels used in gas turbines, diesel engines and other machinery, which contain vanadium or sulfates during combustion can form compounds with a low melting point. These compounds are very corrosive towards metal alloys normally resistant to high temperatures and corrosion, including stainless steel. High-temperature corrosion can also be caused by high-temperature oxidization, sulfidation, and carbonization. The American Society of Metals (ASM) classified various corrosion types as given in Table 11.1.

Table 11.1: ASM Classifications of Corrosion Types

General Corrosion	Localized Corrosion	Metallurgically Influenced Corrosion	Mechanically Assisted Degradation	Environmentally Induced Cracking
Corrosive attack dominated by uniform thinning	High rates of metal penetration of specific sites	Affected by alloy chemistry and heat treatment	Corrosion with a mechanical component	Cracking produced by corrosion, in the presence of stress
• Atmospheric corrosion • Galvanic corrosion • Stray-current corrosion • General biological corrosion • Molten salt corrosion • Corrosion in liquid metals • High – temperature corrosion	• Crevice corrosion • Filiform corrosion • Pitting corrosion • Localized biological corrosion	• Intergranular corrosion • Dealloying corrosion	• Erosion corrosion • Fretting corrosion • Cavitations and water drop impingement • Corrosion fatigue	• Stress – Corrosion Cracking (SCC) • Hydrogen Damage • Liquid metal embrittlement • Solid metal induced embrittlement

11.6 PREVENTION OF CORROSION

Although corrosion is a natural process, it can be controlled by using effective methods and strategies. There are mainly five primary ways to control corrosion. Thus, following methods may be adopted for preventing or reducing corrosion:

(a)   Materials selection

(b)   Design

(c)   Cathodic and anodic protection

(d)   Inhibitors

(e)   Coating

11.6.1 Material Selection

The most common and important method of controlling corrosion is the selection of the right and proper materials for particular corrosive environments. Corrosion behaviour of each metal and alloy is unique and inherent and corrosion of metal and alloy has a strong relation with the environment to which it is exposed. A general relation between the rate of corrosion, corrosivity of the environment and corrosion resistance of materials can be elucidated as follows:

$$\text{Rate of corrosive attack } = \frac{\text{Corrosion resistance of metal}}{\text{Corrosivity of environment}} \qquad \text{... (11.6)}$$

The rate of corrosion directly depends upon the corrosivity of the environment and inversely proportional to the corrosion resistance of the metal. Hence, the knowledge of the nature of the environment to which the material is exposed is very important. Moreover, the corrosion resistance of each metal can be different in different exposure conditions. Therefore, the right choice of the materials in the given environment (metal corrosive environment combination) is very essential for the service life of equipments and structures made of these materials. It is possible to reduce the corrosion rate by altering the corrosive medium. The alteration of the corrosive environment can be brought about by lowering temperature, decreasing velocity, removing oxygen or oxidizers and changing concentration. Consideration of corrosion resistance based on the corrosion behaviour of the material and the environment in which it is exposed is an essential step in all industry. The alternative materials for some of the corrosive materials are listed in Table 11.2.

(a) Pure materials have fewer tendencies towards pitting, but they are expensive and soft. Therefore, only aluminium can be used in pure form.

(b) Improved corrosion resistance can be obtained by adding corrosion resistant elements.

For example, inter-granular corrosion occurs in stainless steel. This tendency can be reduced by addition of small amount of titanium.

(c) Nickel, copper and their alloys are used in non-oxidizing environment, whereas chromium containing alloys are used in oxidizing environment.

(d) Materials those are close in electrochemical series should be used for fabrication.

(e) Corrosive materials are taken with suitable material of construction:

Table 11.2: Corrosive Materials and Their Alternative Metals

Corrosive material	Suitable material
Nitric acid	Stainless steel
Hydrofluoric acid	Monel metal
Distilled Water	Tin
Dilute sulphuric acid	Lead
Caustic	Nickel

11.6.2 Proper Design of Equipment

The structural design of equipment is equally important as that of choice of materials of construction. It greatly reduce the time and cost associated with corrosion maintenance and repair. The proper design of equipment or tools made-up of metals and alloys must consider mechanical and strength requirements along with corrosion resistance. Prior knowledge about the corrosion resistance of the probable material and the environment in which it is supposed to be functioned is very essential for proper design of any equipment. The most common rule for design is avoiding heterogeneity. As corrosion frequently happens in dead spaces or crevices thus it is recommended to eliminate or minimize such areas while designing. All the components of structures should be designed by considering its expected service life. If not, premature collapse of the component or structure is the inevitable and large sum of money should be spent for its repair or replacement or can go waste. The ever-changing environment during the different stages of manufacture, transit and storage as well as the daily and seasonal variations in the environment in which the components are exposed should be taken into consideration for its maximum service life. It is highly important to avoid bimetallic corrosion cells in components by coupling dissimilar metals. The metals involved in coupling should be widely separated in the galvanic series to have a maximum service life of components. Dissimilar corrosion rate can also be minimized by keeping the anodes as large as possible in the particular component or location to reduce the current density. Corrosion using proper design can be minimized in the following conditions:

    (a)   Design for complete drainage of liquids.

    (b)   Design for ease of cleaning.

    (c)   Design for ease of inspection and maintenance

    (d)   A direct contact between two metals should be avoided.

    (e)   They may be insulated from one another.

11.6.3 Coating or Lining

Corrosion resistant coating may be applied on metal surface to improve corrosion resistance. It also separates the metal from corrosive environment. Protective coatings are the most generally used method for preventing corrosion. The function of a protective coating is to provide a satisfactory barrier between the metal and its environment. Coatings can be broadly classified as metallic coatings, inorganic coatings and organic coatings. Usually, an anticorrosive coating system is multifunctional with multiple layers with different properties. A typical multifunctional coating can provide an aesthetic appearance, corrosion control, good adhesion, and abrasion resistance. The functioning of any protective coatings is based upon barrier protection, chemical inhibition and galvanic (sacrificial) protection mechanisms. The metals and alloys can be completely isolated from its environment to achieve barrier protection. Protection of metals through chemical inhibition is achieved by adding inhibitor molecules into the coating system. An active metal is coated on the surface of the metal to achieve sacrificial or galvanic protection.

11.6.4 Cathodic and Anodic Protection

Cathodic protection is an electrochemical way of controlling corrosion. The object to be protected is the cathode. Cathodic protection is achieved by suppressing the corrosion current in a corrosion cell and by supplying electrons to the metal to be protected. The principle of cathodic protection can be explained with the help of a typical corrosion reaction of a metal 'M' in an acid (H^+) medium.

For example, consider an electrochemical reaction in which metal dissolution and hydrogen evolution are taking place;

$$M \rightarrow M^{n+} + ne \qquad \qquad \text{... (11.7)}$$

$$2H^+ + 2e \rightarrow H_2 \qquad \qquad \text{... (11.8)}$$

Equations (11.7) and (11.8) shows that the addition of electrons to the structure would reduce the metal dissolution and increase the rate of evolution of hydrogen.

Cathodic protection of a structure can be achieved by an external power supply and appropriate galvanic coupling. Cathodic coupling by galvanic coupling is realized by using active metal anodes, for example, zinc or magnesium, which is connected to the structure to provide the cathodic protection current. In this case, the anode is called a sacrificial anode, since it is consumed during the protection of the steel structure. In contrast to cathodic protection, anodic protection is one of the more recently developed electrochemical methods for controlling corrosion. Anodic protection is based on the principles of passivity and it is generally used to protect structures used for the storage of sulphuric acid. The difference of anodic protection from cathodic protection is how the metal to be protected is polarized. The component that is to be protected is made as anode in anodic protection. Since the anodic protection is based on the phenomenon of passivity, metals and alloy systems, which exhibit active passive behaviour when subjected to anodic polarization, can be protected by anodic polarization. The corrosion rate of an active-passive metal can be significantly reduced by shifting the potential to the passive range. Anodic protection is used to make a protective passive film on the metal or alloy surface and thereby controlling the corrosion.

11.6.5 Inhibitors

Corrosion inhibitor is a substance that retards corrosion when added to an environment in small concentrations. An inhibitor can be considered as a retarding catalyst that reduces the rate of corrosion. The mechanism of inhibition being complex is not yet well understood. It is established that inhibitors function in following way:

(a)   Adsorption of a thin film on the corroding surface of a metal;

(b)   Forming a thick corrosion product, or

(c)   Changing the properties of the environment and thereby slows down the corrosion rate.

Corrosion inhibitors can be broadly classified as passivators, organic inhibitors and vapour phase inhibitors. The inhibitors can also be classified based on their mechanism of inhibition and composition. A large number of inhibitors fall under the category of adsorption type inhibitors. These are generally organic compounds and function by adsorbing on anodic and cathodic sites and reduces the corrosion current. Another class of inhibitors is hydrogen evolution poisons. Arsenic and antimony are generally used as hydrogen evolution poisons and they specifically retard the hydrogen evolution reactions.

This type of inhibition is very effective only in those environments where hydrogen evolution is the main cathodic reactions and hence these inhibitors are very effective in acid solutions.

The inhibitive substances, which act by removing the corrosive reagents from solution are known as scavengers. Sodium sulfite and hydrazine are these types of inhibitors, which remove dissolved oxygen from aqueous solutions. These inhibitors function very effectively in those solutions where oxygen reduction is the main cathodic reaction. Oxidizers are also a kind of inhibitors. Substances such as chromate, nitrate, and ferric salts act as corrosion inhibitors in certain systems. Generally, they inhibit the corrosion of metals and alloys that exhibits active-passive transitions.

Inorganic oxidizing materials such as chromates, nitrites and molybdates are generally used to passivate the metal surface and shift the corrosion potential to the noble direction. Paint primers containing chromate pigments are widely used to protect aluminum alloys and steel. Inhibitors that are very similar to organic adsorption type with very high vapor pressure are known as vapor phase inhibitors. They are also known as volatile corrosion inhibitors (VCI). VCI's are secondary-electrolyte layer inhibitors that possess appreciable saturated vapor pressure under atmospheric conditions and thus allow vapour-phase transport of the inhibitive substance. These inhibitors are generally placed very near to the metal surface to be protected and they are transferred by sublimation and condensation to the metal surface. Hence, these inhibitors can be used to protect metals from atmospheric corrosion without being placed in direct contact with the metal surface.

Vapour phase inhibitors are very successful, if they are used in closed packages or the interior of equipments.

MATERIALS USED IN CONSTRUCTION OF PHARMACEUTICAL PLANT

Metal is used as structural framework for larger buildings, or as an external surface covering. There are many types of metals used for building and for equipments. Steel is a metal alloy whose major component is iron, and is the usual choice for metal structural construction. It is strong, flexible, and if refined well and/or treated, lasts a long time. Corrosion is metal's prime enemy when it comes to longevity. The lower density and better corrosion resistance of aluminum alloys and tin sometimes overcome their greater cost. Brass was more common in the past, but is usually restricted to specific uses or specialty items today. It requires a great deal of human labour to produce metal, especially in the large amounts needed for the building industries. Other metals used include titanium, chrome, and gold, silver. Titanium can be used for structural purposes, but it is much more expensive than steel. Chrome, gold, and silver are used as decoration, because these materials are expensive and lack structural qualities such as tensile strength or hardness.

Classification of materials used in construction of pharmaceutical plant is as follows.

(A) Metals:

    (i)   Ferrous

        (a)   Cast iron

        (b)   Stainless carbon

        (c)   Stainless steel

(ii)   Non-ferrous
    (a)   Lead
    (b)   Aluminum
(B) Non-metals:
(I)   Inorganic
    (a)   Glass
(II)   Organic
    (a)   Rubber
    (b)   Plastic

11.7 FERROUS METALS

Steels and cast irons are basic materials of construction for the chemical and pharmaceutical industries. Carbonyl iron and electrolytic iron which contain relatively pure low carbon iron are not suitable for structural materials.

11.7.1 Cast Iron

Cast iron consists of more than 1.5% carbon. A different proportion of carbon gives different properties of the steel. Steel is an alloy of iron and carbon, along with small amounts of other alloying elements or residual elements as well. The plain iron carbon alloys contain 0.002 - 2.1% by weight carbon. Steel is manufactured from iron ore. In the blast furnace, pig iron is produced by reducing iron ore. Due to impurities present in pig iron, it becomes hard and brittle. Alloy content are controlled in order to obtain suitable properties of alloy material. In the newer method of producing steel pure oxygen is blown through the molten metal. Steel may be killed (i.e., made to diequietly in the mold by the addition of deoxidants such as silicon or aluminium), to prevent the reaction of residual oxygen with dissolved carbon during solidification. Killed steels are used down to −28.9 °C in thinner sections, because of their improved Nil-Ductility Transition Temperature (NDTT) as compared with ordinary steels. Permissible temperatures varies with thickness and limits of −60 °C are sometimes invoked for vessels in cold temperature service.

Properties:
(i)   Cast iron is resistant to concentrated sulfuric acid, nitric acid and diluted alkali.
(ii)   It is attacked by dilute sulfuric acid, dilute nitric acid and dilute and concentrated hydrochloric acid.
(iii)   It has low thermal conductivity.
(iv)   It is not corrosion resistance hence it is alloyed with silicon, nickel or chromium to produce corrosion resistance.
(v)   It is brittle so it is tough to machine.

Applications:
(i)   It is used as supports for plants.
(ii)   Thermal conductivity is low hence used as the outer wall of steam jacket.
(iii)   It is cheap hence used in place of more expensive materials by coating with enamel or plastic.

11.7.2 Carbon Steel or Mild Steel

Stainless steel has historically been adopted for containment of chemical processing because it is resistant to more chemicals than is iron or mild steel. It is an inorganic chemical combination of essentially iron, chromium, and nickel. Mild steel (or carbon steel) are an iron alloy that contains a small percentage of carbon (less than 1.5%). Iron and carbon is the two prime constituents of carbon steels. Carbon steels also contains small amounts of manganese. Structural membranes, sheet, pipe, plate and tubing are generally made from carbon steel. Steels that have been worked or wrought while hot are covered with a black mill-scale (i.e. magnetite, Fe_3O_4) on the surfaces, and are sometimes called black iron. Cold-rolled steels have a bright surface, accurate cross-section, increased yield and tensile strength. The latter are preferred for bar-stock to be used for rods, shafts etc.

Properties:

(i)   Carbon steel has greater mechanical strength than the cast iron.

(ii)   It is easily weldable.

(iii) It has limited resistance to corrosion. This property can be increased by proper alloying.

(iv)   It reacts with caustic soda, brine (conc. NaCl solution) etc.

Applications:

(i)   Carbon steel is used for construction of bars, pipes and plates.

(ii)   It is used to fabricate large storage tanks for water, sulfuric acid, organic solvents etc.

(iii) It is used as the supporting structures of grinders and bases of vessels.

11.7.3 Stainless Steel

Stainless steel is an alloy of iron usually of nickel and chromium. For pharmaceutical use stainless steel contains 18% chromium and 8% nickel. This steel is called 18/8 stainless steel. Products of stainless steel are strong and their initial cost, though higher than iron or mild steel, are often less than other exotic metallurgical materials of construction. Surface physical chemistry of stainless steel is another significant negative for its use in the pharmaceutical and biotechnology industries as it is wettable by aqueous solutions, a characteristic which enhances not only chemical corrosion, but also biofilm adhesion.

The chemical resistance of stainless steel to certain chemicals can be improved by manipulating the amount of the minor ingredients in the metallurgical formulation. Such improved chemical resistance comes with a corresponding increase in cost. But even such chemical resistance improvement is not sufficient to overcome chemical attack. Stainless steel can be further chemically treated to be made less reactive, i.e., passivated. It is a time consuming and expensive treatment that must be performed regularly to ensure that the iron in this material does not oxidize i.e., rust. Passivation is only temporarily durable. It must be repeated if additional weldments are incorporated into the system. Passivated or not, stainless steel is reactive to many harsh chemicals, particularly chloride and other halides, preventing their beneficial use in pharmaceutical and biotechnological applications.

The surface irregularities of stainless steel ranges from 180 grit to 400 grit and can be improved, although with only temporary beneficial effect, to double digit micro inches by electro polishing. Electropolishing is expensive, non-permanent and needs to be repeated often to maintain such a surface.

Properties:

(i)   Stainless steel has good heat resistant.

(ii)   It exhibits good corrosion resistance.

(iii) Ease of fabrication.

(iv)   Cleaning and sterilization is easy.

(v)   It has good tensile strength.

(vi)   During heat welding the corrosion resistant properties of stainless steel may be reduced due to deposition of carbide that precipitate at the crystal grain boundaries. This steel is stabilized by addition of minor quantities of titanium, molybdenum or niobium.

Advantages:

(i)   Stainless steel has good corrosion resistance.

(ii)   It requires little maintenance, meaning the purchase price is quickly recovered because stainless steel does not require additional coating.

(iii) It is easy to machine, with most types being easy to cut, malleable, ductile, able to be welded etc.

(iv)   It has good heat resistance and resistance to temperature fluctuations.

(v)   Very hygienic properties: unaffected by micro-organisms and easy to clean.

(vi)   Attractive appearance, with a variety of possible finishes

Applications:

(i)   It is used to make storage and extraction vessels, evaporators and fermenting vessels.

(ii)   It is common metal for small apparatus like funnels, buckets, measuring vessels.

(iii) Sinks and bench tops are made of stainless steel..

(iv)   In penicillin production plant nearly all equipment are made of stainless steel.

11.8 NON-FERROUS METALS

11.8.1 Lead

Lead is a weak, heavy metal. It has good resistance to sulfuric acid. In nature, it is usually associated with copper and silver. Applications of lead have been greatly diminished in modern practice, because of toxicity problems associated with its joining.

Properties of Lead:

(i)   Lead is a bluish-white lustrous metal.

(ii)   It is very soft, highly malleable, ductile, and a relatively poor conductor of electricity.

(iii)   It is very resistant to corrosion but tarnishes upon exposure to air.

(iv)   Lead isotopes are the end products of each of the three series of naturally occurring radioactive elements.

1.   **Chemical lead:** Chemical lead is lead with traces of copper and silver left in it. It is costly to recover the silver and copper content from it to improve the corrosion resistance.

2.   **Antimonial lead:** It is an alloy of lead and antimony. Antimony (2 - 6%) is used to improve the mechanical properties. This is effective up to approximately 93°C, above which both strength and corrosion resistance of the antimonial lead rapidly decreases.

3.   **Tellurium lead:** It is an alloy of lead and tellurium. Tellurium is used to improve its strength. It has better resistance to fatigue failure induced by vibration.

Applications:

(i)   Lead pipes are used as drains for the waste water and other liquids.

(ii)   It is used as a coloring element in ceramic glazes, as projectiles.

(iii)   It is used as electrodes in the process of electrolysis.

(iv)   One of their major use is in the glass of computer and television screens, where it shields the viewer from radiation.

(v)   Other uses are in sheeting, cables, solders, lead crystal glassware, bearings, etc.

11.8.2 Aluminium

Aluminium and its alloys are light in weight, strong and quite resistant to natural environments. It is easy to fabricate and join by welding and brazing. Commercially pure aluminium and its alloys have UNS numbers, with identifications derived from the older Aluminium Association designations. The general format is A9xxxx for wrought materials and A0xxxx for castings. The A92000 series of alloys cannot resist contaminated industrial or marine atmospheres. Aluminium is fully compatible with aldehydes, ketones, esters, amines, and organic acids and anhydrides. Chloroform or ethylene dichloride and alcohols can react catastrophically with aluminium. Concentrated nitric acid and hydrogen peroxide are commercially handled in aluminium. The non-oxidizing acids, and alkalis or aqueous ammonia derivatives, are corrosive.

Properties:

(a)   Pure aluminium is soft and more corrosion resistant than its alloys. Small percentages of manganese, magnesium or silicon produces strong, corrosion resistant aluminium alloys (for example, Duralumin).

(b)   It is attacked by mineral acids, alkali, mercury and its salts.

(c)   It is resistant to strong nitric acid.

(d)   It is resistant to acetic acid due to the formation of a gelatinous surface film of aluminium subacetate.

(e)   It has low density and hence is lighter.

Applications:

(a) The salt of aluminium is colorless and non-toxic to microorganisms, hence used for fermenting vessels for biosynthetic production of citric acid, gluconic acids and streptomycin.

(b) Used for making extraction and absorption vessels in preparation of antibiotics.

(c) Used in storage vessels of acetic acid and ammonia.

(d) Used in plants for nitric acid.

(e) Because of its lightness large containers such as drums, barrels, road and rail tankers are made with aluminium.

Copper:

The best known applications of copper are vessels, traditionally used in many breweries and distilleries. Copper is largely applied in the non-product contact area, with its main applications in the tubes in evaporators installed in refrigerators and freezers, electrical wiring, water pipes etc. Copper has shown to restrict bacterial growth. Copper does not really constitute a food safety problem but it is recommended to avoid direct food contact with copper utensils, as it can cause unacceptable organoleptic effects. Moreover, copper can be quickly and severely affected by strong alkaline detergents, sodium hypochlorite, acid and salty food, making it not really suitable in the food contact zone. The rate of attack is slow enough that alkaline detergents can be used for the cleaning of copper vessels. As copper ions may leach from the copper metal, its surface roughness may increase. Oxidation of copper gives rise to the formation of toxic copper (II) oxide.

The copper alloys brass (60 - 70% copper, 30 - 40% zinc) and bronze (80 - 95% copper, 5 - 20% tin) are more prone to corrosion by alkaline and acidic detergents, salty and acid food than the ferrous steels. Brass is susceptible to de-zincification and because cadmium and lead are co-elements to zinc, brass shall never be used in the food contact area. Bronze is widely accepted as material of construction for control valves in gas cylinders, allowing controlling gas pressure and flow without compromising the quality of the gas. Copper alloys, such as brass and bronze, also exhibit antimicrobial activity, albeit of smaller magnitude. Electrical components in bronze or brass should be contained in enclosures.

Nickel:

Nickel alloys have a much higher nickel content showing higher corrosion resistance than the ferrous steels. In alloys, nickel is strongly and micro-structurally bond, because the "alloying elements" react with and dissolve into each other to form a material with new crystalline structures. Strong atomic and chemical binding forces between the constituting alloying elements reduce their migration out of alloys

Nickel usually is evenly worn-off, although pitting and stress-corrosion cracking may occur. Intensive aeration and high temperatures may increase the corrosion rate. Nickel may be attacked by inorganic acids such as nitric, sulfuric and phosphoric acid, but has good resistance to alkaline media and at least at not too high temperatures it is hardly attacked by organic acids, such as vinegar, lemon, and formic acid. Phosphoric acid present in some acid cleaning agents and sodium hypochlorite may leach non-alloyed nickel very easy from pure nickel, causing damage to nickel surfaces during cleaning. Where brass components are nickel-plated, damage to that coating may release physiologically unacceptable amounts of nickel in the food and the product may come in direct contact with brass. In general, pure nickel, nickel-plated steel and nickel-plated brass in the product contact area should better be avoided. The use of stainless steel and nickel alloy utensils does not elicit an allergic reaction by nickel sensitized persons.

Zinc:

Zinc is easily dissolved in diluted acids and by bases, leading to the release of zinc, but also of cadmium and lead. Zinc also reacts with steam to produce zinc oxide and hydrogen gas. Zinc in the formulation contact zone must be avoided, especially where wet or humid acidic formulations are produced. Zinc frequently contains small amounts of the toxic metals cadmium (0.01 - 0.04%) and lead as impurities. Therefore, the use of zinc, zinc alloys or zinc galvanized materials with product contact is banned in some countries.

Titanium:

Titanium has been suggested to be used for corrosive or delicate liquids. It is practically inert, due to the phenomenon of passivation of the titanium surface by the formation of a molecular layer of titanium dioxide. This layer, which is very adherent to the metallic substrate, is scarcely removed at high temperatures even in contact with hypo-chlorites and bleach chemicals, and highly concentrated salt and acid solutions. Titanium is resistant to crevice corrosion, and impingement and pitting attack in salt water. Titanium does not cause health problems, as it is generally considered to be poorly absorbed upon ingestion. Titanium dioxide is also used as white pigment in paints, lacquers, enamels, coatings and plastics. Further titanium compounds (for example, $TiCl_4$) are also found in plastics, as they are used as catalysts in the manufacturing of certain plastics (synthesis of 1-alkene polymers). Recent research has demonstrated that the combined action of UV and titanium dioxide results in photocatalytic disinfection of products, liquids and air.

Titanium alloys are stronger and more resistant to corrosion than the metal itself. Titanium is also used in certain so-called "stabilized" forms of stainless steels, which in general contain less than 1%. In medicine, titanium alloys are used in implants, and they have never indicated any local effects on tissues. However, the use in food contact materials is unknown.

Silver:

Silver is used in the production of cutlery and tableware. Chemically, silver is the most reactive of the noble metals, but it does not oxidize readily; rather it "tarnishes" by combining at ordinary temperatures with sulfur-compounds or H_2S (for example, in eggs). However, migration of silver is limited. Silver may be ingested via consumption in, for example, silver salts used as drinking water disinfectants, and as a colouring agent for decorations of confectionary and in alcoholic beverages. Silver is also used as an antimicrobial in many elastomers, plastics and within coatings of stainless steel.

11.9 INORGANIC NON-METALS

11.9.1 Glass

Glass is composed principally of sand (silica - SiO_2), soda-ash (Na_2CO_3 - sodium carbonate) and lime-stone ($CaCO_3$, calcium carbonate). Glass made from pure silica consists of a three-dimensional network of silicon atoms each of which is surrounded by four oxygen atoms and in this way the tetrahedra are linked together to produce the network. Glass prepared from pure silica require very high temperature to fuse, hence soda-ash and lime is used to reduce the melting point.

Preparation:

    (a) **Glass made of pure silica:** It is very hard and chemically resistant but melting point is very high so it is very difficult to mould.

    (b) **Glass made of pure silica + Na_2O:** The structure of this glass is less rigid so has low m.p. and easier to mould. The glass is too rapidly attacked by water and NaOH is leached out of the glass.

    (c) **Glass made of pure silica + CaO (or BaO, MgO, PbO and ZnO):** The divalent oxides do not break the network of pure silica, but only push the tetrahedron apart. It is more rigid than soda-silica network. Since the bond is stronger, hence chemical reactivity is lowered.

    (d) **Pure silica + Boric (B_2O_3) or aluminium oxide (Al_2O_3):** Boric oxide like silica is acidic and thus it does not disrupt the network of silica but forms tetrahedron itself. However, these are not the same size as the silicon tetrahedra. Hence, the lattice becomes distorted, and this produces flexibility. It is chemically resistant.

Types of Glass:

Type-1 glass:

It is a borosilicate glass, for example, Pyrex, Borosil. It is composed of SiO_2 (80%), B_2O_3 (12%), Al_2O_3 (2%) and $Na_2O + CaO$ (6%). It has high m.p. so can withstand high temperature. It is resistant to chemical substances and has low leaching action. It is used to make laboratory glass apparatus and for storing and packaging of injections and for water for injection.

Type-II glass:

It is known as treated soda-lime glass because it is made of soda lime. Its surface is treated with acidic gas like SO_2 (i.e. de-alkalized) at elevated temperature (500 °C) and moisture. The surface of the glass is fairly resistant to attack by water for a period of time. Sulfur treatment neutralizes the alkaline oxides on the surface, thereby rendering the glass more chemically resistant. It is used for alkali sensitive products, infusion fluids, blood and plasma and for large volume container.

Type-III glass:

It is called as regular soda-lime glass composed of SiO_2, Na_2O and CaO. It contains high concentration of alkaline oxides and imparts alkalinity to aqueous substances. The flakes separate easily and may crack due to sudden change of temperature. It is suitable for all solid dosage forms (for example, tablets, powders), for oily injections but not to be used for aqueous injections and for alkali-sensitive drugs.

Type NP glass:

It is non-parenteral (NP) glass or general purpose soda-lime glass. It is composed of SiO_2 (72-75%), B_2O_3 (7-10%), Al_2O_3 (6%), Na_2O (6-8%), K_2O (0.5 - 2%) and BaO (2-4%). It is softer and can easily be moulded. It has good resistance to autoclaving and alkali-preparations (with pH up to 8). It is cheaper than borosilicate glass. Mainly it is used for storage and packaging of oral and topical preparations but is unsuitable for ampoules.

Neutral glass:

Neutral glass is a borosilicate glass containing significant amounts of boric oxide, aluminum oxide, alkali and/or alkaline earth oxides. It has a high hydrolytic resistance and a high thermal shock resistance. It is used for small vials and large transfusion bottles.

Neutral tubing for ampoules:

It is composed of SiO_2 (67%), B_2O_3 (7.5%), Al_2O_3 (8.5%), Na_2O (8.7%), K_2O (4%), CaO (4%) and MgO (0.3%). In comparison to neutral glass its m.p. is low. After filling the glass ampoules are sealed by fusion and therefore the glass must be easy to melt. It is used to make ampoules for injection.

Coloured glass:

It is composed of glass and iron oxide. This composition produces amber colour glass. It has resistance to radiation from 290 nm to 450 nm. It is used specifically for photosensitive products.

Table 11.3: Typical chemical composition of different glass (approx. % by weight)

Chemical	Borosilicate Glass	Borosilicate Glass (Clear)	Borosilicate Glass (Amber)	Soda-Lime Glass (Amber)	Soda-Lime Glass (Clear)
SiO_2	80.60%	75.00%	70.00%	67.00%	69.00%
B_2O_3	13.00%	10.50%	7.50%	5.00%	1.00%
Na_2O	4.00%	5.00%	6.50%	12.00%	13.00%
Al_2O_3	2.30%	7.00%	6.00%	7.00%	4.00%
CaO	-	1.50%	<1.0%	1.00%	5.00%
Fe_2O_3	-	-	1.00%	2.00%	-
TiO_2	-	-	5.00%	-	-
K_2O	-	-	1.0%	1.00%	3.00%
BaO	-	-	2.0%	<0.5%	2.00%
MnO_2	-	-	-	5.00%	3.00%
MgO	-	-	-	-	-

Advantages:

(i) Glass is quite strong and rigid.

(ii) Being transparent it allows the visual inspection of the contents.

(iii) It can be converted into any shape and size.

(iv) Borosilicate (Type-I) and Neutral glasses are resistant to heat so they can be used in the heating processes and in heat sterilization.

(v) Glass is easy to clean without any damage to its surface for example, scratching or bruising.

(vi) Borosilicate and treated soda lime type of glass is chemically inert.

(vii) As the composition of glass may be varied by changing the ratio of various glass constituents a glass with desired quality features for the purpose can be produced.

(viii) Glass does not deteriorate with age.

(ix) Photosensitive materials may be saved from UV-rays by using amber colour glass.

(x) Glass is cheaper than other materials.

Disadvantages:

(i) Glass is brittle so breaks unexpectedly.

(ii) It could not endure thermal cycling and may crack when subject to sudden changes of temperatures.

(iii) Glass coatings did unpredictably craze (very fine cracks) and thereby expose the underlying iron substrate to the process fluids.

(iv) It leaches elements used to overcome its brittle/crazing shortcomings.

(v) It does tenaciously hold onto biofilms.

(vi) Glass is heavier in comparison to plastic containers thus adds transportation cost.

(vii) Transparent glasses gives passage to UV-light which may damage the photosensitive materials inside the container

(viii) Simple soda-lime glass releases alkali from the surface forming silicate rich layer which sometimes gets detached and can be seen in the contents as 'flakes' and needles.

(ix) Weathering due to moisture condensed on the surface of glass dissolves some silica resulting in loss of brilliance from the surface of glass.

11.10 ORGANIC NON-METALS

11.10.1 Rubber

In earlier days chemical process industries faced perplexing and growing problems as more and more corrosive chemicals and compounds came into use. There was the need for a reliable and durable method of protecting mild steel and concrete storage tanks, process vessels, pickling lines, mixers, reactors, agitators, pipelines, tank trucks, railroad tank cars, ship tankers, and exhaust gas scrubbers against corrosion. Thus it became imperative that the use of rubber as a construction material began to be recognized universally. Acrylonitrile rubber can be used for oil resistance, and the use of neoprene rubber and antioxidants in liberal doses greatly improves resistance to ageing and weathering, ozone attack and attack by flame.

Rubber is exploited through appropriate and more or less conventional equipment design principles. It is an eminently suitable construction material for protection against corrosion in the chemical plant and equipment against various corrosive chemicals, acids and alkalies with minimum maintenance lower down time, negligible scale formation and a preferred choice for aggressive corroding and eroding environment. Rubber is available readily and rapidly, and at a relatively lower cost, and can be converted into usable products, having complicated shapes and dimensions. The terms "elastomer" and "polymer" are synonymous with the term, "rubber".

Advantages:

(i)   It has good mechanical strength and has good adhesion and strength of its bonding to metals and other substrates.

(ii) Its all-round deformability enables it to be used in extension, compression, shear, torsion or combinations.

(iii) Its resilience, resistance to fatigue, resistance to attack by corrosive chemicals and resistance to abrasion is remarkable.

(iv) It has good electrical resistance.

(v)   It has ease of molding or forming to any shape and size.

(vi) Rubber operates in a variety of environments and has usable ranges of deformity and durability.

(vii) Rubber is ablative meaning helps in removal of material from the surface of an object by vaporization, chipping, or other erosive processes.

(viii) It provides passive fire protection and thermal insulation.

Limitations:

(i)   Rubber swells if it is in contact with oil for long time.

(ii) It becomes brittle with ageing.

(iii) It is attacked by ozone and by fire.

Applications:

(i)   Rubber is also used for protection of other materials against fire, heat and wearing.

(ii) It gives excellent performance as a construction material for sealing systems.

(iii) Rubber dampens by transforming kinetic energy into static energy. Thus, provides in protection against explosion and impact and effectively reduces or eliminates noise, vibration and water hammer in pipelines and reaction tanks with agitators.

11.10.2 Plastic

In pharmaceutical plants plastic materials includes components from plastic screws and hinges to bigger plastic parts that are used electric wiring, flooring, wall covering, water proofing and so on. Plastics are defined as shaped and hardened synthetic materials composed of long chain organic molecules called polymers, along with various additives. Additives used facilitates handling and processing (lubricants, mould-release agents, blowing agents etc.), to change or improve properties of the base polymer and to protect plastics from the effects of time and environmental conditions. Plastics are of two types namely thermoplastic and thermosets.

Thermoplastics:

Thermoplastic polymers soften when heated and can be reshaped and the new shape is retained on cooling. The process can be repeated many times by alternate heating and cooling with minimal degradation of the polymer structure. Thermoplastics are largely used in the construction of pharmaceutical and food processing equipment and utilities. Polytetrafluorethylene (PTFE) or Teflon, is inert (to all known chemicals), non-toxic, non-flammable, and has a working temperature range of −270 to 260 °C. It has an extremely low coefficient of friction, and is applied as "non-stick" coating. It is used for machine packings, seals, gaskets, insulators, tubing, vessels for aggressive chemicals, coating in cookware, conveyor belt coating, mechanical and electrical bearings, insulation for coaxial cable, fixture and motor lead wire, industrial signal and control cable etc. Polytetrafluoroethylene (PTFE) is often considered to be a potentially attractive material, because of its high chemical resistance. However, care must be taken, because it can be porous and thus difficult to clean. In addition it may be insufficiently resilient to provide a permanently tight seal, and it is therefore considered unsuitable for aseptic processing.

Thermosets:

Thermosets are cured plastics, meaning that polymer chains within the thermosets are intensively cross-linked, so that they no longer can be softened at higher temperatures and re-shaped by heating. In their final form, they set to a rigid, hard, heat and solvent resistant solid. Thermosets are generally stronger and stiffer than thermoplastics, and have a high modulus of elasticity which is even maintained at high temperatures. With the addition of fillers, the properties of the thermoset resins can be further improved. Inorganic additives such as grinded rock powder, long glass fibres or lamellar mica may give thermosets a higher density, increased strength and thermal resistance, and reduced sensitivity to volume shrinkage. Thermosets are largely used in the construction of pharmaceutical and food processing equipment and utilities.

Properties:

(i) **Durability:** Many plastic materials are as strong as if not stronger than certain metals. Plastic hardware is also frequently corrosion resistant, allowing it to survive outside in inclement weather indefinitely.

(ii) **Cost Effectiveness:** As is the case in most industries these days, cost is an important factor in any construction project. Many plastic materials are very economical.

(iii) **Recycling:** Unlike metals, some plastics can be recycled without losing any chemical properties and hence can be used over

(iv) Energy saving: Plastic consumes less heat than metal. The insulating effects of some plastics can also decrease sound pollution level.

(v) Safety: Plastic materials are typically much lighter than metals. The lightness of the material makes it easier to carry and lift into place.

(vi) Easy to install: The light weight of plastic materials allows for quick and easy installation.

Applications:

(i) Flooring: Plastic materials like polyvinyl chloride (PVC) and polyethylene are used to make flooring less prone to wear and tear. It also decreases the sound pollution level and can be cleaned easily.

(ii) Roofing: To protect the outer surface of the roof from damage, two layers of different plastic materials are required. The upper part is made of coloured thermoplastic olefin or vinyl while the lower part consists of polyurethane foam which consumes less energy and keeps the interior of a house cooler.

(iii) Insulation: Polyurethane spray is frequently used for insulation when constructing green or low energy buildings. Rigid polyurethane foam is known for its high thermal resistance which promotes temperature consistency. Polyurethane foam is also popular because it is lightweight, chemical resistant, and flame retardant. Due to its closed cell nature, polyurethane insulation performs as an air barrier, resulting in significant energy savings.

(iv) Wall: A structural insulated panel (SIP) is a sandwich of expanded polystyrene amidst two slim layers of oriented strand board. This type of pre-fab, composite wall board can be transferred to the work place easily for a particular task and provide good support to columns and other associated essentials during renovation.

(v) Pipes: Commonly made-up of polyvinyl chloride (PVC), CPVC, acrylonitrile butadiene styrene (ABS) or polyethylene, plastic pipes are flexible and very light in weight, making them easy to install. All of these plastic materials are also highly chemical and water resistant, making them suitable for many extreme environments.

(vi) Windows: Polycarbonate is used to manufacture building windows. This plastic material is strong, clear and very light in weight. Polycarbonate windows are considered more burglar-proof than regular glass windows. Two plastics materials, vinyl and fiberglass, are used commonly in the production of window frames. Fiberglass is extremely strong while vinyl is quite durable and also inexpensive.

(vii) Doors: Some construction projects use doors made from a stiff polyurethane foam core with a fiber reinforced plastic (FRP) coating. The sandwich structure of these doors makes them incredibly strong.

11.11 BASICS OF MATERIAL HANDLING SYSTEMS

Material handling involves the basic operations such as movement of bulk, packaged and individual products in a semi-solid or solid state by means of gravity, manually or power-driven equipment and within the limits of individual producing, fabricating, processing or service establishment. Material handling adds to the cost of the product and hence it costs the customer so the handling should be kept at minimum. In Indian industries material handling accounts for nearly 40% of the cost of production. Out of the total time spent for manufacturing a product, 20% of the time is utilized for actual processing on them while the remaining 80% of the time is spent in moving from one place to another, waiting for the processing. Poor material handling leads to delays and idling of equipment. Materials handling can be defined as 'the function dealing with the preparation, placing and positioning of materials to facilitate their movement or storage'. It is the art and science involving the movement, handling and storage of materials during different stages of manufacturing.

11.11.1 Objectives

(i)   To minimize cost of product.

(ii)   To minimize delays and interruptions by making available the materials at the right quantity and at right time.

(iii) To increase the production capacity by effective utilization of capacity.

(iv)   To assure safety in material handling through improvement in working condition.

(v)   To utilize material handling equipment to their maximum level.

(vi)   To prevent damages to materials under handling.

(vii) To lower investment in process inventory.

11.11.2 Principles

The principle of material handling are described as follows. All material handling activities should be planned. Plan a system integrating as many handling activities as possible and co-coordinate the full scope of operations (receiving, storage, production, inspection, packing, warehousing, supply and transportation). Make optimum use of cubic space. The quantity, size, weight of load handled should be increased. Wherever possible, gravitational force should be utilized to move a material. The material flow must be optimized by planning proper operational sequence and equipment arrangement. The unnecessary movement and/or use of equipment must be reduced, combined or eliminated. The measures should be exercised for safety while using handling methods and equipment. Use mechanical or automated material handling equipment. Standardize method, types and size of material handling equipment. Use methods and equipment that perform a variety of task and applications. Consider all aspect of equipment and material to be moved and method to be utilized. Reduce the ratio of dead weight to payload in mobile equipment. Equipment designed to transport material should be kept in use. Reduce idle time/unproductive time of both equipment and man power. There must be a plan for preventive maintenance or scheduled repair of all material handling equipments. Replace obsolete handling methods/equipment when more efficient method/equipment will improve operation. Use handling equipment to help achieve its full capacity and to improve production control, inventory control and other handling. Determine efficiency of handling performance in terms of cost per unit handled which is the primary criterion.

11.11.3 Selection of Equipments

Selection of material handling equipment is a critical decision as it affects both the cost and efficiency of handling system. While selecting a material handling equipment following factors need to be taken into consideration.

1. **Properties of the material:** The type (whether it is solid, liquid or gas), and size, shape and weight or amount of material is to be moved are important issues that help to a preliminary eliminate equipments from the range of available equipments. The nature of material, viz. fragile, corrosive or toxic implies certain handling methods and containers preferable to others.

2. **Layout of the building:** Availability of space for handling is another restricting factor for material movement. Low ceiling heights may restrict the use of hoists or cranes, and the presence of supporting columns in path can limit the size of the material-handling equipment. In multi-storied building for industrial trucks, chutes or ramps are used. Building layout helps to decide type of production operation (continuous, intermittent, fixed position or group) and can indicate the equipment more suitable than the others. Floor capacity as well helps to select the best equipment.

3. **Production flow:** In case of constant material flow between two fixed positions, fixed equipment such as conveyors or chutes can be suitably used. If the flow is not constant and the direction of material movement changes occasionally from one point to another as several products are being produced simultaneously, moving equipment such as trucks would be preferable.

4. **Cost of handling:** Material handling cost help to take a final decision of selecting equipment. Several costs including initial investment and operating and maintenance costs are the major cost to be considered. Comparison of the total costs for each item of equipment under consideration helps to come-up with a more rational decision for most appropriate choice.

5. **Type of operations:** Equipment selection depends on nature of operations like whether handling is temporary or permanent, whether the flow is continuous or intermittent and material flow pattern is vertical or horizontal.

6. **Engineering aspects:** Equipment selection also depends on engineering aspects like door and ceiling dimensions, floor space, floor conditions and structural strength.

7. **Equipment reliability:** Reliability of the equipment and supplier reputation and the after sales service also plays an important role in selecting material handling equipments.

11.11.4 Evaluation of Material Handling System

The factors that help in evaluation of material handling equipment are material handling system costs that include investment cost, labour cost, and anticipated service hours per year, utilization, and unit load carrying ability, loading and unloading characteristics, operating costs and the size requirements. Other factors to be considered are source of power, conditions where the equipment has to operate and such other technical aspects. Therefore, choices of equipments in an organization will improve the material handling system through work study techniques. They usually result in improving the ratio of operating time to loading time through palletizing, avoiding duplicative movements etc. Obsolete handling systems can be replaced with more efficient equipments. The effectiveness of the system can be measured in terms of the time spent in the handling and the total time spent in production. The cost effectiveness can be measured by the expenses incurred per unit weight of material handled. The expenses and time factors as a base for performance help to take remedial measures. Other indices for evaluating the performance of handling systems are:

Equipment Utilization Ratio: Equipment utilization ratio is an important indicator for judging the material handling system. This ratio can be computed and compared with similar firms or in the same over a period of time. In order to know the total effort needed for moving materials, it may be necessary to compute Materials Handling Labour (MHL) ratio. This ratio is calculated as under:

$$\text{MHL} = \frac{\text{Personnel assigned to materials handling}}{\text{Total operating work force}} \qquad \text{... (11.9)}$$

In order to determine material handling system to deliver materials at place with maximum efficiency, it is desirable to compute direct labour handling loss (DLHL) ratio. The ratio is:

$$\text{DLHL} = \frac{\text{Materials handling time lost of labour}}{\text{Total direct labour time}} \qquad \text{... (11.10)}$$

The material movement to operation ratio is calculated by dividing total number of moves by total number of productive operations. This ratio helps to know workers too many unproductive movements because of poor routing. The efficiency of materials handling mainly depends on the following factors:

(i)   Efficiency of handling methods employed for handling a unit weight through a unit distance.

(ii) Efficiency of the layout which determines the distance through which the materials have to be handled.

(iii) Utilisation of the handling facilities.

(iv) Efficiency of the speed of handling.

An effective material handling system depends upon tailoring the layout and equipments to suit specific requirements.

11.11.5 Material Handing Equipments

When a large volume has to be moved from a limited number of sources to a limited number of destinations the fixed path equipments like rollers, belt conveyors, overhead conveyors and gauntry cranes are preferred. For increased flexibility varied path equipments are preferred. Broadly material handling equipment's can be classified into two categories.

(a) Fixed path equipments: Fixed path equipments moves in a fixed path.

For example, conveyors, monorail devices, chutes and pulley drive equipments. A slight variation in this category is the overhead crane can move materials in any manner within a restricted area by virtue of its design. Overhead cranes have a very good range in terms of hauling tonnage and are used for handling bulky raw materials, stacking and at times palletizing.

(b) Variable path equipments: Variable path equipments have no restrictions in the direction of movement. For example, trucks, forklifts, mobile cranes and industrial tractors. The size of these equipments is an important factor to be considered. Forklifts are available in many ranges, they are manoeuvrable and various attachments are provided to increase their versatility.

The choice of material-handling equipment among the various possibilities that exist is not easy. In several cases the same material may be handled by various types of equipments, and the great diversity of equipment and attachments available does not make the problem any easier. In several cases, however, the nature of the material to be handled narrows the choice. Material handing equipments may be classified in following major categories.

(i) Conveyors: Conveyors are useful for moving material either continuously or intermittently between two fixed workstations. They are mainly used for continuous or mass production operations and suitable for most operations where the flow is more or less steady. Examples of conveyors include conveyors with rollers, wheels or belts to help move the material along. These may be power-driven or may roll freely. Although conveyors are costly to install they are less flexible and for two or more converges it is necessary to coordinate the speeds at which these conveyors move.

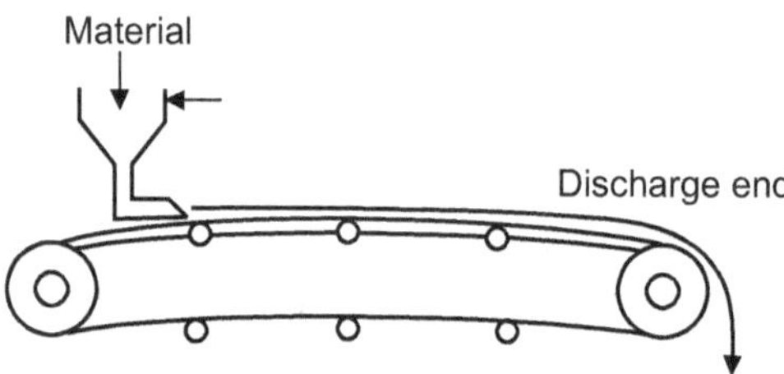

Fig. 11.4: Belt Conveyor

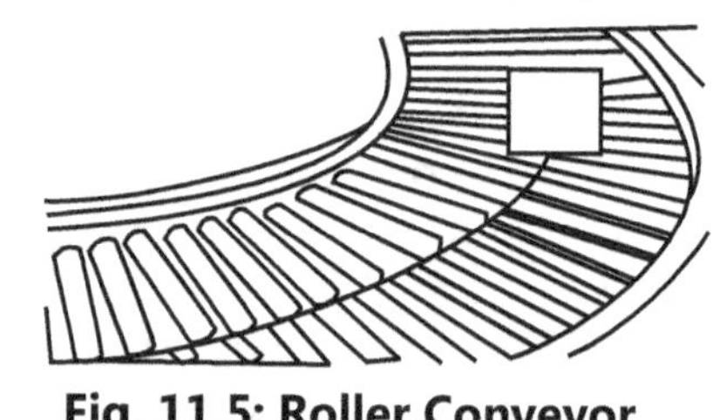

Fig. 11.5: Roller Conveyor

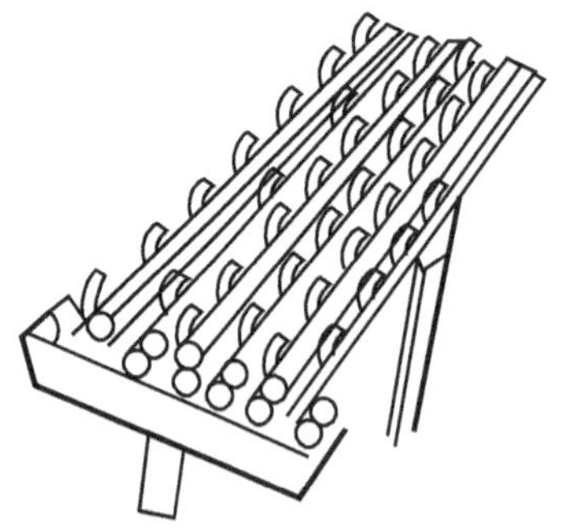

Fig. 11.6: Wheel Conveyor

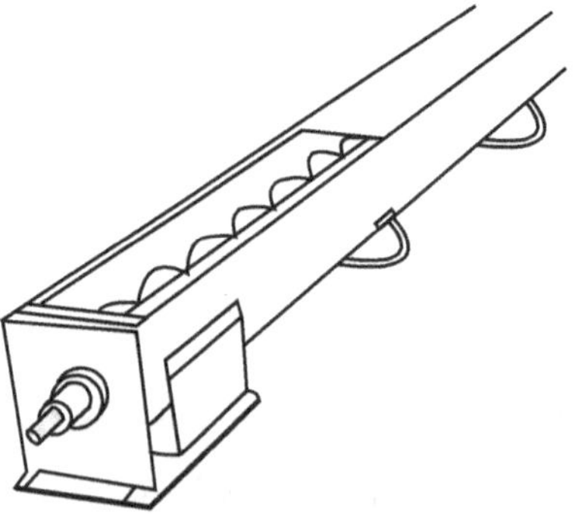

Fig. 11.7: Screw Conveyor

(ii) Industrial trucks: Industrial trucks can move between various points and are not permanently fixed in one place and thus are more flexible in use than conveyors. They are most suitable for intermittent production and for handling various sizes and shapes of material. Different types of truck includes petrol-driven, electric, hand-powered etc. Trucks has advantage that it has wide range of attachments that increase their ability to handle various types and shapes of material.

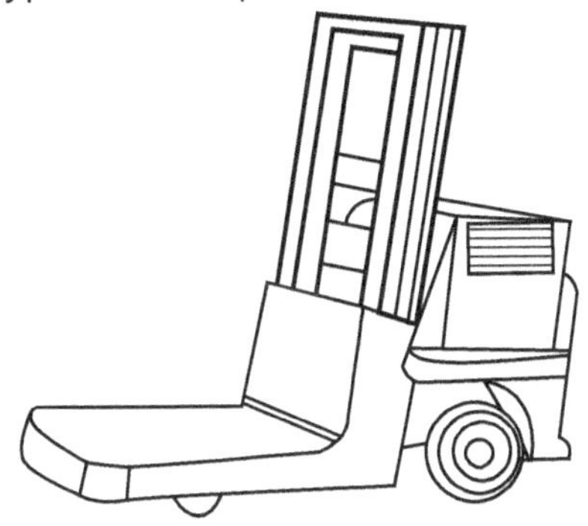

Fig. 11.8: Platform Truck Conveyor

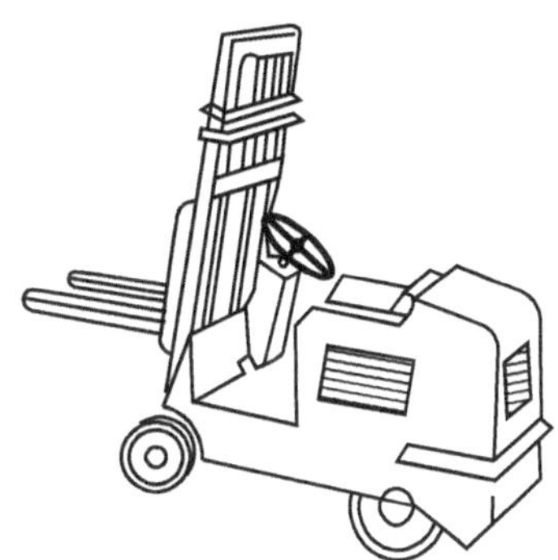

Fig. 11.9: Fork Truck

(c) Cranes and Hoists: The cranes and hoists can move heavy materials through overhead space. They can usually serve only a limited area. There are several types of cranes and hoists with various loading capacities. Cranes and hoists may be used both for intermittent and for continuous production.

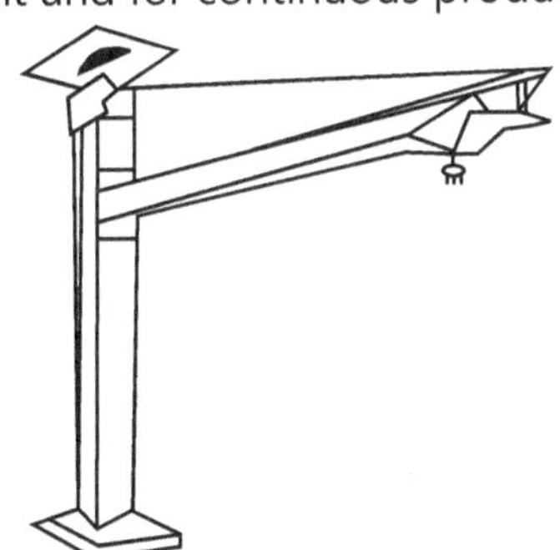

Fig. 11.10: Jib Crane

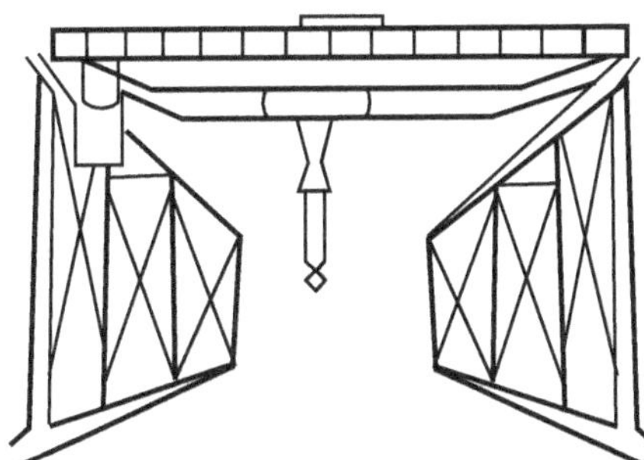

Fig. 11.11: Bridge Crane

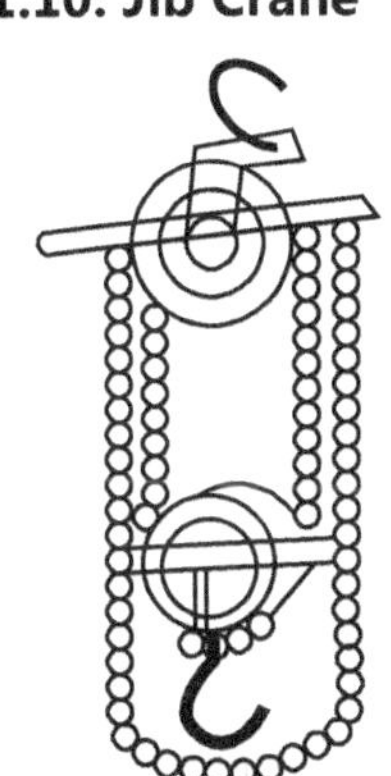

Fig. 11.12: Chain Hoist

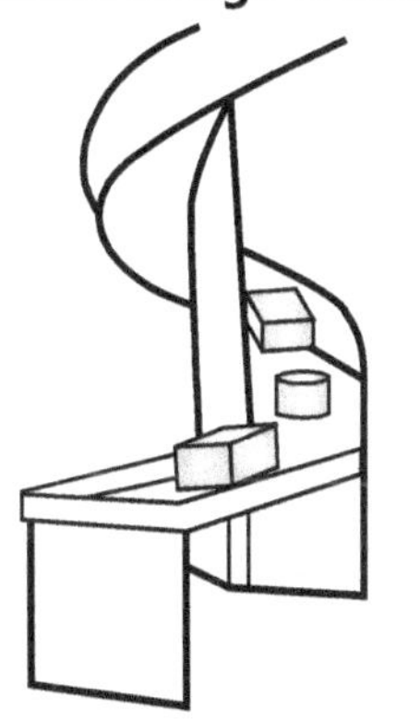

Fig. 11.13: Electric Hoist

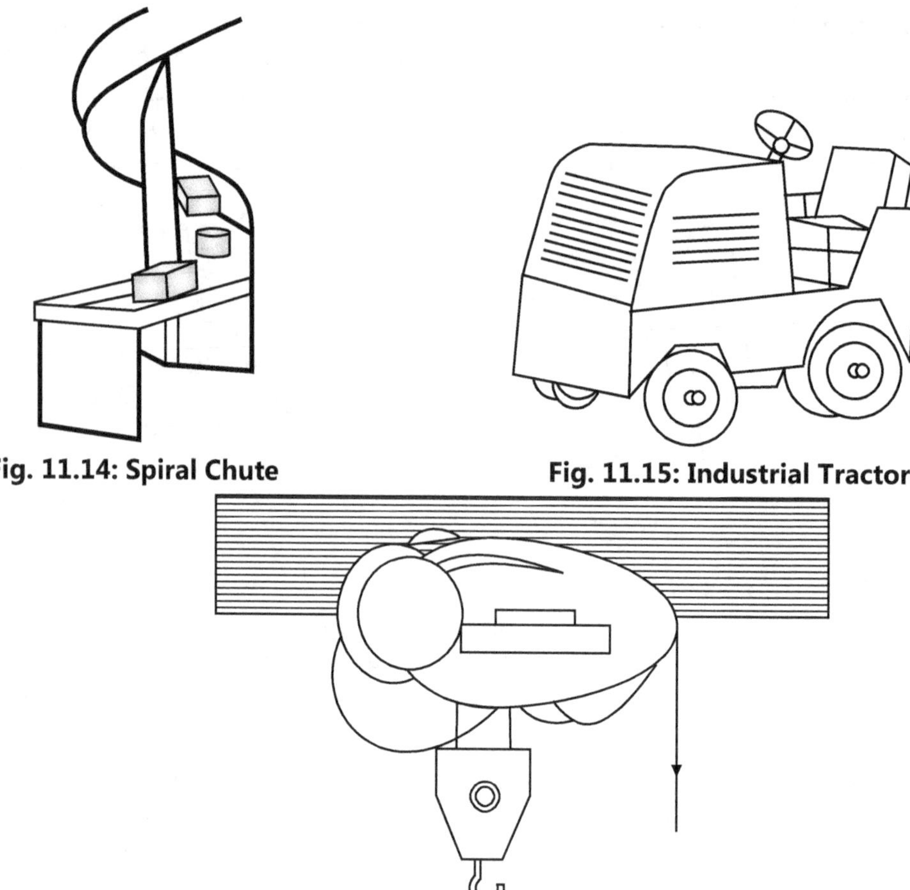

Fig. 11.14: Spiral Chute   Fig. 11.15: Industrial Tractor

Fig. 11.16: Electrical Hoist

(d) Containers: Containers are either 'dead' or 'live'. The dead containers includes cartons, barrels, skids, pallets etc. hold the material to be transported but do not move themselves. The 'live' containers are wagons, wheelbarrows or computer self-driven containers. Handling equipments of these kind can both contain and move the material, and is usually operated manually.

(e) Robots: These days in modern industries many types of robot are used to move materials. They vary in size, and in function and maneuverability. Robots are used for handling and transporting material as well as to perform operations such as welding or spray painting. An advantage of robots is that they can perform in a hostile environment such as unhealthy conditions or carry on arduous tasks such as the repetitive movement of heavy materials.

11.11.6 Effective Utilisation of Equipments

The following guidelines help to design and cost reduction of the materials handling system:

(i)   Material handling increases the production cycle time and thus eliminate handling wherever possible. Ideally there should not be any handling at all.

(ii)   Sequence the operations in logical manner so that handling is unidirectional and smooth.

(iii) Use gravity wherever possible as it results in conservation of power and fuel.

(iv)   Standardize the handling equipments to the extent possible as it means interchangeable usage, better utilization of handling equipments, and lesser spares holding.

(v)   Install a regular preventive maintenance programme for material handling equipments so that downtime would be minimum.

(vi)   The criteria of versatility and adaptability must be the prime factor in selection of handling equipments to ensure investments in special purpose handling equipments will be kept at a minimum.

(vii) Weight of unit load must be maximum so that each 'handling cycle' is productive.

(viii) Elimination of unnecessary movements and combination of processes should be considered while installing a material handling system.

(ix)   Non-productive operations in handling, such as slinging, loading etc., should be kept at a minimum through appropriate design of handling equipment.

(x)   Location of stores should be as close as possible to the plant which uses the materials.

(xi)   Use of queuing technique can be very effective in optimal utilization of materials handling equipments.

(xii) The material handling system should be simple and safe to operate.

(xiii) Avoid any wasteful movements-method study can be conducted for this purpose.

(xiv) Ensure proper co-ordination through judicious selection of equipments and training of workmen.

11.11.7 Plant Layout and Material Handling

There is a close relationship between plant layout and material handling. A good layout ensures minimum material handling and eliminates rehandling in the following ways:

(i)   Material movement does not add any value to the finished product so, the material handling should be kept at minimum though not avoid it. This is possible only through the systematic plant layout. Thus a good layout minimizes handling.

(ii)   The productive time of workers will go without production if they are required to travel long distance to get the material tools etc. Thus, a good layout ensures minimum travel for workman thus enhancing the production time and eliminating the hunting time and travelling time.

(iii) Space is an important criterion. Plant layout integrates all the movements of men, material through a well designed layout with system. It helps to keep material handling shorter, faster and economical. A good layout reduces material handling system.

(iv) Good plant layout helps in building efficient material handling the material backtracking, unnecessary workmen movement ensuring effectiveness in manufacturing. Thus a good layout always ensures minimum material handling.

REVIEW QUESTIONS

1. What are objectives of studying materials of plant construction?
2. Discuss factors affecting materials to be selected for pharmaceutical plant construction.
3. What is corrosion? Classify them. Explain theories of corrosion.
4. Discuss various factors influencing corrosion.
5. Enlist and explain various types of corrosion.
6. Discuss in detail methods of corrosion prevention.
7. Classify materials used in construction of pharmaceutical plant.
8. Discuss ferrous metals used in plant construction with their properties advantages, limitations and applications.
9. Discuss non-ferrous metals used in plant construction with their properties advantages, limitations and applications.
10. Discuss inorganic non-metals used in plant construction with their properties advantages, limitations and applications.
11. Discuss organic non-metals used in plant construction with their properties advantages, limitations and applications.
12. Discuss stainless steel as a choice of material for pharmaceutical plant construction.
13. Discuss glass as a choice of material for pharmaceutical plant construction.
14. Discuss rubber as a choice of material for pharmaceutical plant construction.
15. Discuss plastic as a choice of material for pharmaceutical plant construction.
16. What do you mean by material handling systems? What are its objectives and principle?
17. Enlist and discuss factors involved in selection of equipments for material handling.
18. Discuss evaluation of material handling system. How equipment utilization ratio is calculated? What is its significance?
19. Enlist and explain various material handing equipments used in pharmaceutical industry.
20. Discuss various guidelines used to design and cost reduction of the materials handling system.
21. Discuss relation between plant layout and material handling.

✍ ✍ ✍

SECOND YEAR B.PHARM (SEMESTER-III)

Pharamceutical Organic Chemistry-II	Dr. K.G. Bothara
Pharamceutical Organic Chemistry-II	Dr. Abhishek Tiwari, Dr.Neeaj Upmanyu, Anup K Chakrabarty
Pharamceutical Organic Chemistry-II	Dr. K.S. Jain, Dr. P.B. Miniyar, Dr. L.V.G. Narrgund
Physical Pharmaceutics-I	Dr. Ashok A. Hajare
Physical Pharmaceutics-I	Dr. Vaibhavkumar A. Jagtap, Md. Rageeb Md. Usaman, Atish A. Salunkhe, Basawaraj Bendegumble
Pharmaceutical Microbiology	Chandrakant Kokare
Pharmaceutical Microbiology	Dr. Kuntal Das
Pharmaceutical Microbiology	Dr. S.B.Bhise, M.S. Bhise, Dr. Lalit Lata Jha
Pharmaceutical Engineering	Sunil R. Bakliwal, Dr.Bhushan R. Rane, Dr. Ashish S.Jain
Pharmaceutical Engineering	Dr. Bharat Parashar, Anshu Gupta, Tripti Shukla,
Pharmaceutical Engineering	Md. Rageeb Md.Usman, Dr. Vaibhavkumar A. Jagtap, Atish A.Salunkhe, Neelesh Chaubey, Keerthy H.S.
Pharmaceutical Engineering	Dr. Ashok A. Hajare
A Practical Book of Pharmaceutical Organic Chemistry-II (Combined Book Sem II & III)	Dr. Kishor S. Jain, Dr, Pankaj B. Miniyar, Dr. L.V.G. Nargund
A Laboratory Manual of Pharmaceutical Organic Chemistry-II (Combined Book Sem II & III)	Dr. Abhishek Tiwari, Dr. Anita Singh, Dr. Neeraj Upmanyu, Dr. Varsha Tiwari
A Practical Book of Physical Pharmaceutics-I (Combined book Sem III and IV)	Sudip Das, Dr. Shubhrajit Mantry, Ravi Shankar
A Practical Book of Physical Pharmaceutics-I	Tanvir Y. Shaikh, Rageeb Md. Usman, Siraj N, Shaikh, Basawaraj Bendegumble
A Practical Book of Physical Pharmaceutics-I	Dr. Ashok A. Hajare
A Practical Book of Pharmaceutical Engineering	Md. Rageeb Md. Usman, Prerna K. Mahajan, Dr.Neelesh Chaubey, Dr. Mohammed Z.Shaikh, Keerthy H.S.
A Practical Book of Pharmaceutical Engineering	Dr. Bhushan R. Rane, Dr. Ashish S. Jain, Sunil R. Bakliwal
A Practical Book of Pharmaceutical Engineering	Dr. Suresh G. Sudhe